WHEN CHILDREN DIE

IMPROVING PALLIATIVE AND END-OF-LIFE CARE FOR CHILDREN AND THEIR FAMILIES

Committee on Palliative and End-of-Life Care for
Children and Their Families
Board on Health Sciences Policy

Marilyn J. Field and Richard E. Behrman, Editors

INSTITUTE OF MEDICINE
OF THE NATIONAL ACADEMIES

THE NATIONAL ACADEMIES PRESS
Washington, D.C.
www.nap.edu

THE NATIONAL ACADEMIES PRESS • 500 Fifth Street, N.W. • Washington, DC 20001

NOTICE: The project that is the subject of this report was approved by the Governing Board of the National Research Council, whose members are drawn from the councils of the National Academy of Sciences, the National Academy of Engineering, and the Institute of Medicine. The members of the committee responsible for the report were chosen for their special competences and with regard for appropriate balance.

Major support for this project was provided by the National Institute for Nursing Research (NIH Task Order #79), the Greenwall Foundation, the Project on Death in America of the Open Society Institute, and the National Cancer Institute. Additional support was provided by the Health Services and Resources Administration, the Robert Wood Johnson Foundation, the National Heart Lung and Blood Institute, the National Institute of Mental Health, and the National Institute for Child Health and Development. The views presented are those of the Institute of Medicine Committee on Palliative and End-of-Life Care for Children and Their Families and are not necessarily those of the funding organization.

Library of Congress Cataloging-in-Publication Data

When children die : improving palliative and end-of-life care for children and their families / Committee on Palliative and End-of-Life Care for Children and Their Families, Board on Health Sciences Policy ; Marilyn J. Field and Richard E. Behrman, editors.
    p. ; cm.
Includes bibliographical references and index.
ISBN 0-309-08437-7 (hardcover)
    1. Terminally ill children—Care. 2. Terminally ill children—Family relationships. 3. Palliative treatment.
    [DNLM: 1. Terminal Care—Child—United States. 2. Health Policy—United States. 3. Patient Participation—Child—United States. 4. Professional-Family Relations—United States. 5. Terminal Care—economics—United States. 6. Terminal Care—legislation & jurisprudence—United States. WS 200 W567 2002] I. Field, Marilyn J. (Marilyn Jane) II. Behrman, Richard E., 1931- III. Institute of Medicine (U.S.). Committee on Palliative and End-of-Life Care for Children and Their Families.
RJ249 .W445 2002
362.1'75'083—dc21
                                                            2002014542

Additional copies of this report are available from: The National Academies Press, 500 Fifth Street, N.W., Box 285, Washington, DC 20055; (800) 624-6242 or (202) 334-3313 (in the Washington metropolitan area); Internet, www.nap.edu

Printed in the United States of America

Front cover: Original photograph by Timothy D. Costich, M.D., F.A.A.P.; design and photo manipulation by Francesca Moghari.

"Knowing is not enough; we must apply.
Willing is not enough; we must do."
—Goethe

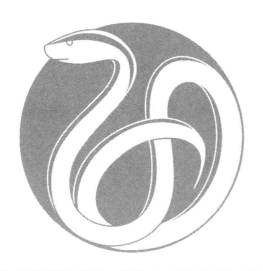

INSTITUTE OF MEDICINE
OF THE NATIONAL ACADEMIES

Shaping the Future for Health

THE NATIONAL ACADEMIES
Advisers to the Nation on Science, Engineering, and Medicine

The **National Academy of Sciences** is a private, nonprofit, self-perpetuating society of distinguished scholars engaged in scientific and engineering research, dedicated to the furtherance of science and technology and to their use for the general welfare. Upon the authority of the charter granted to it by the Congress in 1863, the Academy has a mandate that requires it to advise the federal government on scientific and technical matters. Dr. Bruce M. Alberts is president of the National Academy of Sciences.

The **National Academy of Engineering** was established in 1964, under the charter of the National Academy of Sciences, as a parallel organization of outstanding engineers. It is autonomous in its administration and in the selection of its members, sharing with the National Academy of Sciences the responsibility for advising the federal government. The National Academy of Engineering also sponsors engineering programs aimed at meeting national needs, encourages education and research, and recognizes the superior achievements of engineers. Dr. Wm. A. Wulf is president of the National Academy of Engineering.

The **Institute of Medicine** was established in 1970 by the National Academy of Sciences to secure the services of eminent members of appropriate professions in the examination of policy matters pertaining to the health of the public. The Institute acts under the responsibility given to the National Academy of Sciences by its congressional charter to be an adviser to the federal government and, upon its own initiative, to identify issues of medical care, research, and education. Dr. Harvey V. Fineberg is president of the Institute of Medicine.

The **National Research Council** was organized by the National Academy of Sciences in 1916 to associate the broad community of science and technology with the Academy's purposes of furthering knowledge and advising the federal government. Functioning in accordance with general policies determined by the Academy, the Council has become the principal operating agency of both the National Academy of Sciences and the National Academy of Engineering in providing services to the government, the public, and the scientific and engineering communities. The Council is administered jointly by both Academies and the Institute of Medicine. Dr. Bruce M. Alberts and Dr. Wm. A. Wulf are chair and vice chair, respectively, of the National Research Council.

www.national-academies.org

vi

Ruth Malkinson, School of Social Work, Tel Aviv University, Israeli Center for REBT

Murray M. Pollack, Executive Director, Center for Hospital-Based Specialties; Chief, Critical Care Medicine, Children's National Medical Center; Professor of Pediatrics, George Washington University School of Medicine

J. Donald Schumacher, President and CEO, The Center for Hospice and Palliative Care, Buffalo

Simon Shimshon Rubin, Professor of Psychology, Clinical Psychology Program, University of Haifa, Israel

James Walter Varni, Professor of Psychiatry, University of California, San Diego, School of Medicine

Study Staff

Marilyn J. Field, Study Director
Susan Stefanac, Research Assistant (to June 2001)
Travis Gayles, Research Assistant (from September 2001)
Troy Prince, Senior Project Assistant

Board on Health Sciences Policy Staff

Andrew Pope, Director, Board on Health Sciences Policy
Alden Chang, Board Assistant

DEDICATION

To all the children and families whose lives and whose stories
have helped us to learn and to advocate for changes that will
benefit other children and families

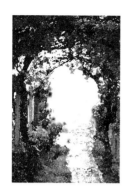

CONTENTS

_____

*Appendices B through H are available only online at http://www.nap.edu/catalog/
10390.html

BOXES, FIGURES, AND TABLES

Boxes

Figures

Tables

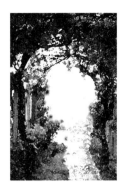

PREFACE

When a child dies, it is always out of season. When a child dies, dreams die and we are all diminished by the loss of human potential. Although dying is a part of life, a child's death, in a very real sense, is unnatural and has a devastating and enduring impact. Over the past century such deaths have been significantly reduced by socioeconomic, public health, and medical advances in developed countries such as the United States. Although with our current knowledge, we could do much more to decrease mortality among children and youth, even our best efforts will not prevent some children from dying. Nevertheless, we all have a mandate to ensure that their young lives do not end in preventable fear, pain and distress and that grieving families are comforted.

This report argues that we can and should do more than we are currently doing to prevent and relieve the physical and emotional suffering of dying children and the psychic pain of their families, to respect the personal dignity of the dying child and grieving family, and to allow all who are affected by a child's death the opportunity to address their feelings and concerns. Although there are many unanswered questions about optimal care in these tragic situations, a great deal is known about what should be done *now* to improve the care of dying children and their families. We can and must reduce the number of those who fail to receive consistent, competent care that meets not only their physical needs, but their emotional, spiritual, and cultural ones as well.

The report also emphasizes the need to improve the professional education of a broad spectrum of groups, develop appropriate supporting public health policies, and provide high quality end-of-life and bereavement services for children and their families. Addressing these needs will require more scientific knowledge and data about the care of children with life-threatening medical conditions, including those of sudden unexpected on-set. Behavioral changes by health providers and administrators, government officials, religious leaders, police and others will be required. Changes in policies at the federal, state, and local level are also critical if systems change in health care is to occur.

By definition, children cannot advocate for themselves. When they are dying, an attuned listener can learn from them, but they are essentially voiceless in the public domain. Add to this the fact that in an end-of-life situation, their families, their most natural advocates, are often paralyzed by grief, and we can perhaps see why their plight has received so little attention.

Although the number of children who die is, thankfully, relatively small, the event can devastate a family. While we cannot relieve all suffering, we can help prepare these children and families for what comes. It is hard to imagine a situation that has a greater imperative for humane caregiving, yet, far too often today, it is not provided. It is time to correct this situation. We hope this report will serve as a call to action.

Richard E. Behrman, M.D., J.D.
Committee Chair

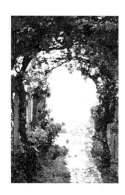

ACKNOWLEDGMENTS

In developing its report, the committee benefited greatly from the assistance of many individuals and groups. Important information and insights came from a public meeting during which the committee heard from many organizations and from individuals with personal experiences that added an invaluable human dimension to our understanding. The committee also learned much from a smaller meeting with families and gives its special thanks to Rosario and Salvador Avila, Gary and Rose Conlan, Deborah Dokken, Winona Kittiko, Tina Heyl-Martineau, and Les Weil for their willingness to discuss their experiences and perspectives. Appendix A includes the meeting agendas and participant lists and also cites the organizations that provided written statements to the committee.

The consultants to the committee, Mildred Solomon, Joanne Wolfe, and Cynda Rushton, provided valuable guidance at many points during the course of the committee's work. The committee appreciates the contributions of the authors of background papers included in the appendixes to the report; Bruce Himelstein often provided help beyond his role as background paper author.

Our project officer at the National Institute of Nursing Research, Anne Knebel, was unfailingly helpful in answering questions about the palliative care research agenda at the National Institutes of Health. Donna Hoyert, Joyce Martini, and others at the National Center for Health Statistics provided guidance on government mortality data. Melissa Harris, Theresa Pratt, and Tammi Levy-Cantor at the Center for Medicare and Medicaid Services helped with the intricacies of Medicaid policies, including those governing demonstration projects.

Nancy Contro, Harvey Cohen, and others at the Lucile Packard Children's Hospital at Stanford University generously shared the knowledge and insights they gained in developing their pediatric palliative care

xvii

program, and Murray Pollack and his colleagues in the Pediatric Intensive Care Unit at Children's National Medical Center in Washington, D.C., also provided insights into the day-to-day reality of caring for seriously ill children. Joan Teno and Sherry Weitzen of Brown University analyzed and provided data on the site of death for children.

Anne-Armstrong Dailey, Kay Scanlon, and others at Children's Hospice International were helpful on many matters and provided extensive information about the Medicaid hospice demonstration projects to test new models of all-inclusive care for children and their families. Among many others who provided information and answered questions are Stephen Connor at the National Hospice and Palliative Care Organization; Elaine Vining and Janis Guerney at the American Academy of Pediatrics; Susan Dull at the National Association of Children's Hospitals and Related Institutions; Stacy Orloff at the Hospice of the Florida Suncoast; and Susan Huff at the Center for Hospice and Palliative Care in Buffalo, New York.

Many within the Institute of Medicine were, as usual, helpful to the study staff. We would especially like to thank Alden Chang, Carlos Gabriel, Francesca Moghari, Sally Stanfield, Christine Stencel, and Bronwyn Schrecker.

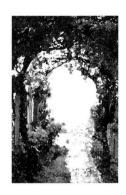

REVIEWERS

This report has been reviewed in draft form by individuals chosen for their diverse perspectives and technical expertise, in accordance with procedures approved by the National Research Council's (NRC) Report Review Committee. The purpose of this independent review is to provide candid and critical comments that will assist the institution in making its published reports as sound as possible and to ensure that the report meets institutional standards for objectivity, evidence, and responsiveness to the study charge. The review comments and draft manuscript remain confidential to protect the integrity of the deliberative process. We wish to thank the following individuals for their review of this report:

KEVIN BERGER, Hospice of the Valley, Phoenix
DEBORAH L. DOKKEN, Consultant/Parent Advocate, Chevy Chase, Maryland
CHRIS FEUDTNER, Child Health Institute, University of Washington
KARIN T. KIRCHHOFF, School of Nursing, University of Wisconsin-Madison
TIFFANY LEVINSON, Palliative Care Consultant, Wilmette, Illinois
STEPHEN LIBEN, The Montreal Children's Hospital
JOANNE LYNN, Center to Improve Care of the Dying, The RAND Corporation
STACY ORLOFF, Hospice of the Florida Suncoast, Largo
JANE TILLY, Urban Institute, Washington, D.C.
ROBERT TRUOG, The Children's Hospital, Boston
GARY WALCO, Center for Tomorrows Children, Hackensack University Medical Center

Although the reviewers listed above have provided many constructive comments and suggestions, they were not asked to endorse the conclusions or recommendations nor did they see the final draft of the report before its release. The review of this report was overseen by **R. DON BLIM**, appointed by the Institute of Medicine, and **ELAINE L. LARSON**, Professor of Pharmaceutical and Therapeutic Research, Columbia University School of Nursing, New York, NY. Appointed by the NRC Report Review Committee, these individuals were responsible for making certain that an independent examination of this report was carried out in accordance with the institutional procedures and that all review comments were carefully considered. Responsibility for the final content of this report rests entirely with the authoring committee and the institution.

WHEN CHILDREN DIE

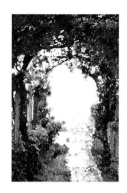

SUMMARY

*We are in need of medicine with a heart. . . . The endless
physical, emotional, and financial burdens that a family carries
when their child dies . . . makes you totally incapable of dealing
with incompetence and insensitivity.*

Salvador Avila, parent, 2001

The death of a child is a special sorrow, an enduring loss for surviving
mothers, fathers, brothers, sisters, other family members and close friends.
No matter the circumstances, a child's death is a life-altering experience.

Except when death comes suddenly and without forewarning, physicians, nurses, social workers and other health care personnel usually play a
central role in the lives of children who die and of their families. At best,
these professionals will exemplify "medicine with a heart," helping all
involved to feel that they did everything they could to help, that preventable
suffering was indeed prevented, and that the parents were good parents. At
worst, families' encounters with the health care system will leave them with
painful memories of their child's unnecessary suffering, bitter recollections
of careless and wounding words, and lifelong regrets about their own
choices. In between these poles of medicine, families will often experience
both excellent care and incompetence, compassion mixed with insensitivity,
and choices made and then later doubted.

Moving the typical experience of children and families toward the best
care and entirely eliminating the worst care is an achievable goal. It is a goal
that will depend on shifts in attitudes, policies, and practices involving not
only health care professionals but also those who manage, finance, and
regulate health care. That is, it will require system changes, not just indi-

1

vidual changes. Improvement will also require more clinical and health services research to fill gaps in our knowledge of what constitutes the "best" palliative, end-of-life, and bereavement care for children and families with differing needs, values, and circumstances.

Viewed broadly, *palliative care* seeks to prevent or relieve the physical and emotional distress produced by a life-threatening medical condition or its treatment, to help patients with such conditions and their families live as normally as possible, and to provide them with timely and accurate information and support in decisionmaking. Such care and assistance is not limited to people thought to be dying and can be provided concurrently with curative or life-prolonging treatments. *End-of-life care* focuses on preparing for an anticipated death (e.g., discussing in advance the use of life-support technologies in case of cardiac arrest or other crises or arranging a last family trip) and managing the end stage of a fatal medical condition (e.g., removing a breathing tube or adjusting symptom management to reflect changing physiology as death approaches). Together, palliative and end-of-life care also promote clear, culturally sensitive communication that assists patients and families in understanding the diagnosis, prognosis, and treatment options, including their potential benefits and burdens.

The death of a child will never be easy to accept, but health care professionals, insurers, educators, policymakers, and others can do more to spare children and families from preventable suffering. Although research is needed to assess systematically the strengths and limitations of different care strategies, promising models exist now in programs being undertaken by children's hospitals, hospices, educational institutions, and other organizations. Some of these programs focus on better preparing pediatricians and other child health specialists to understand and routinely apply the principles of palliative and end-of-life care in their practice. For example, some pediatric residency review committees have added requirements for training in aspects of palliative, end-of-life, and bereavement care. Other innovative programs aim to identify and reform specific clinical, organizational, and financing policies and practices that contribute to care that is ineffective, unreliable, fragmented, or financially out of reach. The federal government is sponsoring several demonstration projects to test modifications in current Medicaid policies to improve care coordination and access, and some private health plans are also making coverage of hospice and palliative care for children more flexible.

This report builds on two earlier Institute of Medicine (IOM) reports— *Approaching Death: Improving Care at the End of Life* (1997) and *Improving Palliative Care for Cancer* (2001). It continues their arguments that medical and other support for people with fatal or potentially fatal conditions often falls short of what is reasonably, if not simply, attainable. Specifically, this report stresses the following themes:

- The death of a child has a devastating and enduring impact.
- Too often, children with fatal or potentially fatal conditions and their families fail to receive competent, compassionate, and consistent care that meets their physical, emotional, and spiritual needs.
- Better care is possible now, but current methods of organizing and financing palliative, end-of-life, and bereavement care complicate the provision and coordination of services to help children and families and sometimes require families to choose between curative or life-prolonging care and palliative services, in particular, hospice care.
- Inadequate data and scientific knowledge impede efforts to deliver effective care, educate professionals to provide such care, and design supportive public policies.
- Integrating effective palliative care from the time a child's life-threatening medical problem is diagnosed will improve care for children who survive as well as children who die—and will help the families of all these children.

The report recognizes that while much can be done now to support children and families, much more needs to be learned. The analysis and recommendations reflect current knowledge and judgments, but new research and insights will undoubtedly suggest modifications and shifts in emphasis in future years.

CONTEXT AND CHALLENGES

In the United States and other developed countries, many infants who once would have died from prematurity, complications of childbirth, and congenital anomalies (birth defects) now survive. Likewise, children who previously would have perished from an array of childhood infections today live healthy and long lives, thanks to sanitation improvements, vaccines, and antibiotics. In the space of a century, the proportion of all deaths in the United States occurring in children under age 5 dropped from 30 percent in 1900 to just 1.4 percent in 1999. Infant mortality dropped from approximately 100 deaths per 1,000 live births in 1915 to 7.1 per 1,000 in 1999. Nonetheless, children still die. Approximately 55,000 children ages 0 to 19 died in 1999.

Patterns of child mortality differ considerably from patterns for adults, especially elderly adults who die primarily from chronic conditions such as heart disease and cancer. Palliative, end-of-life, and bereavement care must take these differences into account. As shown in Figure S.1, about half of all child deaths occur during infancy. Most of these deaths occur soon after birth from congenital abnormalities or complications associated with pre-

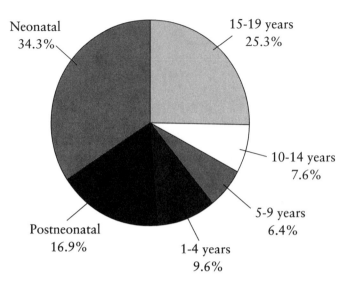

FIGURE S.1   Percentage of total childhood deaths by age group (1999).

maturity, pregnancy, or childbirth. For older infants, sudden infant death syndrome (SIDS) is an important cause of death.

For older children and teenagers, unintentional and intentional injuries are the leading causes of death. Overall, injuries account for approximately 30 percent of child deaths (Figure S.2). Given the importance of sudden and unexpected deaths from injuries and SIDS, efforts to improve care for children and to provide support for bereaved families must extend to emergency first-response personnel, including police, emergency department staff, and staff of medical examiners' offices. Among fatal chronic conditions, the most important are cancers, diseases of the heart, and lower respiratory conditions.

Common Problems Experienced by Both Children and Adults

Some deficits in palliative and end-of-life care for children parallel those experienced by adults. For example, frightened and upset patients and families may receive confusing or misleading explanations of diagnosis, prognosis, and treatment options. They may likewise be provided too little opportunity to absorb shocking information, ask questions, and reflect on goals and decisions, even when no immediate crisis drives decisionmaking. Patients at all ages suffer from inadequate assessment and management of pain and other distress, despite the ready availability of therapies known to help most patients. For both children and adults, physicians may advise and

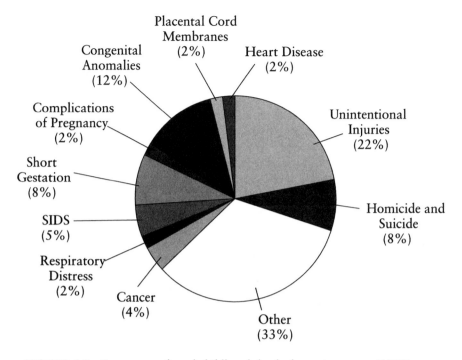

FIGURE S.2 Percentage of total childhood deaths by major causes (1999).

initiate treatments without adequate consideration or explanation of their potential to cause additional suffering while offering no or virtually no potential for benefit. Because clinicians, patients, and families are reluctant to discuss death and dying, opportunities are routinely missed to plan responses for the reasonably predictable crises associated with many fatal medical problems. Failures to prepare for death may deprive families of the chance to cherish their last time with a loved one and say their final good-byes.

Further, if children or adults require complex care from multiple providers of medical and other services, they and their families may find this country's fragmented health and social services systems to be confusing, unreliable, incomplete, and exhausting to negotiate. Even experienced physicians, social workers, and others are frequently frustrated and stymied by these systems. At the same time, patients, families, and providers may feel that they are in a constant battle with health plans over coverage and payment policies that favor invasive medical and surgical procedures, discourage interdisciplinary care, and undervalue palliative services, including the time needed to fully and effectively inform and counsel patients and families facing fatal or potentially fatal conditions. Other children and adults suffer because they lack health insurance altogether.

Issues Unique to or Particularly Evident with Children

Notwithstanding these common problems, certain concerns in palliative, end-of-life, and bereavement care are unique to or particularly evident with children. As is often emphasized, children are not small adults. Clinicians, parents, and others working with ill or injured children must consider developmental differences among infants, children, and adolescents that may affect diagnosis, prognosis, treatment strategies, communication, and decisionmaking processes.

Many children who die are born with rarely seen medical conditions, which creates substantial uncertainty in diagnosis, prognosis, and medical management. Even for common medical problems, children's general physiologic resiliency complicates predictions about their future. In situations laden with fear, anxiety, and desperation, this greater uncertainty adds to the burdens on physicians and families as they try to assess the potential benefits and harms of treatment options and make hard decisions. Further, many communities will not have enough cases of various life-threatening medical conditions in children to generate much local experience and clinical expertise in their evaluation and management, including end-of-life care. As a result, seriously ill children and their families must often travel far from home for treatment, which removes them from their usual sources of emotional support and may disrupt parents' employment and strain family relationships and finances.

While still mentally competent, adults can create advance directives and other binding documents to guide their care if they later suffer significant loss of decisionmaking capacity. In contrast, states, almost without exception, will not recognize a formal advance directive signed by a minor, even a minor living independently. In most situations, parents have legal authority to make decisions about medical treatments for their child.

Many problems facing children with life-threatening medical conditions and their families and many shortcomings in end-of-life care are embedded in broader social, economic, and cultural problems. Unlike virtually all elderly adults, who are covered by Medicare, approximately 15 percent of children lack public or private health insurance. Children with insurance are covered by myriad private and state programs that have widely differing but poorly documented policies and practices for covering palliative, end-of-life, and bereavement services. On the one hand, this diversity of insurance sources could encourage innovation; on the other hand, it makes it extraordinarily difficult to identify and correct deficiencies in any comprehensive way.

In addition, children and young families are disproportionately represented among immigrants and thus are especially vulnerable to misunderstandings related to differences in language, cultural experiences, and values about life, illness, death, and medical or nonmedical therapies. Millions of children, both immigrants and native born, live with their families in unsafe environments that put them at high risk of injury. Such environments can also make it a challenge to get a child to the doctor, pick up a prescription, or persuade a home care provider to come into the neighborhood. These broader problems are not the subject of this report, but their contribution to deficits in care for children and their families should be recognized in strategies to improve pediatric palliative, end-of-life, and bereavement care.

WORKING PRINCIPLES

In general, the basic working principles and starting points set forth in the 1997 IOM report apply to children as well as adults. Some details differ, however, and certain additional values apply either uniquely or with special emphasis to children. Of the principles adopted by this committee (Box S.1), the first three are specific to children; the other four restate earlier principles from the 1997 report in terms of children.

**Box S.1
Working Principles for Pediatric Palliative, End-of-Life, and Bereavement Care**

1. Appropriate care for children with life-threatening medical conditions and their families is designed to fit each child's physical, cognitive, emotional, and spiritual level of development.
2. Good care involves and respects both the child and the family.
3. Families are part of the care team.
4. Effective and compassionate care for children with life-threatening conditions and for their families is an integral and important part of care from diagnosis through death and bereavement.
5. Professionals caring for children have special responsibilities for educating themselves and others about the identification, management, and discussion of the last phase of a child's fatal medical problem.
6. Both individual change and organizational change are needed to provide consistently excellent palliative, end-of-life, and bereavement care for children and their families.
7. More and better research is needed to increase our understanding of clinical, cultural, organizational, and other practices or perspectives that can improve palliative, end-of-life, and bereavement care for children and families.

PROVIDING AND ORGANIZING CHILD- AND FAMILY-CENTERED CARE

Palliative, end-of-life, and bereavement care for children with life-threatening conditions and their families has many objectives and dimensions that relate to the physical, emotional, and spiritual well-being of each child and family and to their frequent need for practical help with coordinating care, preparing for the future, and maintaining as normal a life as possible. Depending on a child's medical condition, his or her plan of care may include a mix of preventive measures, curative or life-prolonging interventions, and rehabilitative services in addition to palliative care. The mix can be expected to change over time as a disease progresses, the goals of care are reconsidered and changed, and the benefits and burdens of therapies are re-evaluated based on guidance and counseling from physicians and others.

When first confronted with the news that their child has a fatal or potentially fatal condition, parents will usually be shocked, perhaps uncomprehending. Initially and thereafter, they may be profoundly reluctant to accept that their child will die and will want to feel that they have tried everything possible to save their child. At the same time, they will want to protect their child from pain and other suffering. Thus, they may simultaneously hold multiple, possibly conflicting goals. This puts an exceptional premium on clear and timely information and sensitive counseling about the potential benefits and harms of different courses of care. Such communication requires not only technical and intellectual skills but also empathy, education, experience, teamwork, time, and reflection—as well as supportive administrative and financing systems.

As parents and clinicians determinedly pursue curative and life-prolonging interventions for an infant, child, or adolescent, they may sometimes fail to appreciate fully the suffering that these interventions may inflict. Not all suffering caused by the pursuit of cure or prolonged life can be prevented, but if the potential sources of distress are not adequately considered, opportunities to prevent or relieve distress will certainly be missed. Care plans should always include steps to assess and prevent physical, emotional, and spiritual suffering. As described by the American Academy of Pediatrics, the goal of palliative care is "to add life to the child's years, not simply years to the child's life."

Formal clinical and administrative protocols are one means of defining expectations and responsibilities for the quality of care provided by health care professionals and institutions. Depending on the aspect of care in question, clinical practice guidelines and institutional protocols may include or be supplemented by ethical guidance, model conversations, checklists, documentation standards, and evaluation plans. They should be based on the best available scientific evidence and expert judgment, including sound guidelines developed by professional societies and other national groups. Careful local review and adaptation may help meet local needs and win support from those who must implement the guidelines and protocols.

Recommendation: Pediatric professionals, children's hospitals, hospices, home health agencies, professional societies, family advocacy groups, government agencies, and others should work together to develop and implement clinical practice guidelines and institutional protocols and procedures for palliative, end-of-life, and bereavement care that meet the needs of children and families for

• complete, timely, understandable information about diagnosis, prognosis, treatments (including their potential benefits and burdens), and palliative care options;
• early and continuing discussion of goals and preferences for care that will be honored wherever care is provided;
• effective and timely prevention, assessment, and treatment of physical and psychological symptoms and other distress, whatever the goals of care and wherever care is provided; and
• competent, fair, and compassionate clinical management of end-of-life decisions about such interventions as resuscitation and mechanical ventilation.

Parents repeatedly cite the frustrations they have experienced in coordinating the care needed by a very ill child. The twin tasks of reducing the burdens of care coordination and improving the continuity of care present formidable challenges. This is especially true for children with complex, chronic problems that require inpatient, home, and community-based services from many different professionals and organizations that may be separated geographically, institutionally, and even culturally from each other and that may be subject to different insurance rules and procedures.

Interdisciplinary care teams (including hospice or palliative care teams), case managers, disease management programs, and "medical homes" for children with special health care needs all have a role to play in improving care coordination and continuity. In addition, those caring for children with life-threatening medical conditions need to collaborate in establishing procedures that support coordination, continuity, and timely transmission of information within and across sites of care. They also should assign specific responsibility to individuals and groups for implementing all policies and procedures related to palliative, end-of-life, and bereavement care.

Recommendation: Children's hospitals, hospices, home health agencies, and other organizations that care for seriously ill or injured children should collaborate to assign specific responsibilities for implementing clinical and administrative protocols and procedures for palliative, end-of-life, and bereavement care. In addition to supporting competent clinical services, protocols should promote the coordination and continuity of care and the timely flow of information among caregivers and within and among care sites including hospitals, family homes, residential care facilities, and injury scenes.

Children with life-threatening medical conditions are often referred to specialized centers for treatment. Some need little follow-up care, but others require considerable attention after they return home. Especially in more rural areas, these children, their families, and the local health care professionals, community hospitals, and other organizations that serve them need additional support. This support may include proven Internet and interactive telemedicine applications as well as telephone consultations and written guidelines and care plans.

Recommendation: Children's hospitals, hospices with established pediatric programs, and other institutions that care for children with fatal or potentially fatal medical conditions should work with professional societies, state agencies, and other organizations to develop regional information programs and other resources to assist clinicians and families in local and outlying communities and rural areas. These resources should include the following:

• consultative services to advise a child's primary physician or local hospice staff on all aspects of care for the child and the family from diagnosis through death and bereavement;
• clinical, organizational, and other guides and information resources to help families to advocate for appropriate care for their children and themselves; and
• professional education and other programs to support palliative, end-of-life, and bereavement care that is competent, continuous, and coordinated across settings, among providers, and over time (regardless of duration of illness).

Parents (or guardians or other designated adults) will, in most cases, have legal authority to make decisions about a child's medical care. Nonetheless, excluding children and, particularly, adolescents from conversations about their diagnosis, prognosis, and treatment strategies can isolate these patients emotionally and prevent parents and clinicians from truly appreciating a child's values, goals, and experience of his or her disease and its treatment.

Recommendation: Children's hospitals, hospices, and other institutions that care for seriously ill or injured children should work with physicians, parents, child patients, psychologists, and other relevant experts to create policies and procedures for involving children in discussions and decisions about their medical condition and its treatment. These policies and procedures—and their application—should be sensitive to children's intellectual and emotional maturity and preferences and to families' cultural backgrounds and values.

After a child dies, friends, neighbors, spiritual advisers, hospice personnel, grief counselors, and others in the local community may provide most of the bereavement and practical support for a family. Parents or siblings may also seek care from their personal physicians or a psychotherapist. Still, the physicians, nurses, social workers, and others who cared for the child can meaningfully "be with" the family in a variety of ways in the days and months following the child's death. An abrupt end to contact can feel like—and be—a kind of abandonment.

Recommendation: Children's hospitals and other hospitals that care for children who die should work with hospices and other relevant community organizations to develop and implement protocols and procedures for

- identifying and coordinating culturally sensitive bereavement services for parents, siblings, and other survivors, whether the child dies after a prolonged illness or after a sudden event;
- defining bereavement support roles for hospital-based and out-of-hospital personnel, including emergency medical services providers, law enforcement officers, hospital pathologists, and staff in medical examiners' offices; and
- responding to the bereavement needs and stresses of professionals, including emergency services and law enforcement personnel, who assist dying children and their families.

FINANCING

Approximately two-thirds of children are covered by employment-based or other private health insurance. About one-fifth are covered by state Medicaid or other public programs, but some 14 to 15 percent of children under age 19 have no health insurance. In this latter group, some children will receive care paid for or provided by "safety-net" providers, private philanthropies, and other sources, but some will go without needed services. The diverse sources of payment for children's health care make it difficult to obtain a comprehensive picture of coverage, reimbursement, and other problem areas, but certain general problems are evident.

For insured children and families, coverage limitations, provider payment methods and rules, and administrative practices can discourage timely and full communication between clinicians and families and may restrict access to effective palliative and end-of-life care. Low levels of payment to providers can make it difficult for health care professionals, hospitals, and hospices to provide certain treatments or even accept some high-cost patients. At the same time, financing policies can promote excessive use of advanced medical technologies and inappropriate transitions between settings of care. In addition, as employers or states restructure their health insurance programs, families are often subject to changes in health plans, provider networks, or terms of coverage (e.g., reduction in home health care benefits). These changes may disrupt continuity of care, including relationships with trusted providers.

Most private health plans, particularly those sponsored by large employers, appear to cover hospice care to some extent, as do nearly all state Medicaid programs. Medicaid programs and some private health plans follow Medicare in limiting hospice care to patients who are certified to have a life expectancy of six months or less and are willing to forgo further curative or life-prolonging care. Such requirements are particularly troublesome for children whose life expectancy is uncertain or whose parents cannot face relinquishing efforts to save or extend their child's life.

Recommendation: Public and private insurers should restructure hospice benefits for children to

- add hospice care to the services required by Congress in Medicaid and other public insurance programs for children and to the services covered for children under private health plans;
- eliminate eligibility restrictions related to life expectancy, substitute criteria based on a child's diagnosis and severity of illness, and drop rules requiring children to forgo curative or life-prolonging care (possibly in a case management framework); and
- include outlier payments for exceptionally costly hospice patients.

In addition to targeting restrictive hospice coverage, this recommendation also is directed at limitations in the current hospice per diem payment method. Research and experience suggest that patients with particularly high-cost needs are often denied hospice or are accepted on the condition that certain expensive services will not be provided by the hospice. An outlier payment system (similar to that adopted by Medicare for inpatient hospital care) for exceptionally high-cost hospice patients should help to reduce access problems by protecting hospices from some financial losses associated with serving these patients.

Even with these changes, additional reforms are needed to promote the integration of palliative care from the time of diagnosis through death and into bereavement and to make palliative care expertise more widely available. If enrollment in hospice is not possible or appropriate for a child, palliative care consultations and counseling for families should be covered.

Further, to recognize the required role of parents in decisionmaking for children, physician reimbursements should be adequate to cover intensive communication and counseling of parents, whether or not the child is present. In addition, bereavement care should be covered as such, whether or not part of a hospice's services. Otherwise, insured parents or siblings who seek counseling generally will be covered only under diagnoses such as depression, which could result in later problems in securing health insurance. Although the committee does not believe that adding these services will be expensive because the number of children who die after extended illnesses is relatively small, it recognizes the cost pressures on private health plans and state Medicaid programs. Thus, the Centers for Medicare and Medicaid Services (CMS) should develop estimates of the cost of adopting these recommendations in Medicaid. As the results of several hospice demonstration projects become available, other adjustments in Medicaid policies may be identified.

Recommendation: In addition to modifying hospice benefits, Medicaid and private insurers should modify policies restricting benefits for other palliative services related to a child's life-threatening medical condition. Such modifications should

• **reimburse the time necessary for fully informing and counseling parents (whether or not the child is present) about their child's (1) diagnosis and prognosis, (2) options for care, including potential benefits and harms, and (3) plan of care, including end-of-life decisions and care for which the family is responsible;**
• **make the expertise of palliative care experts and hospice personnel more widely available by covering palliative care consultations;**
• **reimburse bereavement services for parents and surviving siblings of children who die;**
• **specify coverage and eligibility criteria for palliative inpatient, home health, and professional services based on diagnosis (and, for**

certain services, severity of illness) to guide specialized case managers and others involved in administering the benefits; and

- provide for the Centers for Medicare and Medicaid Services to develop estimates of the potential cost of implementing these modifications for Medicaid.

To implement the recommendations related to improved access to hospice and palliative care, child health professionals, insurers, and researchers will have to work together to define eligibility criteria related to diagnosis and, as appropriate, severity of illness. On a more general level, CMS should take the lead in examining the appropriateness of diagnostic, procedure, and other classification schemes that were originally developed for adult services and are now used by many Medicaid programs and private health plans that cover children. These schemes include diagnosis-related groups (DRGs) for hospital payment and the resource-based relative value scale (RVRBS) for physician payment. Also, given the confusion about billing for palliative care services and the frequent denials of payment for improper coding or documentation, children's access to care may also be improved by providing clearer guidance about accurate coding and documentation of covered palliative services.

Recommendation: Federal and state Medicaid agencies, pediatric organizations, and private insurers should cooperate to (1) define diagnosis and, as appropriate, severity criteria for eligibility for expanded benefits for palliative, hospice, and bereavement services; (2) examine the appropriateness for reimbursing pediatric palliative and end-of-life care of diagnostic, procedure, and other classification systems that were developed for reimbursement of adult services; and (3) develop guidance for practitioners and administrative staff about accurate, consistent coding and documenting of palliative, end-of-life, and bereavement services.

LEGAL AND ETHICAL ISSUES

Questions and disagreements about what constitutes appropriate medical treatment for infants and children with severe and often fatal medical problems are frequent topics in the bioethics literature and occasionally in high-profile litigation. One goal of palliative care is to minimize avoidable conflicts that can arise as a result of failures in communication, insufficient attention to goal setting and care planning, and inappropriate clinical care. Continued efforts at the individual and the organizational level can contribute to the prevention and resolution of conflicts about clinical care, for example, by defining procedures for identifying and managing situations that pose high risks for conflict, developing and testing communication protocols to prevent or defuse conflict, establishing procedures for ethics consultations (or, in some cases, psychological counseling), and developing evidence-based practice guidelines that clarify the benefits and burdens of medical interventions in different clinical situations.

EDUCATION OF HEALTH PROFESSIONALS

Whether the issue is inattention to pain or other symptoms, poor communication, or a clinician's own anxieties about death, children and families suffer when they encounter pediatricians and other professionals who are ill-prepared to provide competent and compassionate palliative, end-of-life, and bereavement care. By itself, education cannot ensure such care or guarantee desired changes in attitudes or behaviors, but it must provide the essential foundation of scientific knowledge, skills, and ethical understanding for all professionals who treat infants, children, and adolescents.

In addition to supporting changes in pediatric generalist and specialist education and consistent with the 1997 IOM report, this committee strongly supports the continued evolution of palliative care as a defined and accepted area of teaching, research, and patient care expertise. The development of a group of specialists in pediatric palliative care has begun, often with support from the larger group of palliative care specialists who care for adults. The numbers of such specialists are still small, but they have a central role not only in providing care but also in enlisting other clinicians, educators, professional societies, research funders, managers, and policymakers to support improvements in pediatric palliative care. Although improved reimbursement will help sustain and expand the ranks of specialists in pediatric palliative care, relevant academic leaders and medical center administrators must also recognize such expertise as essential to meeting their institution's educational and service missions.

Recommendation: Medical, nursing, and other health professions schools or programs should collaborate with professional societies to improve the care provided to seriously ill and injured children by creating and testing curricula and experiences that

- **prepare all health care professionals who work with children and families to have relevant basic competence in palliative, end-of-life, and bereavement care;**
- **prepare specialists, subspecialists, and others who routinely care for children with life-threatening conditions to have advanced competence in the technical and psychosocial aspects of palliative, end-of-life, and bereavement care in their respective fields; and**

• prepare a group of pediatric palliative care specialists to take lead responsibility for acting as clinical role models, educating other professionals, and conducting research that extends the knowledge base for palliative, end-of-life, and bereavement care.

Even for medical conditions that are invariably or often fatal, classroom lectures, clinical rotations, and medical textbooks focus almost exclusively on the pathophysiology of disease and the conventional or experimental interventions that might prolong life—often with little regard for the likelihood of success and with little attention to the burdens experienced by dying patients and their families. In one recent survey of pediatric oncologists, respondents reported that the most common way they learned about end-of-life care was "trial and error." Experience in practice is an important and necessary teacher, but relying on such unstructured and unguided experience puts children and families at risk of much preventable suffering. Even in the crowded undergraduate medical curriculum, opportunities exist to use palliative care and end-of-life issues as powerful illustrations in didactic and clinical teaching.

Recommendation: To provide instruction and experiences appropriate for all health care professionals who care for children, experts in general and specialty fields of pediatric health care and education should collaborate with experts in adult and pediatric palliative care and education to develop and implement

• model curricula that provide a basic foundation of knowledge about palliative, end-of-life, and bereavement care that is appropriate for undergraduate health professions education in areas including but not limited to medicine, nursing, social work, psychology, and pastoral care;
• residency program requirements that provide more extensive preparation as appropriate for each category of pediatric specialists and subspecialists who care for children with life-threatening medical conditions;
• pediatric palliative care fellowships and similar training opportunities;
• introductory and advanced continuing education programs and requirements for both generalist and specialist pediatric professionals; and
• practical, fundable strategies to evaluate selected techniques or tools for educating health professionals in palliative, end-of-life, and bereavement care.

DIRECTIONS FOR RESEARCH

Among the most common phrases in this report are "research is limited" and "systematic data are not available." Research to support improvements in palliative, end-of-life, and bereavement care constitutes only a tiny fraction of research involving children. Likewise, research involving children and their families occupies a small niche in the world of research on palliative and end-of-life care, which itself is small in comparison to other areas of clinical and health services research. Thus, clinicians and parents must often make decisions about the care of children with little guidance from clinical or health services research.

Recommendation: The National Center for Health Statistics, the National Institutes of Health, and other relevant public and private organizations, including philanthropic organizations, should collaborate to improve the collection of descriptive data—epidemiological, clinical, organizational, and financial—to guide the provision, funding, and evaluation of palliative, end-of-life, and bereavement care for children and families.

In the 2001 report *Improving Palliative Care for Cancer*, the IOM's National Cancer Policy Board included two recommendations aimed at stimulating palliative care research in "centers of excellence" designated by the National Institutes of Health and encouraging such centers to take a lead role as agents of national policy in promoting palliative care. This report endorses a similar strategy to use federally funded pediatric oncology centers, neonatal networks, and similar structures to promote attention to palliative, end-of-life, and bereavement care in both pediatric clinical trials and regular patient care. By organizing multiple sites to investigate a common problem using a common methodology, such a strategy should increase the numbers of children involved in studies and increase the credibility of the findings. It should also stimulate the development of investigator expertise in pediatric palliative care research and encourage the formulation and successful completion of more high-quality research projects.

Recommendation: Units of the National Institutes of Health and other organizations that fund pediatric oncology, neonatal, and similar clinical and research centers or networks should define priorities for research in pediatric palliative, end-of-life, and bereavement care. Research should focus on infants, children, adolescents, and their families, including siblings, and should cover care from the time of diagnosis

through death and bereavement. Priorities for research include but are not limited to the effectiveness of

- clinical interventions, including symptom management;
- methods for improving communication and decisionmaking;
- innovative arrangements for delivering, coordinating, and evaluating care, including interdisciplinary care teams and quality improvement strategies; and
- different approaches to bereavement care.

This report also suggests more specific directions for research in a number of areas including symptom control, financing, service organization and delivery, perinatal loss, emergency medical services, and education. Some research in these and other areas will focus narrowly on children who have died or who are expected to die. Other research will include children who have survived or may survive life-threatening medical problems. Both kinds of research should provide knowledge that informs and improves the care of children who survive as well as those who do not. It should likewise help every family that suffers with a seriously ill or injured child. Indeed, all of the recommendations in this report, if implemented, should help create a care system that all children and families can trust to provide capable, compassionate, and reliable care when they are in need.

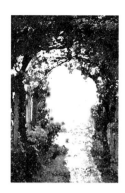

CHAPTER 1

INTRODUCTION

We are the parents of three premature babies—Abigail who died after five and a half months, Jonathan who died soon after being born, and Jeremy who is now 12, tall, athletic, and good in school. . . . I go back to the journals I kept while Abby was in intensive care. . . . It was hard to feel like parents in the ICU. Sometimes there was no room for us, both literally and figuratively. There was no place for parents to hang their coats. The family room closed during the Christmas holidays because of a holiday decorating contest. . . .

No one really talked to us about the possibility that Abigail would die, except in her first week. Even then it was couched in euphemisms that were easy to misunderstand or ignore. I remember being asked one evening, "How far do you live from the hospital?" That was the extent of the inquiry. When Abby coded and died, I was scared and lonely, standing outside, unable to be with her. No one had time to tell me what was happening.

We spent so much time fighting for Abby, getting information, and so forth. Could we have better spent our time just being with her? If we had known better what to expect, would we have just held her? Our second child, Jonathan, died a couple of hours after his birth, largely because we knew some things to ask for after our experience with Abigail.

Looking back, we were professionals, we had contacts, we were used to speaking up for ourselves. What about parents without that?

Deborah Dokken, parent, 2001

The death of a child is a special sorrow, a lifelong loss for surviving mothers, fathers, brothers, sisters, grandparents, and other family members. Some children die after an extended illness; others die suddenly with no forewarning. No matter the circumstances, a child's death is a life-altering experience.

At best, the physicians, nurses, and others who care for a child who dies and for the surviving family will help all involved feel that they did everything they could, that the parents were good parents, that the child and family spent their time together—however limited—forging or reinforcing bonds of love. At worst, families live with memories of possibly needless suffering and with enduring regrets or doubts about their own choices. In between are experiences like that of Abby's family—experiences of good care alternating with unwittingly inflicted pain, of compassion mixed with insensitivity, of choices made and then doubted. Health care professionals may also feel anguished and unsure that they did what was best.

The goal of palliative, end-of-life, and bereavement care for children and their families is to provide them with the best care and support possible and to do so reliably and consistently, no matter how or where a child is cared for. Despite good intentions, that goal is too often not met. Omissions and missteps in care may not be recognized. If they are, health care professionals and organizations may not systematically learn from experience as Abby's and Jonathan's parents did.

Because children are resilient, because they are so cherished, and because advances in medicine and public health have greatly reduced child mortality in the United States, those caring for children with life-threatening medical problems are usually committed to pursuing all curative and life-prolonging options until death is at hand. This intensive but limited focus can expose children and families to unnecessary suffering, particularly if inadequate attention is paid to the potential burdens as well as benefits of these options and to children's physical and emotional distress.

A more comprehensive approach to care is needed. Regardless of the decisions made about curative or life-prolonging treatments, children with life-threatening medical problems and their families should have access to accurate information and excellent supportive care that offers physical, emotional, and spiritual comfort from the time of diagnosis through death and into bereavement—if death is the outcome. Good palliative care should benefit children who survive a life-threatening medical problem as well as those who do not—and should support the families of children in both groups. When they look back, families should feel that everyone did their best to help their child and family.

In recent years, health care professionals, policymakers, researchers, faith communities, and others have paid increasing attention to the needs of people approaching death and those close to them. Because approximately

70 percent of Americans who die each year are elderly adults, most of this attention understandably focuses on their circumstances and needs.

Nonetheless, even in affluent countries, children still die—approximately 55,000 in the United States in 1999. Each of these deaths brings loss, change, and enduring grief to the family. Each death also affects a broader circle of friends, neighbors, schoolmates, and others in the community who may feel distress and a sense of kinship, even if they do not personally know the child or family.

Care for children necessarily differs from care for adults, reflecting children's developing physiological, psychological, and cognitive characteristics and their legal, ethical, and social status. These differences are reflected in the development of pediatric specialties in medicine and other health professions, the creation of pediatric hospitals and other care settings, and the growth of educational programs and research dedicated to improving care for children. Professionals in the evolving fields of palliative and end-of-life care are understanding the need to apply their principles to children and considering how to train palliative care specialists as well as others who regularly care for children and families facing medical problems that are likely to end in the child's death. The importance of such efforts is increasingly being recognized (see, e.g., Armstrong-Dailey and Goltzer, 1993; Armstrong-Dailey and Zarbock, 2002; ChIPPS, 2001; Goldman, 1996; Hilden et al., 2001b; Levetown, 2001; Linke, 2002; Rushton, 2001; Trafford, 2001).

This report examines what is known about the needs of children with life-threatening medical problems and their families and the extent to which these needs are being met. It also presents suggestions and recommendations for strategies to provide more effective, compassionate, and reliable palliative, end-of-life, and bereavement care.

PROBLEMS AND CHALLENGES

When Rosario Maria was born with severe brain injury, she was given two days to live. She survived eight years. . . . It was noticeable that when we finally decided to take the inevitable steps that would lead to her death, the medical staff stopped considering her as a priority.

Rosario Avila, parent, 2001

Many physicians, nurses, social workers, and others provide excellent, sensitive palliative, end-of-life, and bereavement care to children and their families. Nonetheless, as later chapters in this report describe in more depth, shortcomings in care can too frequently be found. Effective, compassionate, reliable palliative and end-of-life care has not usually been a priority for health care providers, managers, researchers, policymakers, or the general public.

Some of the deficits in palliative and end-of-life care for children that are described in this report are similar to those experienced by adults (IOM, 1997). For example, frightened and upset patients and families may receive confusing or misleading explanations of diagnosis, prognosis, and care options. They may likewise be provided too little opportunity to absorb shocking information, ask questions, and reflect on goals and decisions, even when no immediate crisis is driving decisionmaking. Patients of all ages suffer from inadequate assessment and management of pain and other distress, despite the availability of therapies known to help most patients. For both children and adults, physicians may advise and initiate treatments without adequate consideration of their potential to cause additional suffering while offering no or virtually no potential for benefit. Opportunities are routinely missed to plan responses in advance for the reasonably predictable crises associated with many ultimately fatal medical problems.

Certain issues in palliative and end-of-life care are unique to or particularly evident with children. For example, despite 1997 legislation (renewed in 2001, P.L.107-109) that has stimulated increased pediatric drug testing, some drugs used to treat pain, nausea, and other symptoms in adults have yet to be tested or labeled for use in infants, children, or adolescents. Pediatricians thus may have inadequate information to guide their choices of drugs and minimize dangerous side effects, and some may choose not to treat certain children rather than risk such complications and associated liability. To cite another example, although legal issues related to decisionmaking may be somewhat parallel for intellectually and emotionally immature children and for adults who suffer from progressive dementia, the real-life situations may unfold quite differently, particularly in cases of child–parent conflict. While still mentally competent, adults can create advance directives and other binding documents to guide their care if they suffer significant loss of decisionmaking capacity. As discussed in Chapter 8, only one state will recognize an advance directive signed by a minor, although pediatric professionals agree that children should be informed and involved in discussions about their care, consistent with their developmental status.

Many children are born with rarely seen medical conditions, which creates uncertainty in diagnosis, prognosis, and medical management. Even for common medical problems, children's general physiologic resiliency complicates predictions about survival and other outcomes. In situations laden with fear, anxiety, and desperation, this greater uncertainty complicates the physician's and family's efforts to assess and weigh the potential harms and benefits of treatment options.

Further, many communities will not have enough children with life-threatening medical conditions to generate much local experience and clinical expertise. Seriously ill children and their families may, therefore, be more likely than adults to have to travel far from home for treatment. This may remove them from their usual sources of emotional and social support, disrupt parents' employment, and strain family relationships and finances.

Various programs for children with serious disabilities and other special needs help many families obtain and coordinate care for their child. These programs do not, however, cover all such children, especially in middle-income families, and they often require parents to understand and negotiate complicated eligibility and service requirements. Providers likewise may be frustrated by such requirements and by payment methods and levels that favor invasive medical and surgical procedures, discourage multidisciplinary care, and undervalue the time spent assessing children with grave problems, evaluating care strategies, and counseling and assisting their families.

Many problems facing children with life-threatening medical conditions and their families and many shortcomings in palliative and end-of-life care are embedded in broader social, economic, and cultural problems. Large numbers of children and families lack public or private health insurance and have limited access to health services. Even when a child is covered through private or public insurance; some important services may not be reimbursed. If a child requires care from multiple providers of medical and other services, families may find this country's fragmented health and social services systems to be confusing, unreliable, incomplete, and exhausting to negotiate. Even physicians, social workers, and others experienced with sick children and programs to serve them are frequently frustrated and stymied by these systems.

In addition, children and young families are disproportionately represented among immigrants and thus are especially vulnerable to misunderstandings related to differences in cultural experiences and values about life, illness, death, and medical or nonmedical therapies. Many families lack the education or English-language skills that make communication and understanding of clinical and other information easier. Even in communities with large immigrant populations, skilled translators and translated materials tend to be scarce, putting the children and families at greater risk of inadequate or inappropriate care. Many immigrants also lack access to Medicaid or job-based health insurance.

Millions of children, immigrants and native born, live with their families in unsafe environments that put them at high risk of intentional injury and certain kinds of unintentional injury. Such environments also can make it a challenge to get a child to the doctor, pick up a prescription, or persuade a home care provider to come into the neighborhood. These broader problems are not the focus of this report, but those seeking to improve pediatric palliative, end-of-life, and bereavement care must take them into account.

IMPROVING PALLIATIVE, END-OF-LIFE, AND BEREAVEMENT CARE FOR CHILDREN AND THEIR FAMILIES

We took a trip to Florida. It turned out to be just two weeks before Eric died, and he was on multiple medications. And the home health company UPS'd those supplies to Florida so they were waiting for us when we arrived . . . [The very ill mother of] a friend of mine . . . was told that if she left the home, she would lose her home health benefit. . . . I felt very blessed.

Winona Kittiko, parent, 2001

The death of a child will never be easy to accept, and families may resist early explorations or discussions of hospice care, advance decisions about the use of life-support interventions, or other preparations for a child's anticipated death. Nonetheless, health care professionals, insurers, policymakers, and others can do much to save children and families from preventable suffering. Although more research is needed to document the strengths and limitations of different care strategies, the last decade has seen a wide range of initiatives to improve palliative and end-of-life care and focus public attention on the need for individuals and communities to support changes in attitudes, policies, and practices that cause avoidable physical, emotional, and spiritual distress. Some recent initiatives focus specifically on understanding and improving care for children who die and their families and making it easier for families to obtain—and accept—palliative care without forgoing curative or life-prolonging treatments. Many of these projects are at an early stage and have not yet been fully implemented or evaluated.

As discussed in Chapter 6, children's hospitals play a major role in caring for children with medical conditions that are invariably or often fatal. Recognizing this, the Education Development Center in Massachusetts and several children's hospitals—with funding from the Nathan Cummings Foundation, the Open Society Institute, and several other groups—have begun a collaborative project to help improve the quality and consistency of care provided by these specialized institutions to children and their families following the diagnosis of a life-threatening condition (Solomon et al., 2002; see http://www.ippcweb.org). This Initiative for Pediatric Palliative Care promotes the integration of family-centered palliative care with curative or life-prolonging treatments. Related objectives include the development of explicit policies and protocols for symptom management, communication, and decisionmaking and the assessment of performance through routine data collection. Other elements of this project include the development of quality indicators for family-centered pediatric palliative care and the creation of curriculum materials and learning strategies to improve practitioner competence.

As wider use of sonograms and other diagnostic technologies has expanded the number of families who receive a prenatal diagnosis of a lethal or potentially lethal congenital anomaly, several organizations have developed perinatal hospice programs for parents who choose to or have no option but to continue the pregnancy (Sumner, 2001). For example, in 1995, the Madigan Army Medical Center began a program of support for families from the time of diagnosis through fetal death, stillbirth, or infant death and into bereavement (Calhoun and Hoeldke, 2000; see also Sumner, 2001).

The American Academy of Pediatrics recently issued its first explicit policy statement and recommendations on palliative and end-of-life care for children (AAP, 2000g). The American Academy of Hospice and Palliative Medicine has designed a series of self-study modules for physicians who care for dying patients and their families that can be used in undergraduate and medical as well as continuing medical education (AAHPM, 2000). A new module will focus specifically on children. In 2001, the National Hospice and Palliative Care Organization began distributing a compendium of educational and practical resource materials on pediatric palliative care intended for clinicians and others in both hospices and hospitals (ChIPPS, 2001). A recent Institute of Medicine (IOM) report on palliative care for cancer included a chapter on children and families (IOM, 2001c). Several hospices and children's hospitals have begun or are starting palliative care programs.

One recent initiative comes as the result of congressional action directing the Centers for Medicare and Medicaid Services (CMS; formerly the Health Care Financing Administration) to support several demonstration projects to help Medicaid programs, hospices, and other organizations in five specified states develop and evaluate a Program for All-Inclusive Care for Children and their Families (PACC). The program is administered by Children's Hospice International (CHI, 2002; see also http://www.chionline.org). These projects focus on children living with life-threatening medical conditions and their families. The idea is to develop and test models of continuous, integrated, and comprehensive pediatric palliative and end-of-life care similar to the Program of All-Inclusive Care for Elders (PACE) program, which was pioneered for older adults by OnLok Senior Health Services in California. As explained in Chapter 7, waivers of certain federal or state Medicaid requirements for the projects will remove some of the financial and regulatory barriers to such comprehensive care.

A number of public and private organizations including the National Institute of Nursing Research, the National Cancer Institute, the Open Society Institute, and the Robert Wood Johnson Foundation are supporting various efforts by individuals and research coalitions (e.g., the Children's Oncology Group) to strengthen the research base for palliative and end-of-life care for children and their families. These efforts involve clinical research as well as policy, organizational, educational, and behavioral research. For example, three studies have helped clarify the extent and limitation of Medicaid and private insurance coverage for palliative and end-of-life care (e.g., Gabel et al., 1998; Huskamp et al., 2001; Tilly and Wiener, 2001). Other research has assessed clinicians' knowledge and effective use of therapies for children's pain and other distress (see Chapter 3). Congress has substantially increased the incentives for research by pharmaceutical companies to tests drugs in children so that pediatricians, families, and child patients will have better information on which to base therapy decisions (see Chapter 10).

STUDY ORIGINS AND REPORT OVERVIEW

In 1993, the Institute of Medicine convened a small group to discuss the value and content of a study of end-of-life care. That group recommended that the IOM undertake to stimulate discussion and encourage consensus on directions for change in the care of dying patients (IOM, 1993). The IOM launched the study in 1995. The resulting report, *Approaching Death: Improving Care at the End of Life* (IOM, 1997), assessed the knowledge base for providing effective and compassionate end-of-life care and recommended steps that clinicians, educators, researchers, policymakers, and others could take to improve such care.

Although the 1997 report was intended to address care across the age spectrum, this proved difficult in practice given that the overwhelming majority of deaths occur in adults, primarily those age 65 and over. Those under age 20 account for approximately 2 percent of deaths each year. Thus, most of the programs, policies, and research cited in the earlier report focused on older adults.

This second study, which began late in 2000, examines the special needs and circumstances of children and their families and, again, suggests steps that clinicians, educators, researchers, policymakers, and others can take to improve care. The IOM, which is the health policy arm of the National Academy of Sciences, appointed an expert committee of 14 members to prepare this report. Their charge was to

- describe the major causes and settings of death for children;
- review what is known about (1) the medical and other services

provided to dying children and their families and (2) the education of physicians and other professionals who care for gravely ill children;

• assess the state of knowledge about clinical, behavioral, cultural, organizational, legal, and other important aspects of palliative and end-of-life care for children and their families;

• examine methods for communicating information, determining family and child/ patient preferences, resolving conflicts, and evaluating the quality of palliative and end-of-life care as experienced by children and their families; and

• propose a research and action agenda to strengthen the scope and application of the knowledge base for providing effective and compassionate palliative and end-of-life care for children and their families.

This report presents the committee's analysis and recommendations. The committee recognizes that while much can be done now to support children and families, much more needs to be learned. The analysis and recommendations included here reflect current knowledge and judgments, but new research and insights will undoubtedly suggest modifications and shifts in emphasis in future years.

Appendix A describes the committee's information-gathering strategies, which included a public meeting at which interested professional, family, and advocacy groups presented statements and a smaller meeting with families of children who had died or were living with life-threatening medical conditions. The remainder of this chapter describes some of the basic principles that guided the committee's work and reviews a number of concepts important in an examination of palliative and end-of-life care for children and their families.

Chapter 2 presents a profile of death in childhood. That profile and the concepts and principles discussed in this chapter provide a foundation for subsequent examination of the clinical, social, financial, and other practices and policies needed to support effective, flexible, and compassionate palliative and end-of-life care for children and their families.

To underscore the variability in the pathways followed by children who die and their families and set the stage for the discussion in Chapters 4, 5, and 6, Chapter 3 reviews several prototypical trajectories of death in childhood. It also presents a number of case histories that further illustrate this variability and the challenges it presents for families, health care providers, policymakers, and others. The last part of the chapter reviews the limited research investigating the nature and adequacy of palliative and end-of-life care for children and their families.

Chapter 4 considers several questions of concern to children and families faced with a child's serious medical problem: What is happening to me?

What is happening to my child? What are our choices? How will you help us? Chapter 5 considers the basic dimensions of palliative and end-of-life care: physical, emotional, spiritual, and practical as they should engage all those who regularly care for children with life-threatening medical problems and their families. The chapter also discusses bereavement care. In Chapter 6, the focus is on caregivers and care settings. The availability and elements of palliative and end-of-life care in the hospital and at home are reviewed as are strategies for reducing the burdens that families experience in coordinating care for their child within this country's fragmented health care system.

Chapter 7 examines the financing of palliative and end-of-life care for children and their families. It discusses how financing policies and their implementation can create obstacles to effective and compassionate care. Chapter 8 presents an overview of ethical and legal issues that health care professionals, administrators, policymakers, and families may confront in deciding about care for children with life-threatening medical conditions. Chapter 9 discusses what is known about how health care professionals are or can be educated to care for children and families living with a child's life-threatening medical condition. Because the knowledge base for effective pediatric palliative and end-of-life care is so limited, Chapter 10 describes directions for clinical and health services research and examines some of the ethical and practical issues in involving children, especially seriously ill children, in research.

In addition, the report includes several appendixes that explore certain issues in greater detail. Appendix B discusses efforts to develop quantitative tools that provide more accurate estimates of prognosis, especially for infants. The challenge of measuring quality of life for seriously ill or dying children is examined in Appendix C. Appendix D reviews issues of cultural sensitivity in palliative, end-of-life, and bereavement care for children and families, and Appendix E discusses bereavement following the death of a child. A large fraction of children's deaths result from sudden and unexpected events, and Appendix F discusses the role of emergency medical services providers in caring for these children and their families. Appendix G reviews the current state of education in pediatric palliative care. Appendix H describes the planning for one of the PACC projects mentioned earlier. These appendices are available only online (http://www.nap.edu/catalog/10390.html).

GUIDING PRINCIPLES

Early in the course of this study, the committee concluded that the basic working principles or starting points set forth early in the 1997 IOM report applied to children as well as adults, although the specifics sometimes

---

Box 1.1
Working Principles for Pediatric Palliative, End-of-Life, and Bereavement Care

1. Appropriate care for children with life-threatening medical conditions and their families is designed to fit each child's physical, cognitive, emotional, and spiritual level of development.
2. Good care involves and respects both the child and the family.
3. Families are part of the care team.
4. Effective and compassionate care for children with life-threatening conditions and for their families is an integral and important part of care from diagnosis through death and bereavement.
5. Professionals caring for children have special responsibilities for educating themselves and others about the identification, management, and discussion of the last phase of a child's fatal medical problem.
6. Both individual change and organizational change are needed to provide consistently excellent palliative, end-of-life, and bereavement care for children and their families.
7. More and better research is needed to increase our understanding of clinical, cultural, organizational, and other practices or perspectives that can improve palliative, end-of-life, and bereavement care for children and families.

---

differ. The committee also recognized additional values that apply either uniquely or with special emphasis to children. The working principles that guided this committee are summarized in Box 1.1 and discussed below. The first three are specific to children; the remainder restate the earlier principles from the 1997 report in terms of children.

Appropriate care for children with life-threatening medical conditions and their families is designed to fit each child's physical, cognitive, emotional, and spiritual level of development. As is often emphasized, children are not small adults. From birth to adulthood, their physical, intellectual, spiritual, and emotional characteristics, needs, and capacities change in relatively predictable ways, although individual children may vary in the pace and details of their development. For children and families living with life-threatening medical problems, developmental science should guide both the formulation and adaptation of care plans appropriate for the individual child and the information and support provided to the family.

Good care involves and respects both the child and the family. For clinicians who care for children, it is a norm of practice to consider the family as the unit of care. *Family* most commonly means parents, siblings, and other close relatives, but it may be used more broadly to include legal guardians as well as close friends such as godparents, neighbors, and schoolmates. For families, respect means being sensitive to their culture, values, and resources. It also means understanding and supporting the need of mothers and fathers to be "good parents" as they provide and make decisions about medical care for their child. For children, respect means being sensitive to their goals and values, their suffering, their maturity and desire to participate in decisions about their care, and the ways in which different care strategies may help them live as normally as possible given their circumstances.

Families are part of the care team and need full information and support to perform well. Parents are key decision makers and usually are key providers of physical and emotional care for their child, not only at home but also in hospitals. Like other caregivers, parents need appropriate training and information to function effectively. At the same time, for physicians and the rest of the health care team, parents are also part of the unit of care—along with their child. Although parents may cherish every minute of care they provide to an ill child, other caregivers should be alert to excessive strain on parents from a physically, emotionally, or technically demanding regimen of caregiving.

Competent, consistent, and compassionate palliative, end-of-life, and bereavement care is an integral and important part of pediatric care in all settings, from diagnosis of a child's life-threatening medical problem through death and bereavement—if death is the outcome. As stated in the 1997 IOM report, those who are dying "deserve attention that is as thorough, active, and conscientious as that provided to those for whom disease prevention, diagnosis, cure, or rehabilitation are still dominant goals. Individual and system failures to care humanely for dying patients—including failures to use existing knowledge to prevent and relieve distress—should be viewed as clinical and ethical failures" (IOM, 1997, p. 22). All those who care for children who may die should examine their own practices and their institutional context to identify areas for improvement. To guide their own judgments and those of the families that depend on them, clinicians must have a solid scientific and clinical understanding of appropriate symptom assessment and management and of the potential benefits and harms of life-prolonging technologies. They then must help families develop the understanding of these issues that they need to make informed decisions.

Good communication skills and compassion are critical. Parents of children with life-threatening medical conditions are unusually vulnerable to misunderstanding communication that is not attentive to their shock, fear, numbness, confusion, grief, and need for hope. Children's ability to understand their situation and their interest in participating in care decisions will vary depending on their intellectual and emotional maturity and personal characteristics.

Professionals caring for children have special responsibilities for educating themselves and others about the identification, management, and discussion of the last phase of a child's fatal medical condition. Much of the emotional, practical, spiritual and other support needed by children who die and their families will come from within the family. Friends and neighbors, members of their faith community or other social groups, schoolmates and teachers, coworkers, and others outside the medical world may also offer significant support. Nonetheless, perhaps more than for aged adults, physicians, nurses, and other medical personnel play a central role for children who die, in part because parents usually want every medical option to save or extend the life of their child. Clinicians have a moral responsibility to educate themselves about what constitutes good physical and emotional care for dying children and appropriate and sensitive support for their families.

Both individual change and organizational change are needed to provide more effective and consistent palliative, end-of-life, and bereavement care. The commitment of clinicians, researchers, and policymakers to saving children's lives and restoring them to health is powerful and beneficial. Acceptance that cure or meaningfully prolonged life is not possible is painful and difficult—so difficult that some clinicians and parents may not recognize that they are pursuing treatments that bring suffering without benefit. Physicians and other professionals may not commit themselves fully to understanding, assessing, preventing, and relieving pain and other distress. They may even draw away from children and families when death is inevitable and fail to support grieving family members after a child's death. Efforts to change individual attitudes, knowledge, and behavior are essential, but they are unlikely to succeed without supportive organizational, professional, legal, and financial structures. It should not be so difficult—as it is today—to provide timely, coordinated, reliable, effective, and compassionate palliative care for children and adults alike.

More and better research is needed to improve palliative, end-of-life, and bereavement care for children and families. For children even more than for adults, the knowledge base for good palliative and end-of-life care is limited in all areas including physiological, psychosocial, and policy research. Research involving infants, children, and adolescents often involves particular practical and ethical challenges. Still, researchers and research funders have a responsibility to identify questions important to improving pediatric palliative and end-of-life care that can be feasibly and ethically studied. Although protection of children and close oversight of potential risks and burdens are essential, research involving children is also essential and can be undertaken ethically and responsibly. Such research is critical to fill gaps in clinicians' understanding of steps that can help prevent or relieve the suffering of children and their families and also to provide them with tested medications and other strategies for doing so.

CONCEPTS AND DEFINITIONS

This section considers a number of terms widely used in discussions of childhood and in discussions of death. Other concepts are defined and discussed in later chapters (e.g., child- and family-centered care in Chapter 6).

Child

This report uses the terms *child* and *children* very generally to cover the age spectrum from birth through the teenage years. Without taking a position in the moral and legal debate over what constitutes personhood, the report also considers efforts to support families facing a prenatal diagnosis of a lethal congenital condition. Further, although it is not the focus of this report, the committee recognizes the grief of parents who suffer the death of an adult daughter or son.

As they move from birth into adulthood, children are constantly changing and developing physiologically, intellectually, and emotionally. Chronological age is often less important than an understanding of a child's physical, cognitive, emotional, and spiritual development and the medical, social, and other support appropriate to different stages of development.

Definitions of the periods of childhood vary somewhat and reflect a mix of biological and social considerations (see, e.g., Needlman, 2000). In general, a *neonate* is a child from birth through 4 weeks of age (under 28 days). An *infant* is a child from 4 weeks of age through the end of the first year of life. (See Chapter 2 for more terminology related to infants and fetuses.) A *toddler* is often described as a 1 to 3-year old. Preschool children—ages 2 or 3 through 4 or 5 years—are often distinguished from school-age children. An adolescent is sometimes described as a child from 13 through 17 or 19 years of age, but children 10 through 14 may be described as pre- and early adolescents and those 15 through 19 as middle and late adolescents.[1] At 18, a person may make his or her own decisions about matters such as health care and advance directives without parental consent. The need for clarity in the definition of age groupings is obvious for statistical comparisons and analyses involving, for example, leading causes of death among different demographic groups.

---

[1]Some of those involved with adolescent health services identify the transition period to adulthood as extending into the third decade of life (SAM, 1995; Stepp, 2002). The spectrum of pediatric or adolescent care may also be stretched to cover the situation of children with conditions such as congenital heart disease or cystic fibrosis who survive into adulthood and continue to benefit from care and support provided by their pediatric care team.

Family

As noted earlier, *family* generally refers to parents (or legal guardians), siblings, grandparents, and other close relatives. It sometimes is used more broadly to include godparents, playmates, girlfriends or boyfriends, and others close to the child or immediate family. In certain contexts, particularly those involving decisionmaking, family may occasionally be used as a synonym—when the meaning is clear—for parents or legal guardians. As noted earlier, even people who have no personal tie to a child who dies or to the surviving family may experience a sense of loss when they learn of a child's death and feel a strong connection with the family's grief.

Palliative Care, End-of-Life, and Hospice Care

Although some use palliative care and hospice or end-of-life care interchangeably, the committee views *palliative care* more broadly as care that seeks to prevent, relieve, reduce, or soothe the symptoms produced by serious medical conditions or their treatment and to maintain patients' quality of life.[2] The benefits of such care are not limited to people thought to be dying or those enrolled in hospice programs. Rather, "palliative care is a model of caring for patients and their families who suffer from life-threatening illnesses" (AAP, 2000g, p. 351). As used in this report, palliative care also considers the needs of patients and families for timely, accurate, and compassionate provision of information about their diagnosis, prognosis, and treatment options, including the benefits and burdens of treatments. Such information assists patients and families in making decisions.

Palliative care does not itself focus on cure, but it can be provided concurrently with curative or life-prolonging care. Effective anticipation,

---

[2]See, for example, *American Heritage Dictionary* (1992); *Stedman's Medical Dictionary* (1995). In contrast, the World Health Organization defines palliative care more narrowly as "the active total care of patients whose disease is not responsive to curative treatment . . . [when] control of pain, of other symptoms, and of psychological, social and spiritual problems is paramount" (WHO, 1990, p.11). Another source refers to the "appropriate medical care of patients with advanced and progressive disease for whom the focus of care is quality of life and in whom prognosis is limited (although sometimes it may be several years)" (Association of Palliative Medicine of Great Britain and Ireland, cited in ABIM, 1996a). Similarly, the definition prepared in Great Britain in 1987 when palliative care was first recognized as a specialty defines palliative medicine as the "study and management of patients with active, aggressive, far-advanced disease for which prognosis is limited and the focus of care is quality of life" (Doyle et al., 1998, p.3). Billings defines palliative care as an interdisciplinary approach to the comprehensive management of physical, psychological, social and spiritual needs for patients who have progressive incurable illnesses (Billings, 1998).

prevention, and relief of pain and other physical and emotional distress may, in fact, be essential for patients to tolerate demanding treatment regimens. For children who live into adulthood with difficult chronic conditions and experience periodic medical crises, palliative care is also important to prevent unnecessary physical and emotional suffering. In sum, good palliative care following the diagnosis of fatal or potentially fatal condition should help children who survive as well as children who die. All those regularly involved in caring for patients with life-threatening medical problems have roles to play in the delivery of palliative care as defined here.

In addition to the meticulous management of pain and other physical symptoms, palliative care emphasizes the emotional, spiritual, and practical needs of patients and those close to them—from the time of diagnosis through death and bereavement. Helping people live well in the presence of life-threatening medical conditions (and their treatments) requires both compassion and sophisticated strategies and tools for measuring, preventing, and reducing the physical, psychological, and other burdens often associated with such conditions and their treatment.

End-of-life care has no precise meaning (see the discussion below of end-of-life, dying, and death). The term is used in this report to describe care that focuses on preparing for an anticipated death (e.g., advance discussion about using life-support technologies in case of cardiac arrest or other crises, arranging a last family trip, notifying relatives and friends) and managing the end stage of a fatal medical condition (e.g., removing a breathing tube, adjusting symptom management to reflect changing physiology as death approaches).

The term *hospice* may be used to describe a philosophy, a program of care, or a site of care (e.g., a unit in a hospital or other facility). Most commonly, and in this report, hospice refers to an organization or program that provides, arranges, coordinates, and advises on a wide range of medical and supportive services for dying patients and those close to them. The great majority of hospice care is provided at home to elderly adults with chronic conditions, although hospices also provide care for residents of nursing homes and, less commonly, assist with hospitalized patients.

Most hospice services that are provided to elderly people are financed by Medicare. For this reason, hospice care and the Medicare hospice benefit are often, but incorrectly, considered synonymous. As discussed in Chapter 7, the Medicaid hospice benefit follows the Medicare model, but private insurance coverage sometimes is more flexible. Hospice care may also be covered by philanthropy or direct payments from families.

Terms such as *comfort care* or *supportive care* are sometimes used as synonyms for palliative or hospice care by those who believe that they are more understandable and acceptable to patients and their families. Because hospice is so closely associated with end-of-life care and because a child's death is especially hard to accept, hospices may similarly devise different names for their pediatric programs as well as rethink their models of care. As noted later in this report, parents may dread—even hate the thought of—hospice care and may be reluctant to participate in explicit discussions about their child's prognosis, recognize the burdens of certain treatments, or prepare for their child's death.

The broad principles of palliative and end-of-life care apply to children as well as adults. Nonetheless, differences in children's anatomy, physiology, psychosocial and cognitive development, and social and legal status require that assessment, treatment, communication, prognostic, and decisionmaking strategies be adapted to each child's level of development.

Grief and Bereavement

Grief is the term usually used to describe people's feelings and behaviors in response to death. Sadness, numbness, anger, sleep disturbances, inability to concentrate, fatigue, and similar feelings and behaviors are normal responses to a loved one's death. Research suggests that the death of a child prompts more intense grief than the death of a parent or spouse. (See Appendix E.)

Anticipatory grief often occurs in advance of an expected loss. Such losses may include not only death but also losses of expectations for a "normal" life, for example, following diagnosis of a child's serious physical or cognitive disability. Anticipatory grief may be experienced by children with potentially fatal medical problems as well as by those close to them.

Bereavement describes the situation or fact of having experienced loss through death rather than to the emotional content of the experience. *Mourning* sometimes refers to the social rituals and expressions of grief (IOM, 1984) and sometimes to the psychological process of adapting to loss (Silverman, 2000). Rather than talk of recovery or closure following bereavement, experts in grief and bereavement prefer the concepts of emotional reconstruction or reconstitution. *Complicated grief or bereavement* refers to a response to loss that is more intense and longer in duration than usual (Prigerson and Jacobs, 2001).

Although bereavement is a term usually applied to family members, feelings of grief may be shared by many others who have known the child or who feel close to the family. The physicians, nurses, and others who care for a child who dies may grieve, whether or not they feel able to express it. Families may feel comforted and supported when these caregivers communicate that they too grieve the child's death, even as they also offer other support including follow-up information about the child's death (e.g., after a pathologist's or medical examiner's report), referrals to bereavement support groups, and inquiries about the physical and emotional status of parents, siblings, and other family members. Increasingly, researchers and others are considering the grief experienced by those who care for children who die and their families (see, e.g., Rushton, in press; Browning, in press).

The End of Life, Dying, and Death

The end of life can come at any age, including infancy. Nonetheless, because death now typically comes in old age, it is natural for Americans to think of that time as life's end. Today, life ended in childhood seems an affront to the natural order of things, different from the sad but commonplace fate of children in earlier times or distant places.

The IOM's 1997 report noted that *dying* is not a precise descriptive or diagnostic term. Usually, people referred to as dying have a condition from which they are likely to die within a few days to several months. Nonetheless, concern also extends to people with progressive conditions expected to end in death but perhaps not for years.

The definition of *death* is less important for this report than the identification of clinically, ethically, and legally appropriate ways to make decisions and manage care at the end of life. Nonetheless, some concerns do surround the definition of death and application of criteria for declaring death—in particular, brain death (or death by brain criteria). Today, there is widespread but not complete consensus that death occurs either with the irreversible cessation of circulatory and respiratory functions or with the irreversible cessation of all functions of the brain, including the brain stem (see, e.g., President's Commission, 1981; Capron, 2001). Generally accepted criteria for determining brain death require a series of neurological and other assessments, although some jurisdictional and institutional differences exist in details such as who can determine brain death and how long a patient must be observed (Wijdicks, 2001). For children, special guidelines apply. They generally specify two assessments separated by an interval of at least 48 hours for those 1 week to 2 months of age, 24 hours for those ages 2 months to 1 year, and 12 hours for older children; additional confirmatory tests may also be advisable under some circumstances. (Brain death criteria are normally not applied to infants less than 7 days old.[3]) Researchers have found inconsistencies in the application of pediatric brain death criteria (Lynch and Eldadah, 1992; Mejia and Pollack,

---

[3]Because of the unique physiologic changes of brain blood flow during the period of transition from fetus to newborn infant, the brain death criteria developed for adults and older infants and children have not proven useful for infants less than a week old. Currently, no clinically applicable criteria for brain death for newborn infants less than 1 week of age are available.

1995), and professional and parental confusion about the concept has been documented (see, e.g., Harrison and Botkin, 1999). Declaration of brain death, particularly following traumatic injuries, often permits organ donation, an option that allows many parents to feel that some good will come from their tragic loss. Sometimes, the declaration of death may be somewhat delayed beyond the period required by protocols to provide families more time to understand their child's situation and to say their good-byes.

Life-Threatening and Fatal Conditions

The term *life-threatening* condition has no common definition. For purposes of this report, life-threatening conditions are those that (1) carry a substantial probability of death in childhood, although treatment may succeed in curing the condition or substantially prolonging life, and (2) are *perceived* as potentially having a fatal outcome. For example, children with Down syndrome have lower-than-average life expectancy, but the condition is not usually viewed as life threatening unless a child has associated anomalies likely to prove fatal in infancy or childhood.

As used in this report, a *life-shortening or fatal medical condition* is one that is not curable and will end in premature death, especially during childhood.[4] Although such a prognosis for some medical problems may be very clear to clinicians, parents may not accept that their child will die, even when death is very near.

Determination of prognosis is not, however, a precise science, and it is often not possible to identify far in advance which children with life-threatening problems will die. (See Appendix B.) For example, although the fatality rate is high for extreme prematurity, many infants survive after being near death. Whether or not the eventual outcome of a child's medical problem is death, the needs of children and their families for physical, emotional, spiritual, and practical support and for accurate information will often be similar and substantial during much of the time following diagnosis of a life-threatening medical problem. The combination of medical uncertainty and families' need to maintain hope reinforces the principle that palliative care should be integrated with curative and life-prolonging care from the time a life-threatening problem is diagnosed.

---

[4]Some use the term *life limiting* to refer to these conditions (see, e.g., ACT, 1997). This term is potentially confusing because various nonfatal conditions can be life limiting in the sense that they limit people's quality of life or limit their ability to undertake activities of daily living.

Pathways or Trajectories of Dying

Chapter 2, which reviews mortality data for children, makes clear that death comes to children in many different ways, although certain pathways are more common than others. For many infants born very prematurely or with lethal birth defects, death usually comes soon after birth. For many other children, death comes suddenly and with no forewarning following intentional or unintentional injuries. (Even for children with progressive fatal conditions who experience and survive several medical crises, death from a final crisis may still be regarded by parents as unexpected.) Some children die of serious but potentially curable illnesses such as cancer, perhaps after an extended period of apparent recovery. The demands on physicians and others will vary for each of these and other pathways. Chapter 3 includes case histories that further illustrate this point.

For an increasing number of conditions, technologies such as bone marrow and organ transplantation have blurred the pathways of dying. They offer a last chance, possibly very small, of significantly prolonged survival, often with a diminished but—for many—still acceptable quality of life. For inherited genetic conditions such as cystic fibrosis or neurodegenerative disorders, parents may hope their child will live long enough to benefit from gene therapy or some other as yet unproven or undiscovered treatment. These hopes affect discussions with physicians about treatment goals and sometimes interfere with preparations for death, including decisions about resuscitation in the event of cardiopulmonary arrest.

Extending Life, Prolonging Death

Life-extending or *life-prolonging* interventions can add decades, years, months, weeks, days, or minutes of life for a child with a serious medical problem. At some point, the balance of the expected benefits and burdens of efforts to cure or prolong life may shift decisively. The intervention cannot meaningfully extend life but can only prolong dying and suffering. As discussed later in this report, both clinicians and parents may be reluctant to recognize or accept such a shift in the balance of benefits and burdens and may continue nonbeneficial treatments, sometimes to their later regret. Differences in understanding or perceptions of benefits and harms are at the heart of many difficult discussions among family members, clinicians, and others involved in decisions about end-of-life care.

This report uses the terms *life support* and *life-sustaining treatment* to describe interventions or technologies such as cardiopulmonary resuscitation or mechanical ventilation that can maintain vital functions temporarily during and after major surgery or following medical crises. In some situations, these interventions may only prolong a patient's dying. Antibiotics, artificial hydration, and other common therapies may likewise, in some situations, merely prolong dying and suffering.

Quality of Life, Quality of Dying

Many clinicians, researchers and policymakers are now familiar with the concept of health-related *quality of life*, which emphasizes health as perceived and valued by people for themselves (or, in some cases, for those close to them) rather than as seen by experts (see, e.g., Cohen and Mount, 1992; Patrick and Erickson, 1993; Gold et al., 1996). Measures of health-related quality of life include physical, mental, social, and role functioning; sense of well-being; freedom from bodily pain and other physical distress; satisfaction with health care; and overall sense of general health. Many people who have medical problems that are likely to cause their death can spend months or years living well despite the boundaries posed by their condition and its treatment. Increasingly, those who are working to improve palliative and end-of-life care for children and adults emphasize the goal of living as fully or normally as possible in the face of death.

The still-evolving concept of the *quality of dying* focuses on a person's experience of living as death comes near (Wallston et al., 1988; Byock, 1997; Patrick et al., 2001). In the special world of the dying patient, some physical outcomes become increasingly less possible, while other outcomes, such as a sense of peace or spiritual transcendence, may become more meaningful. The world of the dying child is less understood, particularly the ways in which goals, concerns, and perceptions relate to developmental changes. Nonetheless, as discussed in this report, even young children may have spiritual and existential concerns, seek meaning in their short lives, and have goals to achieve before they die.

Efforts to measure these concepts present many challenges. As Appendix C describes, measuring quality of life for children, especially very young or developmentally delayed children, presents special difficulties related to their ability to communicate their needs or feelings. Regardless of age, measuring the quality of dying is difficult because it is often unclear when someone is "dying" and because patients may be unable to respond to questions as a result of their condition or medications. Researchers and others frequently rely on reports from parents, especially through after-death interviews, but family members and patients may diverge in their ratings of a patient's pain, anxiety, and other physical or psychological distress.

Good and Bad Deaths

References to "good" deaths appear less commonly in discussions of children who die than in recollections of the deaths of elderly family members or friends. This undoubtedly reflects, in part, the different cultural perception of death at a young age that has come with the last century's sharp reductions in child mortality in this country. Nonetheless, the committee believes that, in general, an earlier IOM committee's characterizations of "good" and "bad" deaths apply when death comes to a child (IOM, 1997, p. 24):

> A *decent or good death* is one that is: free from avoidable distress and suffering for patients, families, and caregivers; in general accord with patients' and families' wishes; and reasonably consistent with clinical, cultural, and ethical standards. A *bad death*, in turn, is characterized by needless suffering, dishonoring of patient or family wishes or values, and a sense among participants or observers that norms of decency have been offended.

As noted by the earlier committee, notions of a good death may reflect values of a dominant culture that some may not share. Thus, it proposed that "a humane care system is one that people can trust to serve them well as they die, even if their needs and beliefs call for departures from routine practices or idealized expectations of caregivers" (IOM, 1997, p. 24). This kind of trustworthiness—and the competence, sensitivity, and flexibility it demands—is integral to good palliative, end-of-life, and bereavement care for both children and adults.

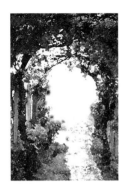

CHAPTER 2

PATTERNS OF CHILDHOOD DEATH IN AMERICA

A simple child, that lightly draws its breath, And feels its life in every limb, What should it know of death?
William Wordsworth, 1798

In 1999, children aged 0 to 19 accounted for 29 percent, or 77.8 million, of the U.S. population of 272.7 million (U.S. Census, 2001). Reflecting their generally good health, children accounted for only 2 percent of all deaths—about 55,000 compared to more than a half million deaths for adults aged 20 to 64 and 1.8 million for those age 65 and over (NCHS, 2001a).[1] Wordsworth's implicit hope is far more a reality today than during the time 200 years past when the poet's two youngest children died.

This chapter summarizes information about the death rates and leading causes of death for children of different ages. It also reviews information about where children die. The discussion begins, however, by briefly putting life-threatening illness and death during childhood in the broader context of child health and illness in the United States. The chapter ends with a short discussion of conclusions and implications for health care providers and policymakers.

CHILDHOOD DEATH IN THE CONTEXT OF IMPROVED CHILD HEALTH

Any discussion of death in childhood and the experience of children

---

[1]Unless otherwise indicated, data are from the National Center for Health Statistics report *Deaths: Final Data 1999* (NCHS, 2001a).

and families living with life-threatening medical problems has to be put in the context of child health as it has improved during the last century. First, in the United States, death in childhood is now rare rather than commonplace. Second, causes of death in childhood have changed. Third, children have different patterns of mortality than adults. Fourth, although most children are now healthy, a significant fraction lives with serious health problems.

Death in Childhood Is No Longer Expected

In 1900, 30 percent of all deaths in the United States occurred in children less than 5 years of age compared to just 1.4 percent in 1999 (CDC, 1999a; NCHS, 2001a). Infant mortality dropped from approximately 100 deaths per 1,000 live births in 1915 (the first year for which data to calculate an infant mortality rate were available) to 29.2 deaths per 1,000 births in 1950 and 7.1 per 1,000 in 1999 (CDC, 1999b; NCHS, 2001a).[2]

This decrease in mortality reflects a century's worth of advances in public health, living standards, medical science and technology, and clinical practice. Many infants who once would have died from prematurity, complications of childbirth, and congenital anomalies (birth defects) now survive. Children who previously would have perished from an array of childhood infections today live healthy and long lives thanks to sanitation improvements, vaccines, and antibiotics. In the United States, the average life expectancy at birth rose from less than 50 years in 1900 to more than 76 years in 1999, due in considerable measure to continuing reductions in infant and child mortality (NCHS, 2001c).

Nonetheless, each year in this country, thousands of parents lose their children to conditions such as prematurity, congenital anomalies, injuries, and diseases such as cancer and heart disease. Thousands more siblings, grandparents, other family members, friends, neighbors, schoolmates, and professional caregivers are touched by these deaths. Instead of being a sad but common family experience, death in childhood now stands out as a particular tragedy, at least in developed nations such as the United States.

---

[2]Despite such progress, the United States ranked twenty-seventh in infant mortality among 38 countries in 1997, lower than such nations as the Czech Republic and Portugal and tied with Cuba (NCHS, 2001c). The relatively high infant mortality rate in the United States has been attributed in part to this country's large number of low birth weight infants, which in turn, reflects underlying social and economic problems and disparities (see, e.g., Guyer et al., 2000; Hoyert et al., 2001).

Leading Causes of Death in Childhood Have Changed

In 1900, pneumonia and influenza, tuberculosis, and enteritis with diarrhea were the three leading causes of death in the United States, and children under 5 accounted for 40 percent of all deaths from these infections (CDC, 1999a). Today, only pneumonia (in combination with influenza) is among the top 10 causes of death overall or for children. Substantial declines in mortality have continued in recent decades. During the past 40 years, infant deaths due to pneumonia and influenza fell from 314 per 100,000 live births in 1960 to 8 per 100,000 in 1999 (Singh and Yu, 1995; NCHS, 2001b). As infectious disease mortality has declined in significance, unintentional and intentional injuries have emerged as leading causes of death, especially for children past infancy.

In 1960, infant deaths from short gestation/low birth weight and congenital anomalies (described in federal reports as "congenital malformations, deformations, and chromosomal abnormalities") occurred at rates of 457 and 361 per 100,000 live births, respectively (Singh and Yu, 1995). By 1999, these rates had dropped to 111 and 138 per 100,000, respectively (NCHS, 2001b).

More recently, mortality from sudden infant death syndrome (SIDS), which was first reported as a separate cause of death in 1973, has dropped substantially—by more than a third between 1992 and 1996, with continuing decreases since then (Willinger et al., 1998; NCHS, 2000b). SIDS is still, however, the third leading cause of infant death in this country.

Children Have Different Patterns of Mortality Than Adults

As shown in Table 2.1 (which uses broader age categories than those used later in this chapter) the leading causes of death differ considerably for children compared to adults, especially elderly adults. For infants, the leading causes of death include congenital anomalies (a highly diverse group of malformations and other conditions), disorders related to short gestation and low birth weight, and sudden infant death syndrome. For older children and teenagers, mortality from unintentional and intentional injuries grows in importance. Among adults, as age increases, the relative contribution of injuries decreases, and death rates related to chronic conditions such as heart disease increase sharply. Beginning in adolescence, increasing age also brings increases in causes of death linked to individual behaviors involving diet, exercise, smoking, alcohol use, and similar factors.

Figure 2.1 shows the percentages of all deaths in childhood accounted for by leading causes of child mortality. Table 2.2 shows the proportion of all deaths for given age groups accounted for by the top five leading causes of death. For most age groups, a few causes of death account for two-thirds

TABLE 2.1 Top Ten Causes of Death, Numbers of Deaths by Cause and Total, and Total Death Rates, by Age Group (1999)

Rank	Age Group (years)		
	Infant (<1)	1–4	5–14
1	Congenital anomalies[a] 5,473	Accidents[b] 1,898	Accidents 3,091
2	Short gestation and LBW[c] 4,392	Congenital anomalies 549	Malignant neoplasms 1,012
3	SIDS 2,648	Malignant neoplasms 418	Homicide 432
4	Complications of pregnancy 1,399	Homicide 376	Congenital anomalies 428
5	Respiratory distress syndrome 1,110	Diseases of the heart 183[4]	Diseases of the heart 277
6	Placental cord membranes 1,025	Pneumonia and influenza 130	Suicide 242
7	Accidents 845	Perinatal period[e] 92	Chronic lower respiratory diseases 139
8	Newborn Sepsis 691	Septicemia 63	Benign neoplasms 101
9	Diseases of the circulatory system 667	Benign neoplasms 63	Pneumonia and influenza 93
10	Atelectasis[f] 647	Chronic lower respiratory diseases 54	Septicemia 77

15–24	25–44	45–64	>65
Accidents 13,656	Accidents 27,121	Malignant neoplasms 135,748	Diseases of the heart 607,265
Homicide 4,998	Malignant neoplasms 20,737	Diseases of the heart 99,161	Malignant neoplasms 390,122
Suicide 3,901	Diseases of the heart 16,666	Accidents 18,924	Stroke 148,599
Malignant neoplasms 1,724	Suicide 11,572	Stroke 15,215	Chronic lower respiratory disease 108,112
Diseases of the heart 1,069	HIV infection 8,961	Chronic lower respiratory diseases 14,407	Pneumonia and influenza 57,282
Congenital anomalies 434	Homicide 7,437	Diabetes mellitus 13,832	Diabetes mellitus 51,843
Chronic lower respiratory diseases 209	Diseases of the liver 3,709	Diseases of the liver 12,005	Alzheimer's Disease 44,020
HIV 198	Stroke 3,154	Suicide 7,977	Accidents 32,219
Stroke 182	Diabetes mellitus 2,524	HIV 5,056	Nephritis 29,938
Pneumonia and influenza 179	Pneumonia and influenza 1,402	Septicemia 4,399	Septicemia 24,626

continued next page

TABLE 2.1   Continued

	Age Group (years)		
Rank	Infant (<1)	1–4	5–14
Total deaths (all causes)	27,937	5,249	7,595
Death rate per 100,000 (all causes)	705.6^g	34.7	19.2

NOTE: The rank order of leading causes of death changed somewhat between 1998 and 1999, reflecting in part changes in the coding rules for selecting underlying cause of death between the ninth and tenth editions of the International Classification of Diseases.
^{a}Congenital malformations, deformations, and chromosomal abnormalities.
^{b}Most vital statistics reports now use the term "unintentional injury" rather than accidents.
^{c}LBW = low birth weight.

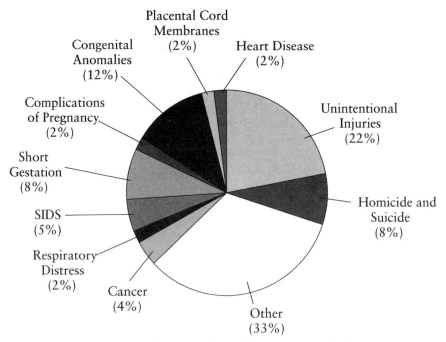

FIGURE 2.1   Percentage of total childhood by major causes (1999).
SOURCE: NCHS, 2001a.

15–24	25–44	45–64	>65
30,656	130,322	391,953	1,797,331
81.2	157.5	662.2	5,203.6

*d*Deaths related to congenital malformations of the heart are included with congenital anomalies.
e Certain conditions originating in the perinatal period.
f Pulmonary collapse or, more generally, absence of gas from part or all of the lung.
g Death rate calculated per 100,000 population (under 1 year) rather than per 1,000 live births, which is the infant mortality rate (see Table 2.4)

SOURCE: NCHS, 2001a, b.

to three-quarters of all deaths. The major exception involves infants who die from a broader array of medical problems, as discussed in more detail below.

Most Children Are Healthy, but Many Live with Serious Health Problems

Although experts worry about the long-term health consequences of common problems such as juvenile obesity and lack of exercise, most children are healthy. Nonetheless, many children live with special health care needs, in part because medical and clinical advances make it possible to save and prolong the lives of children who in earlier times would have died from prematurity, congenital anomalies, injuries, and other problems.

As defined by the Maternal and Child Health Bureau of the U.S. Department of Health and Human Services, children with special health care needs "have or are at increased risk for a chronic physical, developmental, behavioral or emotional condition and . . . also require health and related services of a type or amount beyond that required by children generally" (McPherson et al., 1998, p. 138).[3] These conditions include cerebral palsy,

---

[3]The definition is not yet consistently used, even by the government. For example, one federal government web site (www.childstats.gov) uses the term to describe children who are "limited in their activities because of one or more chronic health conditions."

TABLE 2.2   Percentage of All Deaths Due to
Top Five Leading Causes, by Age (1999)

Age (years)	Percentage of Total
<1	53
1–4	65
5–9	71
10–14	69
15–19	84
20–24	81
25–44	66
45–64	74
>65	73

SOURCE: NCHS, 2001a,b.

vision loss, sickle cell anemia, asthma, mental retardation, autism, and serious learning disorders (NRC, 1996; Newacheck et al., 1998).

Newacheck (2000) has estimated that some 18 percent of children (more than 12 million) have special health care needs, which range from modest to extraordinary. Most have conditions that are not expected to lead to death in childhood. Of the estimated 12.8 million individuals with needs for long-term care at home or elsewhere, approximately 384,000 were children (National Academy on Aging, 1997).

A study by Feudtner and colleagues (2001) found that complex chronic conditions such as cancer and cardiovascular problems accounted for nearly 15,200 deaths among individuals 0 to 24 years of age in 1997. (Note that this estimate spans an additional five years beyond the 0 to 19 age range discussed in this chapter.) The researchers estimated that on any given day, about 5,000 of these individuals were in their last six months of life and potentially could have benefited from hospice care based on restrictive Medicaid eligibility criteria.

A working group on pediatric palliative care has estimated that about 8,600 children would benefit on any given day from palliative care services because of their limited life expectancy and serious needs (ChIPPS, 2001). This estimate did not link the potential for benefit to an assumed life expectancy of six months or less, a criterion for Medicare or Medicaid hospice benefits.

Some children who die from critical acute problems might need intensive palliative or hospice services for a few days or even hours, whereas children with complex chronic problems might need mostly intermittent services over a period of months or years. A substantial percentage of children would not benefit from palliative or hospice services because they die suddenly and unexpectedly, leaving caregivers to tend to the bereaved family.

The next three sections of this chapter review death rates and major causes of death for children by broad age groups. Later sections consider socioeconomic and other disparities in death rates and causes of death.

INFANT, FETAL, AND PERINATAL DEATHS

Because so many deaths occur during pregnancy and in the first year after birth and because understanding the causes of such deaths is of particular interest, a number of terms have been developed to describe and differentiate these deaths. Table 2.3 lists the most widely used terms and their definitions and also includes other common terms and definitions relating to this period.

Death Rates and Numbers

Table 2.4, which shows trends in infant, fetal, and perinatal mortality rates since 1950, reveals continuing mortality decreases in the last half-century. In 1999, the infant mortality rate in the United States reached a low of 7.1 infant deaths per 1,000 live births, or 28,371 total infant deaths. After infancy, the mortality rate drops significantly and does not rise again to similar rates until people reach their mid-50s.

More children die in the first year of life than in all other years of childhood combined (27,937 infants compared to 26,622 children aged 1 to 19 years in 1999) (see Figure 2.2). Two-thirds of infant deaths occur in the neonatal period (18,728 of 27,937 deaths).

Of some 6.2 million pregnancies each year, about 63 percent result in a live birth, 20 percent in an induced abortion, and 15 percent in a fetal death (Martin and Hoyert, 2001). Ninety percent of spontaneous fetal losses occur within the first 20 weeks of pregnancy. A large percentage of these end so early that the pregnancy is unrecognized. Most of the decline in fetal death rates in recent decades has occurred in the late fetal period.

Leading Causes of Infant Death

Understanding the common causes of infant death is important in understanding the potential role of supportive care for these children and their families. Table 2.5 reports the five leading causes of infant, neonatal, and postneonatal death. These causes account for approximately 54 percent of all infant deaths. In contrast, the next five causes (complications of placenta, cord, and membranes; infections; unintentional injuries; intrauterine

TABLE 2.3   Terminology Relating to Infants and Fetuses

Term	Definition
Infant	Child less than 1 year of age
Full-term infant	Infant born between 37 and 42 weeks' gestation
Premature infant	Infant born before 37 weeks of gestation
Neonatal period	First 27 days of life[a]
Early neonatal period	First 6 days of life[a]
Postneonatal period	Days 28–365 of life[a]
Low birth weight	Birth weight less than 2,500 grams (5.5 pounds) at birth
Very low birth weight	Birth weight less than 1,500 grams (3.3 pounds) at birth
Extremely low birth weight	Birth weight less than 1,000 grams (2.2 pounds) at birth
Miscarriage or spontaneous abortion	Naturally occurring, spontaneous expulsion of a human fetus, especially between the twelfth and twenty-seventh weeks of gestation
Antepartum fetal death	Death of a fetus before labor begins
Intrapartum fetal death	Death of a fetus during labor
Fetal death	Death of fetus prior to complete expulsion or extraction from the mother of a product of human conception (irrespective of duration of pregnancy) that is not an induced termination of pregnancy.[b] Some states use the term "stillbirth" for such fetal deaths
Late fetal deaths	Fetal deaths of 28 weeks' or more gestation[b]
Perinatal mortality	Late fetal deaths plus infant deaths within 7 days of birth. (definitions of perinatal mortality vary and sometimes include fetal and infant deaths from the twentieth or the twenty-eighth week of gestation through the seventh or twenty-seventh day of life)
Infant mortality rate	Number of infant deaths per 1,000 live births

[a]NCHS, 2001c, Table 23.
[b]NCHS, 1997. The federal government recommends that state governments, for vital statistics reporting purposes, report fetal deaths of 350 grams or more or, if the weight is unknown, 20 weeks' or more gestation; 13 U.S. jurisdictions follow this recommendation, but the majority (25) use only the 20 weeks' gestation criterion. Fetal mortality rates are based on deaths of 20 or more weeks' gestation.

hypoxia and birth asphyxia; and pneumonia and influenza) account for approximately 14 percent of deaths.

Congenital anomalies and disorders relating to short gestation and unspecified low birth weight dominate as causes of neonatal deaths. During the postneonatal period, SIDS and unintentional injuries and intentional

TABLE 2.4 Infant, Fetal, and Perinatal Mortality Rates, Selected Years 1950–1999

Year	Infant(All)	Neonatal		Post-neonatal	Fetal	Late Fetal	Perinatal
		<28 Days	< 7 Days				
1950	29.2	20.5	17.8	8.7	18.4	14.9	32.5
1970	20.0	15.1	13.6	4.9	14.0	9.5	23.0
1990	9.2	5.8	4.8	3.4	7.5	4.3	9.1
1999	7.1	4.8	3.8	2.4	6.7	3.4	7.2

NOTES: Infant, neonatal, and postneonatal rates are based on deaths per 1,000 live births.
Fetal mortality rate = number of fetal deaths of 20 weeks or more gestation per 1,000 live births plus fetal deaths (at 20 weeks or more).
Fetal deaths are sometimes called stillbirths, but terms and criteria (e.g., gestation period, weight) vary among jurisdictions (NCHS, 1997).
Late fetal mortality rate = number of fetal deaths of 28 weeks' or more gestation per 1,000 live births plus late fetal deaths. Perinatal
mortality rate = number of late fetal deaths plus infant deaths within 7 days of birth per 1,000 live births.
SOURCE: NCHS, 2001c.

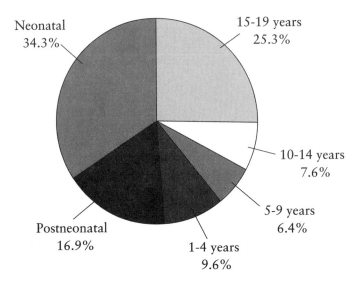

FIGURE 2.2   Percentage of total childhood deaths by age group (1999).
SOURCE: NCHS, 2001b.

injuries increase in relative importance, although the mortality rate overall is substantially lower. Congenital anomalies also cause deaths among children past infancy, but they do so to a lesser extent because most children with problems likely to prove fatal have already died.

Feudtner and colleagues (2001) reported that about one-quarter of all infant deaths in Washington state during 1980 to 1998 were linked to complex chronic conditions such as cardiac, brain, and spinal malformations, with the rest relatively evenly divided between injuries and other acute events (e.g., extreme prematurity, SIDS, respiratory distress syndrome). For the entire group of children, approximately one-fifth of all deaths were linked to chronic complex conditions.

Congenital Anomalies

Congenital anomalies, whether detected before or after birth, can involve any part of an infant. (Federal mortality reports refer to "congenital malformations, deformations, and chromosomal abnormalities" [NCHS, 2001b, p. 71].) Definitions vary. For example, one source defines them as "structural defects present at birth" (*Merck Manual*, 2001, Chapter 261). Another definition is "existing at birth, referring to certain mental or physical traits, anomalies, malformations, diseases, etc. which may be either

TABLE 2.5 Top Five Causes of Infant, Neonatal, and Postneonatal Mortality and Total Deaths (1999)

Rank	Infant Mortality	No.	Neonatal Mortality	No.	Postneonatal Mortality	No.
1	Congenital anomalies	5,473	Short gestation and LBW	4,320	SIDS	2,440
2	Short gestation and LBW	4,392	Congenital anomalies	3,892	Congenital anomalies	1,581
3	SIDS	2,648	Complications of pregnancy	1,391	Accidents and adverse effects	743
4	Complications of pregnancy	1,399	Respiratory distress syndrome	1,050	Pneumonia and influenza	399
5	Respiratory distress syndrome	1,110	Complications of placenta, cord, membrane	1,010	Homicide	288
Total (all causes)		27,937		18,728		9,209

SOURCE: NCHS, 2001b.

hereditary or due to an influence occurring during gestation up to the moment of birth" (*Stedman's Medical Dictionary*, 1995). Congenital anomalies may be inherited or sporadic (for example, arising de novo during embryonic development). Some are readily evident during physical examination at birth, whereas others are detectable only by radiologic, genetic, or other testing. Many defects may be detected before birth by ultrasound examination or examination of fluid or tissue samples.

Congenital anomalies can arise from fetal environmental causes (e.g., drug exposure, infection, maternal nutritional deficiencies, injury) or from chromosomal or genetic abnormalities (which may be inherited or spontaneous). About one newborn in 100 has a hereditary malformation, and about 1 in 200 has an inherited metabolic disorder or an abnormality of the sex chromosomes (Shapiro, 2000). Most anomalies are not lethal, and most (for example, an extra finger, toe, or nipple) have little effect on infant health. The most serious structural anomalies affect the formation of the heart, brain, or other vital organs, and many fatal inherited disorders involve neuromuscular or metabolic functions. Congenital heart disease is the major cause of death in children with congenital anomalies, but it still occurs in only 0.5 to 0.8 percent of live births. The incidence of cardiac anomalies is higher in fetal deaths (10 to 25 percent) and premature infants (about 2 percent, excluding patent ductus arteriosis, a common heart problem that results from the persistence of a fetal circulatory pattern, not from a malformation) (Bernstein, 2000). Advances in surgical procedures, in particular, have significantly improved outcomes for infants with congenital heart problems, but survival is still limited for infants with uncorrectable malformations or coexisting defects in other vital organs.

Congenital disorders of the nervous system that are often or always fatal include anencephaly (absence of all or a major part of the brain) and severe spina bifida (especially rachischisis, a completely open spine) among others. Anencephaly and spina bifida (all degrees of severity) each occur in approximately 1 in 1,000 live births. Virtually all children with anencephaly die within days after birth. The overall risk of mortality for children with spina bifida is 10 to 15 percent, and death usually occurs within the first 4 years of life. Children with severe spinal cord defects who survive often have major chronic care needs (e.g., assistance in eating, bathing, toileting, and dressing). Even with surgical repair of the spinal opening, the spinal cord injury is permanent. The extent of paralysis or mental retardation depends on the location and extent of the defect (Haslam, 2000). Congenital anomalies can also affect the gastrointestinal tract, skeletal system, genitourinary system, circulatory system, and pulmonary system, with varying prognoses depending on the severity of the anomaly and its susceptibility to surgical correction.

Genetic abnormalities may be inherited or arise sporadically. For example, trisomy 13 (Pateau syndrome), trisomy 18 (Edward's syndrome), and trisomy 21 (Down syndrome), conditions in which an extra chromosome is present, are typically not inherited in the usual sense but tend to arise from age-linked errors in the division of ova. Trisomy 13 and 18 are almost always fatal, with less than 10 percent of children surviving more than one year (*Merck Manual,* 2001, Chapter 261). In contrast, trisomy 21 (Down syndrome) rarely leads to death in childhood, but associated problems (e.g., cardiac and skeletal anomalies and a propensity to leukemia) generally cause death by middle age. Duchenne muscular dystrophy and Tay-Sachs disease are among a number of nonchromosomal genetic disorders that are inherited and usually or always lead to death in childhood.

Low Birth Weight and Prematurity

Short gestation and low birth weight are the leading causes of neonatal mortality and handicaps in infants (Stoll and Kliegman, 2000b; see also Sowards, 1999). Most very low birth weight infants are premature, rather than simply small for their gestational age. Only 20 percent of infants weighing 500 to 600 grams at birth survive, compared to 85 to 90 percent of those weighing between 1,250 and 1,500 grams. Similarly, very few infants born at 22 weeks' gestation survive, but more than 95 percent of those born at 30 weeks do.

Most extremely low birth weight (<1,000 grams at birth) infants who die do so within a few days of birth, although some survive for weeks or months before dying (see, e.g., Meadow et al., 1996; Lemons et al., 2001; Tommiska et al., 2001). A study by Meadow and colleagues (1996) reported that the survival rate at birth for these infants was 47 percent but rose to 81 percent by the fourth day of life. After the fourth day of life, an infant's overall severity of illness was a more important factor in survival than the original birth weight. Mortality for premature infants results primarily from conditions associated with immature organs (e.g., respiratory distress related to immature lungs and intraventricular hemorrhage, bleeding into the brain related to underdeveloped cerebral blood vessels) or infection (e.g., sepsis [infection of the blood], necrotizing enterocolitis [an inflammation that causes injury to the bowel], pneumonia) that are complicated by an insufficiently developed immune system.

Sudden Infant Death Syndrome

SIDS is the most common cause of death in infants after 1 month of age. It is a diagnosis of exclusion when a postmortem examination, death scene investigation, and review of case records fail to reveal a specific cause of death. Deaths typically occur between 2 and 4 months of age, and 90 percent of SIDS deaths occur before the child is 6 months old (AAP, 2001c). Environmental factors such as the baby's sleeping position, soft bedding, and cigarette smoke have been implicated as risk factors. An immaturity of the infant's innate ability to control his or her breathing, heartbeat, blood pressure, or arousal level may also contribute to these deaths (AAP, 2001c). Educational programs encouraging parents to put infants to sleep on their backs (the "Back to Sleep" campaign) have been credited as an important factor in the reduction of SIDS rates (Willinger et al., 1998; AAP, 2000b).

The vast majority of unexpected and unexplained infant deaths are caused by SIDS. Experts estimate, however, that between 1 and 5 percent of deaths that are diagnosed as SIDS may actually result from intentional suffocation or other abuse (AAP, 2001c). For this reason and, more generally, to learn more about sudden unexplained infant deaths, death scene investigations of all such deaths are recommended (AAP, 1999c), although no uniformly accepted standards for such investigations now exist (NMRP, 1999). Autopsies are performed in approximately 90 percent of sudden infant deaths that occur without evident explanation (Iverson, 1999). In addition, although the details vary, an increasing number of jurisdictions routinely require an assessment of child deaths by multidisciplinary child fatality review teams that attempt to determine the circumstances surrounding child deaths and identify preventable causes of death, including child abuse and neglect. As discussed later, police investigations, although necessary when the cause of a child's death is unexplained, add extra stress for parents and warrant extra sensitivity by investigators who meet parents.

MORTALITY FOR CHILDREN AGED 1 TO 4 AND 5 TO 9

Death Rates and Numbers

Children in these age groups are much less likely to die than infants. The death rate for infants is more than 751 per 100,000 population (and 7.2 per 1,000 live births) whereas the death rate for children aged 1 to 4 is 34.6 per 100,000 and for children aged 5 to 9 is 17.7 per 100,000 (Tables 2.2 and 2.6). Of the age groups reviewed in this chapter, children aged 5 to 9 have the lowest death rate, with lower rates of death from most leading causes including unintentional and intentional injuries.

TABLE 2.6   Top Five Causes of Death in Children Aged 1–4 and 5–9 Years, Death Rates, and Total Deaths (1999)

Rank	Mortality Ages 1–4	No.	Rate[a]	Mortality Ages 5–9	No.	Rate[a]
1	Unintentional injury	1,898	12.6	Unintentional injury	1,459	7.3
2	Congenital anomalies	549	3.6	Malignant neoplasms	509	2.6
3	Malignant neoplasms	418	2.8	Congenital anomalies	207	1.0
4	Homicide	376	2.5	Homicide	186	0.9
5	Diseases of the heart	183	1.2	Diseases of the heart	116	0.6
Total (all causes)		5,249	34.7		3,474	17.4

[a]Per 100,000 population in age group.

SOURCE: NCHS, 2001a.

Leading Causes of Death for Children 1 to 4 and 5 to 9

Not only death rates but also causes of death differ significantly for children who survive their first year. In particular, unintentional and intentional injuries become more important. The diseases that kill so many older adults—heart disease and cancer—kill relatively few children in these age groups. As shown in Table 2.6, more children aged 1 to 4 were murdered in 1999 than died of heart disease.

Unintentional Injuries

Unintentional injuries are the leading cause of death in children ages 1 to 9. In 1999, they accounted for 36 percent of deaths in the 1 to 4 age group and 42 percent of deaths in the 5 to 9 age group.

Among children aged 1 to 4, motor vehicle occupant injury is the leading cause of unintentional injury-related death, followed by drowning, fire and burns, airway obstruction injuries (choking and suffocation), and motor vehicle pedestrian injuries. Among children aged 5 to 9, motor vehicle occupant injury is again the leading cause of unintentional injury-related death, followed by drowning, fire and burns, airway obstruction injuries, and other transportation fatalities (NCHS, 2001b). Failure to wear seat belts is an important factor in motor vehicle deaths. Nearly 6 out of 10 children under the age of 15 killed in a motor vehicle crash in 2000 were not restrained by a seat belt or child safety seat (NHTSA, 2000).

Congenital Anomalies

Congenital anomalies continue to be a leading cause of death for children in the 1 to 4 age group and, to a lesser extent, the 5 to 9 age group. The total deaths from this cause were, however, slightly more than 800 in 1999 for both age groups combined compared to more than 5,000 for the infant group.

Malignant Neoplasms

Cancer is the leading disease-related cause of death for children more than 1 year of age.[4] In 1999, 2,244 children aged 0 to 19 died of malignant neoplasms (NCHS, 2001a). Analyses by the National Cancer Institute show

---

[4]Cancer is not a leading cause of infant death (see Table 2.1). Nonetheless, although it causes only 0.2 percent of infant deaths, the peak incidence of childhood cancer occurs in the first year of life. Infants fare worse than older children for some diagnoses (e.g., acute lymphoblastic leukemia) but better for others (e.g., neuroblastoma) (Ries et al., 1999, 2001).

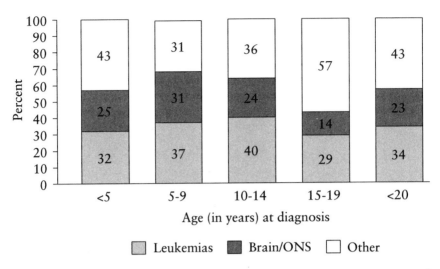

FIGURE 2.3   Percentage distribution of childhood cancer mortality by type and age group, age <20 (1995).
NOTE: ONS = other nervous system.
SOURCE: Ries et al., 1999.

that leukemias and cancers of the brain and central nervous system are the most frequent causes of cancer-related deaths in those under age 20 (Figure 2.3) (Ries et al., 1999, 2001). For adults, lung cancer, breast cancer, and prostate cancer dominate as cancer-related causes of death (Reis et al., 2001).

Survival rates for most childhood cancers have improved dramatically over the past three decades. Age-adjusted mortality dropped by nearly 44 percent from 1975 to 1998 (Ries, 2001). For leukemias in childhood, the decrease was more than 55 percent, but for brain and other nervous system tumors, it was considerably smaller, 24 percent.

According to the National Cancer Institute, the death rate between 1994 and 1998 from all cancers was 2.7 per 100,000 for children aged 0 to 4 and 5 to 9 years (Ries, 2001). Leukemias and brain and other nervous system cancers were the most common types of cancer in these two age groups (as well as in the 10- to 14-year group). They also accounted for more than half the cancer mortality for these age groups. Five-year relative survival rates for children in all age groups for these cancers were fairly similar—between 76 and 79 percent—for the period 1992 to 1997.

Intentional Injuries

In 1990 to 1995, the homicide rate for children aged 1 to 14 in the United States was five times the rate in other industrialized countries (CDC, 1997). The rate of suicide was twice as high for the United States. Although the overall death rate for children decreased substantially during 1950 to 1993, homicide rates tripled and suicide rates quadrupled. More recently, child deaths due to homicide have been declining (NCHS, 2001c). Firearms are the major cause of homicide deaths among children in the United States. Gunshot wounds account for 5 percent of pediatric injuries seen in emergency departments and produce the highest death rate due to injury (NPTR, 2001).[5]

In 1999, homicide was the fourth leading cause of death for children aged 1 to 4 years and was also the fourth leading cause for 5- to 9-year-olds, who had the lowest rate among children. Homicide mortality was nearly threefold higher (2.5 deaths per 100,000, or 376 deaths) for children aged 1 to 4 years than for the 5 to 9 age group (0.9 per 100,000, or 186 deaths). As discussed below, homicide mortality rates vary not only by age but by sex and other characteristics.

Although young children are less likely to be victims of violence than are adolescents, when they are victims, parents and other caretakers are more likely than acquaintances and strangers to have inflicted the abuse, especially for children aged 1 to 4. Within the category of parents and other caretakers, analyses of data from the Federal Bureau of Investigation indicate that parents accounted for 60 percent of the abuse reported to the police, and stepparents and boyfriends or girlfriends of parents accounted for 19 percent (Finkelhor and Ormrod, 2001). As discussed in Chapter 8, such abusive situations present ethical and legal problems related to normal parental responsibilities for decisions about children's medical care.

MORTALITY FOR CHILDREN AGED 10 TO 14 AND 15 TO 19

Death Rates and Numbers

The age groups 10 to 14 and 15 to 19 include the adolescent years. Adolescents can, however, be categorized differently based on social, biological, or developmental criteria. For example, those age 18 and older are legally adults. In most states, they can obtain a driver's license at age 16. Still, pediatricians may continue to care for patients with complex chronic conditions even after they have entered early adulthood.

---

[5]The National Pediatric Trauma Registry is a multicenter nationwide registry established in 1985 to study the etiology of pediatric trauma and its consequences.

TABLE 2.7 Top Five Causes of Death for Adolescents (1999)

Rank	Mortality Ages 10–14	No.	Rate[a]	Mortality Ages 15–19	No.	Rate[a]
1	Unintentional injury	1,632	8.3	Unintentional injury	6,688	33.9
2	Malignant neoplasms	503	2.6	Homicide	2,093	10.6
3	Homicide	246	1.3	Suicide	1,615	8.2
4	Suicide	242	1.2	Malignant neoplasms	745	3.8
5	Congenital anomalies	221	1.1	Heart Disease	463	2.3
	Total (all causes)	4,121	21.1	Total (all causes)	13,778	69.8

[a]Per 100,000 population in the age group.

SOURCE: NCHS, 2001b.

Leading Causes of Death for Children 10 to 14 and 15 to 19

Table 2.7 reports the leading causes of death for children aged 10 to 14 and 15 to 19. Overall, 10- to 14-year-olds have death rates similar those of 5- to 9-year-olds. For older teenagers, however, death rates rise sharply—more than tripling compared to the 10 to 14 age group. This increased mortality reflects developmental changes, including increased risk-taking behaviors as adolescents accelerate their independence from their parents.

Unintentional Injuries

Unintentional injuries are the leading cause of death for both younger and older adolescents, but the rate for older adolescents is almost four times that of the younger group. Not surprisingly, given that younger children are not legally allowed to drive, the rate of unintentional deaths involving motor vehicles increases dramatically with age, from 5.0 deaths per 100,000 children aged 10 to 14 to 26.3 deaths per 100,000 in those aged 15 to 19 in 1999 (NCHS, 2001e). Almost three-quarters of all unintentional traumatic deaths in the older adolescent group involved motor vehicle crashes, including collisions between vehicles, single-car crashes, collisions with fixed objects (e.g., telephone poles, trees), pedestrians, and trains. Older teens also have higher death rates for other kinds of injuries (7.3 per 100,000 for those aged 15 to 19 compared to 3.5 per 100,000 for those aged 10 to 14 in 1998) (NCHS, 2001e).

The teens who die in motor vehicle crashes are passengers 86 percent of the time, but in 68 percent of those crashes, the driver is also a teenager. Alcohol is a significant factor when teens are killed in motor vehicle crashes, with more than half of the teenaged victims found to have blood alcohol levels 0.1 mg/dL or greater (Jones et al. 1992).

Intentional Injuries

Homicide and suicide mortality rates increase as children move through adolescence, with greater than an eight-fold difference between the younger and older adolescent groups for homicide and about seven-fold difference for suicide. Among 10- to 14-year-olds, homicide was the third leading cause of death in 1999, and suicide ranked fourth. For those aged 15 to 19, homicide was the second leading cause of death with suicide ranking third. The majority of suicide and homicide deaths in both age groups were linked to firearms (NCHS, 2001e).

Malignant Neoplasms

Adolescents tend to suffer from different types of cancers than younger children (Ries et al., 1999). Embryonal cancers (e.g., neuroblastoma, Wilms' tumor) are uncommon cancer diagnoses in this age group; germ cell cancers (e.g., testicular cancer) are more common. In 1995, the top four causes of cancer mortality in 10- to 14-year-olds were leukemia, brain and central nervous system (CNS) tumors, bone and joint tumors, and non-Hodgkin's lymphoma (Ries et al., 1999). In 15- to 19-year-olds, the top causes of mortality due to malignant neoplasm were brain and CNS tumors, leukemia, bone and joint tumors, sarcomas, and non-Hodgkin's lymphoma.

Overall, malignant neoplasms are the second leading cause of death in 10- to 14-year-olds and the fourth leading cause of death in 15- to 19-year-olds. The cancer death rate is, however, slightly higher in the older teens than in the younger group (3.8 per 100,000 versus 2.6 per 100,000 in 1999) (NCHS, 2001b). Between 1973 and 1992, the incidence of cancer rose the most and the death rate decreased the least in the 15- to 19-year age category compared to any other child or adult age group (Bleyer et al. 1997).

GENDER, SOCIOECONOMIC, AND OTHER DIFFERENCES AND DISPARITIES IN CHILD MORTALITY

Whether the objective is preventing deaths or planning programs to improve palliative and end-of-life care for children and their families, one useful step is examining demographic and other data for risk factors or variables associated with different rates or causes of child death. Variables typically examined include geographic location, age, sex, socioeconomic and ethnocultural characteristics, and community characteristics such as density, average income or income inequality, and rates of violence.[6]

Differences and Disparities by Region

Reflecting social, economic, physical, and other differences, states and regions show considerable variation in child mortality by cause. One stark contrast involves infant mortality. In 1999, the District of Colombia had the highest infant mortality rate (15.0 per 1,000 live births), followed by South Carolina (10.2 per 1,000 live births). Maine and Utah had the lowest rate in 1999 at 4.8 deaths per 1,000 live births (NCHS, 2001e).

In 1999, for those aged 0 to 19, Wyoming led the nation in motor vehicle fatality rates (23.5 per 100,000), followed by Mississippi (20.9 per 100,000). The lowest fatality rates were for Hawaii (3.6 per 100,000) and Rhode Island (3.8 per 100,000) (NCHS, 2001e). For motor vehicle fatalities involving all ages, factors contributing to differences in rates appear to include population density, proportions of light and heavy trucks in use, alcohol use, and delayed medical care (see, e.g., Muelleman and Mueller, 1996). Two single-state studies, one in Colorado (Hwang et al., 1997) and one in Alabama (King et al. 1994), reported higher death rates from motor vehicle crashes and unintentional injuries for children in rural areas. Another study reported that rural children ages 1 to 19 had a 44 percent higher death rate from injuries than their urban counterparts in 1992, with the greatest differences found in the 15 to 19 age group (Ricketts, 2000). (Reported differences in urban and rural death rates may vary depending on how rural and urban are defined [Farmer et al., 1993]).

Juvenile homicide rates also differ substantially among states. Maryland led the nation in 1999 with a homicide rate of 7.8 per 100,000, followed by Illinois at 7.25 per 100,000. Hawaii and Utah had the lowest

---

[6]Reporting categories for published information from various data sets that include mortality are not completely standardized. For example, the federal government's primary mortality report provides information by Hispanic origin and by race (white and black non-Hispanics (NCHS, 2001a). In contrast, published information from the NCHS linked data set of births and infant deaths subdivides infants by Hispanic origin (black and white) and by race (white, black, American Indian, and Asian or Pacific Islander (NCHS, 2000b). Because death information is linked to information collected at birth, the latter data set also includes more detailed individual data such as the mother's age, educational attainment, marital status, place of birth (U.S. or foreign), and smoking during pregnancy. Information about the infant includes birth order, birth weight, period of gestation, and trimester when prenatal care began.

TABLE 2.8 Death Rates for Selected Causes by Geographic Region (1999)

Region	Infant Mortality	Motor Vehicle (ages 15–19)	Suicide (ages 15–19)	Homicide (ages 15–19)
Northeast	13.6	19.0	5.9	8.0
South	32.8	33.3	8.5	11.8
Midwest	30.8	26.3	8.7	10.7
West	23.5	30.0	8.8	11.0

NOTE: Infant mortality rate is per 1,000 live births. Other death rates are per 100,000 children aged 15 to 19. Homicide deaths include deaths from homicides and legal interventions.

Regions: Northeast (Connecticut, Maine, Massachusetts, New Hampshire, New Jersey, New York, Pennsylvania, Rhode Island, and Vermont); South (Alabama, Arkansas, Delaware, District of Columbia, Florida, Georgia, Kentucky, Louisiana, Maryland, Mississippi, North Carolina, Oklahoma, South Carolina, Tennessee, Texas, Virginia, and West Virginia); Midwest (Illinois, Indiana, Iowa, Kansas, Michigan, Minnesota, Missouri, Nebraska, North Dakota, Ohio, South Dakota, and Wisconsin); and West (Alaska, Arizona, California, Colorado, Hawaii, Idaho, Montana, Nevada, New Mexico, Oregon, Utah, Washington, and Wyoming).
SOURCE: NCHS, 2001e.

rates at 0.6 and 0.75 per 100,000, respectively[7] (NCHS, 2001e). For homicide rates across all age groups, factors contributing to variations appear to include level of urbanization and socioeconomic conditions (see, e.g., Cubbin et al., 2000).

On a regional basis (Table 2.8), the South led the nation in infant mortality, homicides, and motor vehicle-related mortality rates for ages 15 to 19. The West Coast led in suicide rates for this age group. The Northeast region had the lowest death rates for all categories reported here.

Gender Differences

Across all age ranges and for most causes of death, boys have a higher death rate than girls. The disparity increases with age and ranges from a 20 percent higher death rate for male children less than 5 to a 130 percent greater death rate for older adolescent boys compared to girls (NCHS, 2001a).

Male gender is a major risk factor for all injury-related deaths (NPTR, 2001; Hussey, 1997). The most dramatic gender difference is seen in the homicide rate for older adolescents. Boys are more than five times as likely

---

[7]Rates are based on fewer than 20 deaths throughout the year.

to be victims of homicide than girls (1,748 boys aged 15 to 19 were killed compared to 345 teen girls in 1999 aged 15 to 19). Thus, homicide prevention efforts typically focus on young males. For those concerned about support for survivors, special attention to the psychological impact on young male siblings and friends of teen homicide victims may serve dual goals of support for the grieving and preventing further violence.

Socioeconomic and Ethnocultural Differences

A number of studies have examined the association between socioeconomic variables—including income, education, and social status—and variations in mortality among geographic areas and population subgroups (see, e.g., IOM, 2002). Nonetheless, the validity of racial categories and their relevance in clinical and health care research and decisionmaking are sometimes controversial.[8] Concerns about the appropriate use of such categories without adequate attention to underlying differences in access to health care, poverty, and other factors are reasonable. Nonetheless, racial and ethnic disparities in health outcomes and health care access are troubling and cannot be ignored in health care research, planning, and delivery. For example, in addition to considering underlying sources of disparities and developing programs to counter them, advocates of palliative care must consider disparities in the help available to and desired by families for themselves and their children.

---

[8]For example, a recent editorial in the *New England Journal of Medicine* argues that race is a social not a scientific construct and that "attributing differences in a biological end point to race is not only imprecise but also of no proven value in treating an individual patient," although it may be important in the formulation of "just and impartial public policies" (Schwartz, 2001, p. 1392). A second editorial argues that "racial differences . . . have practical importance for the choice and dose of drugs" but emphasizes the clinical importance of identifying and understanding "the genetic determinants of the reported racial differences" rather than relying on self or other reports (Wood, 2001, p. 1395). In the same issue, authors of an article reporting outcomes by racial categories note that such categories may be "only a surrogate marker for genetic or other factors" (Exner et al., 2001, p. 1355). Brosco (1999) suggests that the American habit of separating statistics based on race, especially infant mortality statistics, has led to a policy in children's health that focuses on welfare and reducing poverty rather than on improving all children's health. He argues that such policy allows for bias against certain races, or moral character judgments against socioeconomically disadvantaged groups, and may contribute to resistance to policies that would benefit all children, such as universal health care coverage for children. Others argue that the collection of information on race, ethnicity, and primary language is necessary to guide social policy to reduce racial and ethnic disparities in health status (Perot and Youdelman, 2001). The AAP (2000h) has concluded that it "is no longer sufficient to use [racial, gender, and socioeconomic] categories as explanatory. If data relevant to the underlying social mechanisms have not been collected and are otherwise unavailable, researchers should discuss this as a limitation of the possible conclusions of the presented research."

At all ages, the death rate for black children is higher than for white or Hispanic children. Even before birth, black fetuses have higher mortality rates than white fetuses. In 1998, the fetal mortality rate was more than twice as high for blacks as for whites (12.3 versus 5.7 per 1,000)[9] (NCHS, 2001, Table 23).

In the United States, disparities in infant mortality rate are related to maternal variables such as the mother's age, level of education, amount of prenatal care, marital status, or smoking habits and also differ depending on the infant's age at death, sex, birth weight, or period of gestation. Nonetheless, even when adjusted for these risk factors, racial disparities in mortality remain (Guyer, 2000).

Black infants have a 150 percent higher mortality rate than white infants (1,456 compared to 577 deaths per 100,000 live births, respectively) (NCHS, 2001b). Puerto Rican, Hawaiian, and American Indian infants also experienced higher mortality rates than white infants (26, 33, and 55 percent higher, respectively) (Singh, 1995). In contrast, Chinese, Japanese, and Filipino infants had 30 percent, 23 percent, and 16 percent lower infant mortality rates, respectively, than white infants. Cuban, Central and South American, and Mexican infants had mortality rates that were 12 percent, 10 percent, and 6 percent lower, respectively, than those of whites (Singh, 1995).

Low birth weight is the primary cause of infant mortality in black infants and occurs at a rate of 280.9 per 100,000 live births compared to 72 per 100,000 for white infants.[10] Infants born to black American women are more likely to have low birth weights than those born to either white American women or African-born black women in the United States, which suggests the role that social and cultural factors may play in this difference (Stoll and Kliegman, 2000a,b).

Over the past 50 years, infant mortality has declined at a relatively lower rate for black than for white infants (2.9 percent per year for the former compared to 3.2 percent per year for the latter [Singh and Yu, 1995]). The result is lower rates for both but a greater relative difference. Between 1964 and 1987, racial disparity in infant mortality generally increased across all levels of education and was wider at the highest levels of education (Singh, 1995).

---

[9]Race determined by using the race of the mother.

[10]The number of low birth weight infants, however, increased in white, American Indian, and Asian or Pacific Islander women between 1990 and 1999. Guyer suggests that this increase, for white women in particular, is likely due to the increased use of in vitro fertilization leading to more multiple births, which have a higher likelihood of premature delivery and low birth weights (Martin and Parks, 1999; Guyer et al., 2000).

A study of injury-related mortality attempted to identify socioeconomic factors linked to racial differences in injury rates (Hussey, 1997). When compared to white children, black children were twice as likely to live with a head of household who had not completed high school, more than four times as likely to live in a household in the lowest income bracket, almost four times as likely to live in a female-headed household, and almost three times as likely to live in an inner city. Of these socioeconomic factors, however, the educational attainment of the head of household was the single independent factor related to mortality of children related to injuries. When the head of household had less than a high school diploma, the injury-related death rate of children in the family was 3.5 times greater than for children living with a college-educated head of household. Income and other disparities interact to account statistically for almost two-thirds of the overall difference in injury-related death rates.

Older black children have higher death rates than whites for both injury-related and other causes of death (Table 2.9). For other causes of death, in 1999, HIV/AIDS was not among the top 10 among white children, but it ranked tenth among causes of death for black children 1 to 4 years old, seventh for those aged 5 to 14, and sixth for ages 15 to 24 (NCHS, 2001e).

The greatest disparity in death rates between races is seen in the adolescent homicide rate. Black adolescents between the ages of 15 and 19 years are killed at six times the rate for white adolescents (37.5 per 100,000 versus 5.7 per 100,000). In contrast, suicide and motor vehicle death rates are almost half again as high among white adolescents, ages 15 to 19, compared to black adolescents in this age group (8.6 per 100,000 versus 5.9 per 100,000 for suicide and 28.4 versus 18.2 per 100,000 for motor vehicle deaths) (NCHS, 2001e).

A number of factors appear to underlie racial differences in homicide rates including socioeconomic disparities and age structure of racial subgroups. For example, in a study of domestic homicides in black and white neighborhoods in New Orleans and Atlanta, Centerwall (1995) reported that differences in relative risk of homicide essentially disappeared when controlled for socioeconomic variables such as household crowding. As noted earlier, the United States has substantially higher homicide mortality for children than other developed countries, and explanations for this difference (and similar differences across all age groups) generally focus on handgun availability (CDC, 1997).

WHERE CHILDREN DIE

Based on analysis of 1997 national mortality data, more than 56 percent of child deaths (under age 19) occurred in inpatient hospital settings

TABLE 2.9 Deaths Due to Injury Compared to Other Conditions, by Age and Race (1999)

Age (years)	Injury Rate (number) [a]			Other Conditions Rate (number) [b]		
	Black	White	Black/White Ratio	Black	White	Black/White Ratio
1–4	27.4 (609)	13.4 (1,605)	2.0	30.6 (693)	16.1 (1,936)	1.9
5–9	14.8 (465)	7.2 (1,129)	2.1	13.2 (418)	8.2 (1,278)	1.6
10–14	13.8 (426)	10.7 (1,650)	1.3	13.9 (416)	9.1 (1,385)	1.5
15–19	69.6 (2,119)	51.2 (8,009)	1.4	22.9 (692)	13.9 (2,156)	1.6

[a]Unintentional and intentional injuries.
[b]All noninjury causes.

SOURCE: NCHS, 2001e.

and another 16 percent in outpatient hospital sites (primarily the emergency department).[11] Approximately 5 percent of children were declared dead on arrival at a hospital. Almost 11 percent of children died in home, and the site of death was unknown for a similar percentage. Only a tiny fraction of children (0.36 percent) died in nursing homes. For the population overall, an estimated 52 percent of deaths occurred in hospitals, 22 percent at home, and 21 percent in nursing homes. The percentage of those dying in nursing homes rises steeply with age, increasing from 11 percent among those aged 65 to 74 to 43 percent among those aged 85 or older.

For children who died of cancer in 1997, about 58 percent of deaths occurred in hospital inpatient units, about 36 percent occurred at home, and 2.8 percent occurred in hospital outpatient settings (see footnote 11). In contrast to these national data, a study at Boston Children's Hospital and Dana-Farber Cancer Center found that of 103 child patients who died of cancer during the period September 1997 to August 1998, about half (49 percent) died in the hospital and about half died at home (Wolfe et. al., 2000b). Of those who died in the hospital, nearly half died in the pediatric intensive care unit (PICU) and an additional third in the oncology ward. Regional variations in medical practice, health care resources, urban or rural place of residence, and other factors could account for the different pattern in the national data.

A recent analysis of deaths of individuals less than 25 years old in Washington state from 1980 to 1998 found that 52 percent occurred in the hospital, 17 percent at home, 8 percent in the emergency department or during transport, and 22 percent at other sites (Feudtner et al., 2002). When only deaths from complex chronic conditions and only individuals between ages 1 and 24 were considered, the picture changes. Between 1980 and 1998, the proportion of these deaths occurring at home rose from 21 to 43 percent. Although those who resided in more affluent areas and those with congenital, genetic, neuromuscular, and metabolic conditions were more likely to die at home, considerable regional variation in site of death remained unexplained.

Nearly all SIDS deaths occur in the home. In contrast, most babies who die during the neonatal period never leave the hospital. Some die in the delivery suite shortly after birth; others die within hours to months after being transferred to the neonatal or pediatric intensive care unit. A few

---

[11]This information was provided by Joan Teno, M.D., and Sherry Weitzen, M.H.A., Center for Gerontology and Health Care Research, Brown University, based on an analysis of a database of all deaths in 1997 reported to the National Center for Health Statistics. For more detailed information on site of death data, see http://www.chcr.brown.edu/dying/siteofdeath.htm.

hospitals and hospices have worked together so that families, if they wish and the infant survives long enough after birth, can take infants with fatal conditions home, if only for a day or two before the child's expected death (Sumner, 2001).

According to the National Pediatric Trauma Registry, the most common sites for injuries to children are the road (41 percent) and the home (31 percent). One study of children who died of injuries in an urban county during 1995 and 1996 found that most were pronounced dead at hospitals (although some of these deaths actually occurred outside the hospital) (Bowen and Marshall, 1998), but 10 percent of the children were pronounced dead at home and 4 percent on roads.

Although data are limited, children who die of complex chronic conditions such as AIDS, cystic fibrosis, and muscular dystrophy usually die in the hospital, typically following several earlier hospitalizations for crises that they survived. One multicenter study of children with AIDS who died reported that nearly 65 percent died in the hospital and almost one-quarter died at home (Langston et al., 2001). Another study of children with AIDS reported that nearly three-quarters died in the hospital, either in the pediatric ward (38 percent), the PICU (29 percent), or the emergency department (7 percent) (Oleske and Czarniecki, 1999). Forty percent of these children were orphans living in foster care, adoptive care, or with extended families prior to their deaths.

Clinicians from cystic fibrosis centers in Canada and the United States have reported that the majority of their patients with cystic fibrosis died in the hospital. Of the 45 patients who were reported to have died of the disease in Canada in 1995, 82 percent died in the hospital (Mitchell et al., 2000). A U.S. study, which examined 44 deaths over a 10-year period (1984–1993) in a children's hospital, found that 43 of the children died in the hospital (5 in intensive care) and 1 died at home under hospice care (Robinson et al., 1997). The typical length of stay in the hospital prior to death was two to three weeks, with a range of several hours to several months.

Very few studies describe the deaths of children who suffer from other congenital or genetic conditions. Records of patients admitted to Helen House, the first pediatric hospice in England, between 1982 and 1993 indicate that the largest group of child patients (127 children, 41 percent) had a neurodegenerative disease. By the end of the study period, 77 (58 percent) of the children had died: 49 percent at home, 23 percent at Helen House, and 20 percent in the hospital (8 percent died in "other situations") (Hunt and Burne, 1995). A very small Australian study indicated that six of the nine patients who died from muscular dystrophy and spinal muscular atrophy died in the hospital, some in the emergency department (Parker et al., 1999). The majority of children with congenital heart disorders die in an intensive care setting, often after or while awaiting a heart transplant (Rees in Goldman, 1999). Regardless of the specific cause of death, many patients who die in the hospital die in the PICU after a short hospitalization for an acute problem. In a study of a diverse set of 16 pediatric intensive care units, Levetown and colleagues (1994) found that of 5,415 consecutive admissions to the PICUs, 265 (5 percent) of the patients died. Of the group that died, 248 (94 percent) died in the PICU. The average length of stay in the PICU before death was 3 days (range 0 to 82 days), and the average total length of stay in the hospital prior to death was only 4 days (range 0 to 305 days). The majority (61 percent) of children who died in the PICU suffered from an acute condition such as brain damage due to lack of oxygen (for instance, in drowning), infection, and trauma. Thirty-five percent of the children who died in the PICU had chronic conditions such as congenital malformations, acquired neurologic problems, cancer, metabolic disease, immune deficiency, and respiratory disease. A recent Canadian study, which examined end-of-life care for children who died anticipated deaths (77 of 236 deaths) following admission to one hospital, reported that more than 80 percent died in intensive care (McCallum et al., 2000).

IMPLICATIONS

The profile of childhood death presented in this chapter has a number of implications for those providing or supporting care for children who die and their families. First, children who die and their families are clearly a diverse group. Many children die suddenly and unexpectedly from injuries. Many others die in infancy from complications of prematurity or congenital defects. Some children need care for a few days, whereas others, particularly those with severe neurological deficits, require care for years before death. Further, some children have conditions that are inevitably fatal, whereas other children die from conditions that may be survivable. These differences suggest that palliative and end-of-life care must be flexible if it is to meet child and family needs. Chapter 3 further illustrates the differences in the paths that lead to death in childhood and the different challenges presented by these varied pathways.

Second, unintentional and intentional injuries are important contributors to death in childhood. Emergency medical services dominate in these situations, but many children die before care arrives or without awareness of care. They leave shocked and bereft parents, siblings, grandparents, and others needing support in their bereavement.

Third, particularly for infants and very young children, a varied array of rare, fatal disorders generates a relatively small number of deaths individually, although collectively their impact is more significant. The combination of diversity and small numbers adds to the complexity of determining prognosis, recognizing the end stage of illness, assessing the appropriateness of shifts in the emphasis and goals of care, and helping children and their families prepare for death. Small numbers and diversity can also complicate the development of successful programs to provide and fund palliative and end-of-life care for children and their families. Further, the combination of these characteristics with children's changing developmental needs suggests that palliative care and hospice programs designed for adults will require significant modifications to help children and their families.

Fourth, many important causes of death in childhood—including those due to injuries, low birth weight, and SIDS—are linked to socioeconomic disparities. In addition to encouraging preventive health services and other policies and programs to counter or reduce socioeconomic inequalities, advocates of pediatric palliative care need to consider how their programs can best serve disadvantaged and troubled families and how they can best identify the kinds of support desired by these families for themselves and their children.

Fifth, hospitals, especially their neonatal and pediatric intensive care units, play a particularly important role in care for children who die of complex chronic problems. Discussions of end-of-life care for older adults tend to emphasize practices and policies intended to allow more people to die at home without unwanted "rescue" efforts. Although similar efforts adapted to children and their families may be desirable, more flexible attitudes about the role of hospital care including intensive care at the end of life may be appropriate for this young population.

Sixth, no single protocol for palliative and end-of-life care will fit the varied needs of children who die and their families, and no single focus of research will build the knowledge base to guide such care. The diversity of circumstances and the relatively small numbers of child deaths will challenge researchers and policymakers as well as clinicians.

Chapter 3 builds on this chapter's epidemiologic and quantitative focus by adding a more qualitative perspective on the pathways to death in childhood. It reinforces the conclusion that care for children who die and their families must be adjusted to their specific circumstances and needs, although the fundamental principles outlined in Chapter 1 will broadly apply.

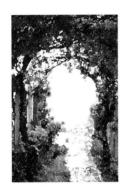

CHAPTER 3

PATHWAYS TO A CHILD'S DEATH

. . . I ran downstairs . . . out into the pouring rain. . . . "For God's sake, where is the ambulance?" . . . [At the hospital,] Dr. Stillman came back looking devastated, and utterly drained. . . . He said that Alexander had died of SIDS. . . . The whole thing was sick. I would know if Alexander was dead. Wasn't I his mother?
Esmeralda Williamson-Noble, parent, no date

My twenty-year-old brother died 8 months ago from cancer. When he became ill, our whole family changed, and my parents didn't have time to think of anything else. . . . It still seems as if Michael's death is all my mother thinks about.
High school junior (Paulson, 2001)

Since birth [our son's] medical needs have increased, and his health has deteriorated. . . . Our goal has been to try to provide him with the best quality of life he could have. . . . We live every day not knowing when will be our son's last. . . . [For emergencies] we carry around a sheaf of papers—about 12 pages—that detail all of our wishes as we know them to this point, because we don't know what every situation will bring.
Tina Heyl-Martineau, parent, 2001

Children who die follow many different pathways to death. Their families accompany them and then follow their own pathways of grief beyond the child's death, even to the end of their own lives. Understanding the similarities and differences in pathways to a child's death and in the experi-

72

ences of their families is a helpful foundation for considering the range of palliative, end-of-life, and bereavement services needed to assist children and families. In addition, it is important to keep in mind that for life-threatening conditions that are not invariably fatal, children who eventually die and children who survive often cannot be predictably distinguished at the time of diagnosis, during initial treatment, or sometimes even after initial treatments have failed. This unpredictability increases the challenges and the importance of understanding how to integrate aspects of palliative care from the time of diagnosis.

The first section of this chapter discusses prototypical trajectories of dying that depict in graphic form the different ways that death may come to children. The second section presents illustrative stories or vignettes that attempt to represent—in ways that epidemiologic data and charts cannot—the human dimensions of death in childhood. These stories, although they inevitably and greatly simplify real life, suggest how the varied circumstances that surround the deaths of children may affect the child, the family, and the health professionals who care for them.

The third section discusses prototypical patterns of care that illustrate traditional and newer perspectives on the relationship between curative or life-prolonging care and palliative and end-of-life care. The newer perspective, stressed in this report, encourages the integration of certain aspects of palliative care from the time a child is diagnosed with a fatal or potentially fatal medical condition. The section also discusses how the emphasis of care may vary depending on the medical circumstances and may, given similar medical "facts," be affected by differences in family values and circumstances as well as differences in the resources available to them.

Documentation of the focus and adequacy of pediatric palliative and end-of-life care is very limited. The final section of the chapter reviews this small literature.

TRAJECTORIES OF DYING

To help illuminate differences in the paths that people follow to death, Glaser and Straus introduced the concept of a trajectory of dying. They proposed that "the dying trajectory of each patient has at least two outstanding [and variable] properties . . . duration and shape" (Glaser and Straus, 1965, p. 6). The shape of the trajectory depends on time and on the person's level of functioning or health status. Figure 3.1 presents four simplified trajectories of death in childhood that depict time along the horizontal axis and health status along the vertical axis. These trajectories underscore the reality that no single model of care and support will apply to all dying children and their families. The trajectories do not, however, necessarily map in a straightforward fashion to specific models of palliative care.

a. Sudden, unexpected death

b. Death from potentially curable disease (e.g., brain cancer)

c. Death from lethal congenital anomaly

d. Death from progressive condition with intermittent crises (e.g., muscular dystrophy)

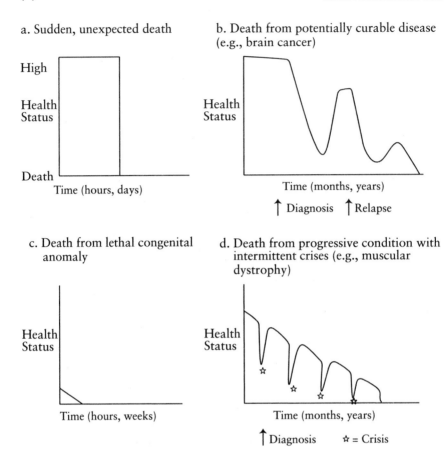

FIGURE 3.1   Prototypical trajectories of child death.
SOURCE: Adapted from IOM, 1997.

The most abrupt trajectory, Figure 3.1a, represents the unexpected, sudden death—for example, that of a child killed instantly in a car crash or discovered dead in his crib at home. Such events account for more than a third of childhood deaths. Although children who have died can themselves experience no medical or supportive care, first-response emergency medical personnel commonly follow protocols that require efforts at resuscitation. When a child is involved, only rarely is death actually declared "in the field" rather than in the hospital. If the declaration is based on criteria for brain death, protocols require a period of assessments and observation that may take from 12 to 48 hours or longer (see Chapter 1).

Figure 3.1b depicts the experience of children who respond positively to initial, sometimes difficult and possibly life-threatening treatment for a potentially fatal condition, for example, certain brain cancers, but who eventually die of their disease or its further treatment. At diagnosis and during the early stages of initial treatment, these children may not be uniformly distinguished either from children who will not respond or from children who will eventually be cured. (Overall, 70 percent of children with cancer are cured.) Even when an initial positive response to treatment is followed by a return of the disease, determining prognosis is not automatic. From a palliative care perspective, at least three tasks follow diagnosis—each adapted to the situation of the individual child and family. One task is to provide the family—and the child, as appropriate—with accurate and timely information on diagnosis, prognosis, and treatment options and to help them make informed decisions and prepare for a future that includes the hope of cure. A second task is to provide comfort to the child (in particular, by preventing or relieving symptoms of the disease or its treatment) and support to the family. If initial or subsequent treatment fails the child, families will need information about the benefits and burdens of remaining treatment options and about prognosis. When further curative or life-prolonging interventions fail, the additional task for the care team is to help the child and family through the dying phase of the child's illness and then support the family at death and after.

Figure 3.1c depicts the brief trajectory of an infant born with problems incompatible with extended life. As described in Chapter 2, extreme prematurity, severe congenital anomalies, and other life-threatening conditions affecting infants account for a significant fraction of child deaths. With modern prenatal care, some families know in advance that their child will not survive, and some know that they are at significant risk of premature delivery. Extremely premature infants and infants with severe congenital anomalies have produced high-profile disagreements about appropriate care, but care to comfort the infant and the family is always appropriate. As illustrated later in this chapter and discussed further in Chapters 4 and 5, actual support for families may be very limited.

Figure 3.1d abstracts the experience of children who suffer from a fatal progressive illness—for example, muscular dystrophy—that is characterized by periods of slowly deteriorating health status that are interrupted by potentially fatal medical crises, which the child repeatedly survives until one crisis ends in death. In some situations, a child's past favorable response to treatment may leave parents and even clinicians unprepared for and surprised by a subsequent failure of treatment. In other situations, clinicians and parents recognize that the child has reached the final stage of his or her illness and focus on physical and emotional comfort, accepting that resuscitation and other life-sustaining interventions will be more burdensome than beneficial.

Various other trajectories for progressive conditions and for some chronic conditions could be mapped. For example, children with severe asthma and appropriate treatment may have mostly normal functioning without disease progression, but a sudden life-ending crisis may occur and be almost as unexpected as a death from injury.

The illustrative vignettes presented next describe experiences of a child's death that approximate the four trajectories presented above. In addition to the two dimensions of health status and time, they depict other dimensions of a child's death including the individuality of the child and family and the competence and compassion of health care professionals.

ILLUSTRATIVE STORIES OF CHILDREN AND THEIR FAMILIES

During the course of its work, the committee heard many compelling stories from parents whose child had died. In the details of their experiences and in their expectations, the families differed, but they made clear that parents long remember how health care professionals helped or hurt them.

Most parents reported a mix of good and bad experiences. Some told of exemplary care. Others reported insensitive and even cruel behavior from physicians, nurses, or others involved in their child's care. Some found that insurers or health plans were supportive; some had no insurance; others had continuing and exhausting difficulties trying to get care approved—and then suffered with their child when coverage of hospice or other supportive services was denied. Often faced with uncertainty about their child's prognosis and treatment options, some parents anguished over decisions about how far to pursue experimental treatments or whether and when mechanical ventilation or other life-support interventions should be withheld or withdrawn.

Beyond his or her medical condition, a child's experience of dying will depend on many factors, including the family's circumstances, values, and responses to the illness and the kind of medical and other services that are available to meet the child's physical, psychological, spiritual, and other needs. The brief stories presented below suggest how the complex interplay of these factors may affect the level of distress experienced by children and their families.

None of the following stories depicts a specific child and family exactly, although each is based on real experiences. Some are fairly typical of childhood deaths, whereas others represent more unusual or particularly challenging situations. The stories are clearly simplified, but they highlight differences in the needs of children and families and differences in the extent to which the care provided met these needs. Most depict deficits in some aspects of the care provided the child or family.

"Ana Rivera"

When death comes to children, it often is sudden and unexpected (Figure 3.1a). In this case, 3-month-old Ana's father finds her lifeless body in her crib one morning. Her parents' grief is complicated and intensified when they realize that a police officer's questions are probing the possibility of homicide. This story also illustrates the special difficulties facing immigrant parents whose language abilities and resources are limited.

Jorge and Maria Rivera had emigrated from El Salvador two years prior to Ana's birth, leaving their three children behind with Maria's mother and promising to send money to support the family. Maria's first husband and two older brothers had been killed during the war, but her cousin had escaped to the United States and urged Maria and her second husband Jorge to follow him. Jorge got a job at a fast-food restaurant and Maria cleaned houses, and they scrimped on everything so that they could send a little money back to their family in El Salvador. They felt isolated but were overjoyed when they learned that Maria was pregnant. A neighbor brought Maria to a clinic that provided prenatal care to poor women. The Riveras were proud to give this new baby—Ana—such a good start.

After an uneventful pregnancy, delivery, and first few months, Jorge found 3-month-old Ana cold, blue, and motionless in her crib one morning. The Riveras rushed Ana to the public hospital where she was immediately taken into a treatment room. In a short while, the Riveras were led into a small sitting room in the emergency department where a physician informed them, through a janitor who spoke both English and Spanish, that Ana had died. The janitor did not understand all of the words the physician said but assured the Riveras that everything had been done to help Ana. After the physician left, a police officer came into the room and began to ask Jorge questions about how he had found Ana, what he was doing prior to finding her, what her health had been like prior to that morning, and whether Jorge had ever hurt either Ana or Maria. Jorge remembered that he had been angry the night before and yelled at Ana when she wouldn't stop crying, but he was afraid to tell the police officer this information. No charges were brought against Jorge and Maria, but they lived in fear that they would be arrested and sent back to El Salvador. Both had intense feelings of loss for Ana and for their three other children who were still in El Salvador. A hospital social worker told the Riveras about bereavement support groups, but none was nearby and none had groups for Spanish speakers. The social worker really helped in one way. She helped make sure that the Riveras qualified for free care under a community program for the medically indigent, so at least they did not face medical bills that they could not possibly pay.

"Jimmy Marshall"

In this case, which involves another leading cause of child mortality, a car–bicycle collision set off a frantic effort to save an injured child's life. To the parents, the emergency department and intensive care unit are frightening and strange. Despite the help of several social workers, there is much they do not understand and that is never explained. They are unwittingly misled by one clinician who is satisfied with the technical success of a procedure but not focused on what is still a very grim, likely fatal situation. One result is a father's lifelong regret that he was not with his wife and son when the boy died.

While riding his bicycle with a friend, Jimmy Marshall, an 11-year-old boy, was struck by a car. Emergency personnel found him semiconscious with obvious head injuries and rushed him to the nearest trauma center, which treated but did not specialize in pediatric trauma. In the emergency department (ED), Jimmy was taken to a large, open resuscitation bay while the trauma team, including nurses, surgeons, neurosurgeons, emergency physicians, and pediatricians, cared for him. His condition was clearly very serious.

Friends rushed Jimmy's mother to the hospital. In a small, windowless room, the social worker provided some brief information and comforting words. Then, the ED "attending" came in to explain that Jimmy had suffered a serious brain injury and they were doing everything they could to help him. Later, a "pediatric resident" said that Jimmy was being taken to x-ray for special scans of his brain and that the team was very worried. Fighting tears and hysteria, Mrs. Marshall asked, "But he is going to be all right isn't he?" The resident appeared to almost shrug as she said, "I can't tell you that." The rest was a blur.

Just after Jimmy was taken to the intensive care unit, his father arrived. The attending physician gave a brief, grim update. Both Marshalls started to weep. The family would have welcomed the support of a hospital chaplain, but no one thought to see if someone was available. As they waited, the conversation around them sounded ominous, but the terminology was mysterious, and both parents were too bewildered or intimidated to ask many questions. Told that neurosurgeons needed to put a hole in their son's skull in order to monitor dangerous swelling, Mr. Marshall protested that this might injure Jimmy's brain. A doctor replied, "You have more important things to worry about right now."

After the procedure, the neurosurgeon approached, smiling and commenting that things went "great." For the first time, Jimmy's parents felt relieved and somewhat confident. The father, afraid that he would lose his job, then left to return to his construction work. However, when the doctor who appeared to be in charge returned, he told Mrs. Marshall that they needed to talk and that she should try to reach her husband.

In the interim, the doctor told Jimmy's mother that there had been increasing brain injury and that the task was to prevent the brain from swelling and "crushing itself." Her son might die. This seemed impossible given that only a few minutes earlier someone else had seemed so cheerfully pleased.

Suddenly, a nurse rushed in to say that the doctor was needed. Jimmy's heart had stopped and CPR (cardiopulmonary resuscitation) had been initiated. The doctors knew that the likelihood of resuscitating Jimmy was negligible but were obligated to try. The doctors subsequently had to tell the Marshalls that they had done everything, but Jimmy had died. Later, Mr. Marshall agonized that he hadn't been told enough to realize that he should stay with his wife and boy, and he sometimes felt angry at how the neurosurgeon misled them. He and his wife got a piece of paper with information about bereavement support, but it was laid aside and then lost in all the turmoil. There was no further contact from those who were with Jimmy when he died. At least, they had qualified for "free" hospital care.

"Melissa Devane"

As children mature, their intellectual and emotional understanding of serious illness and the prospect of death evolves. This story describes the complex relationships between a severely ill adolescent and her parents and physician and the different concerns she has as she moves from diagnosis and treatment, to recurrences and further treatment, to death (Figure 3.1b). The adolescent is in conflict with her parents and physician about undergoing burdensome experimental treatment but eventually persuades them to respect her wishes.

When Melissa was 13 years old, she was an excellent softball player who hoped some day to play on the Olympic softball team. Late one summer, her knee began to hurt severely and kept hurting. When Melissa's primary care physician thought an x-ray suggested a tumor, she referred her to Dr. Garcia, a pediatric oncologist. After a biopsy, Dr. Garcia diagnosed osteogenic sarcoma, an invasive bone cancer. As Dr. Garcia recommended, Melissa had several weeks of chemotherapy followed by surgical removal of the tumor and then several months more of chemotherapy plus physical therapy. Although the hospitalizations for chemotherapy and episodes of fever were no fun, what bothered Melissa most was losing the ability to play her sport ever again. Also, her hair fell out just as school was starting. The social worker on her oncology team helped Melissa to get a wig and, as part of the team's attention to school reentry issues, explained Melissa's situation to classmates and teachers.

The family celebrated the end of Melissa's chemotherapy with a big party. Melissa was sad that only half of her former teammates made it to the party. She commented to the social worker that she had learned through the experience "who her real friends were." The yearbook club and her younger sister's softball games became new focal points.

At a follow-up appointment 13 months after the end of chemotherapy, Dr. Garcia found a spot on the CT (computed tomography) scan of Melissa's right lung. He recommended surgical removal of the suspected tumor to confirm the diagnosis. The surgery was uneventful, and Melissa was pleased there would be no chemotherapy. Six months later, however, scans showed tumors in both lungs. This time, intensive chemotherapy followed surgery. Family and friends and an occasional tutor supported Melissa through the months of hospitalization.

Now almost 17 years old and hoping to plan for college, Melissa did her best to look to the future and regain her strength. By the winter of her senior year, she was back in school full time, working on the yearbook, and seeing a new boyfriend. Then, routine scans showed another recurrence in the lung, but this tumor was too big to remove surgically. Dr. Garcia proposed experimental chemotherapy that would require long hospitalization. Melissa reacted by saying, "I'd rather die than have more chemotherapy" and "you're unreal—I'm going to die anyway." This surprised everyone. Melissa had been "such a perfect patient." Melissa's dad felt the issue was settled. ("It's our decision. She's a child.") Her mother felt that "since it is her body and her life," Melissa should be part of the decision-making and that Dr. Garcia ought to be clearer about what could be expected. The subsequent discussions were emotional but less anger filled as they went along and Dr. Garcia acknowledged that it was unlikely that the experimental treatment would help meaningfully prolong her life and would be arduous.

Melissa explained that she wanted to live what time she had left by doing what she wanted to do: attend the prom, finish the yearbook, and coach her sister in softball a bit more. Melissa was able to do those things. She and her parents and Dr. Garcia ultimately agreed on palliative chemotherapy that was given by mouth. The Devanes' health plan quickly approved referral to a local hospice. Because Melissa was likely to die within six months and because the family had opted for palliative care only, there was no issue of appealing the plan's limits on hospice coverage. The hospice care team gave the family the help it needed to keep Melissa at home with minimal pain. Dr. Garcia continued to keep in regular touch with Melissa and her parents. Melissa died peacefully at home in July in her mother's arms, having lived longer than Dr. Garcia predicted and having seen her sister have a championship season with Melissa's support and coaching.

"Sean Riley"

This story illustrates the increasingly common situation in which a fatal congenital anomaly is diagnosed prenatally and the families await a birth that likely will be followed by death within hours or days (Figure 3.1c). Although many mothers and fathers opt for abortion when faced with such a tragic diagnosis, others—for religious, philosophical, or emotional reasons—choose to continue the pregnancy. A few innovative programs have recently been developed to provide extensive clinical information and preparation and emotional, spiritual, and practical support (e.g., help with coordinating services) to these families following diagnosis and through and after the infant's death (see, e.g., Sumner, 2001). Most parents, however, have limited access to such information, preparation, comfort, and assistance from health care professionals. They may be able to rely on families and friends, and some discover parent-to-parent support groups or other resources.

Catherine and Kevin Riley were delighted to learn that they were expecting a new baby to join their 4-year-old daughter, Caitlin. In Catherine's sixteenth week of pregnancy, she had an ultrasound examination. From the reactions of the technicians, she knew immediately that something was wrong, but no one was willing to tell her anything except that she should contact her obstetrician.

Told initially that the ultrasound results would be reviewed at Catherine's next regularly scheduled visit in four weeks, Kevin called the obstetrician's office to explain the extreme stress they were under and their need to know the results. The obstetrician explained that the fetus had anencephaly (failure of the brain to develop), that he had little training in managing such pregnancies, and that they should consider termination of the pregnancy "because the baby would not live." The Rileys were unwilling to consider termination and requested a referral to a new obstetrician who specialized in high-risk pregnancies. The second obstetrician said that there was nothing to be done for mother or fetus and that if they did not want to terminate the pregnancy, he would see Catherine again when she was ready to deliver (in about five months).

Without access to regular obstetrical visits for further information and preparation, the Rileys drifted in fear, uncertainty, and grief during the following weeks and months. They sought information from the Internet where they found stories from other families about anencephalic infants who had survived "for years" but learned little to answer their questions about why this problem had happened and how they should prepare for what was to come.

Catherine went into labor at 38 weeks' gestation. The Rileys found delivery room nurses who were unaware of her fetus's diagnosis and an unfamiliar obstetrician who was covering for the obstetrician she had last seen. As Catherine's contractions increased in intensity, the nursing staff on the delivery floor became concerned about the fetus's heart rate. The obstetrician suggested delivery by cesarean section. Kevin questioned this recommendation, but the obstetrician and nursing staff both insisted it was needed and that if they refused both parents would have to sign a form stating their refusal. Confused by these demands given the diagnosis and prognosis, Kevin and Catherine requested a second opinion. Before the opinion could be obtained, the fetus's heart rate dropped to dangerously low levels, and the baby was delivered by cesarean section with Catherine under general anesthesia. The obstetrician and anesthesiologist confirmed the diagnosis of anencephaly. Kevin was not allowed in the delivery room because Catherine was under general anesthesia. Neither saw their son, Sean, during his brief moments of life.

After delivery and her baby's death, Catherine was placed on a floor in the hospital to recover where there were no babies or other postpartum women. She noticed that nursing staff avoided her, and she felt very isolated. Her obstetrician saw her once, inquired about her pain control, and said she could go home "when she was feeling better." She was discharged three days later, after receiving an envelope with a lock of Sean's hair, a handprint, and a Xeroxed paper about "grief." Many of the Riley's friends avoided any contact when news about Sean's birth and death became known. Her employer refused postpartum leave or paid bereavement leave because "she had no baby."

Kevin never spoke about Sean again, although he noticed that he became extremely sad unexpectedly for years afterward. Daughter Caitlin had stayed with relatives during the delivery. No one told her much about Sean's birth and death. She began to think that her parents were angry with her. Expectations of both Kevin and Catherine for Caitlin increased significantly, which added more pressure for an already vulnerable child. Five years after Sean's death, the Rileys remain a sad and troubled, though loving, family.

"Johnny Gabrielle"

Although caring for a child with a serious chronic condition is always demanding, the burden is significantly increased when the child is developmentally delayed and cannot communicate his or her needs directly. Most children and families can be helped to lead fairly normal lives for extended periods, but they may face major financial, bureaucratic, and other problems in actually obtaining such assistance. When death approaches, systems focused on chronic medical conditions may not be prepared to help families face the end stage of illness. In some cases, a child's medical problems severely test the ability of very experienced clinicians and others to identify effective therapies and relieve the suffering of the child and the family.

Shortly after Johnny Gabrielle was born, the doctors caring for him noted that his head was smaller than expected and that he had certain unusual facial features. A number of specialists examined him and eventually they diagnosed a rare genetic disorder. A pediatric neurologist informed Peter and Laura Gabrielle that Johnny would most likely be developmentally delayed and ultimately mentally retarded and probably would have a shortened life span. Although she tried to prepare the family for what lay ahead, the neurologist could only talk in general terms because so few children with his condition had been treated and their history documented. The neurologist became Johnny's primary physician, assuring the Gabrielles that she would "be there" for them whatever the future brought, would bring other specialists in as needed, and would do everything she could to keep Johnny comfortable and free of pain and other distress.

As predicted, Johnny's development was far behind that of his older brother. He never talked or achieved normal milestones, but his parents learned to recognize his cues. His sunny disposition brightened the lives of all who encountered him. Johnny's main problem was that he never slept through the night but instead awakened repeatedly. Johnny's physicians tried many drugs to induce sleep, but none were reliably successful. The Gabrielles developed a system of shared responsibility for his care at night but always felt tired. They felt fortunate to qualify for assistance under their state's generous and well-managed programs for children with special health care needs. As time went by, they became acquainted with families from other states who had terrible financial problems and even had to sell their homes to pay medical bills.

At about age 5, Johnny became increasingly irritable and was diagnosed with gastroesophageal reflux. Medication and position did not seem to help nor did surgery. Physicians eventually placed a tube directly into Johnny's stomach so he could be fed. Shortly thereafter, Johnny's personality began to change. He became inconsolable at times and would scream out and tighten his body throughout the day. His sleeping became even more disrupted, lasting only an hour at a time before he screamed again. He was hospitalized frequently, but physicians could find no specific explanation for his problems. Morphine slightly reduced his crying and irritability, which led his care providers to believe that he might be experiencing pain at times. Even with pain medications, he was still inconsolable much of the time. His physicians, who now included a specialist in pediatric pain, managed a fine line between relief and excessive sedation and were alert to other potential complications of his treatments. Although the Gabrielles had written documents that listed Johnny's medications and described their preferences for the use of certain life support technologies should Johnny's condition suddenly deteriorate, it was hard for either Johnny's parents or physicians to know what to expect in the near term (days, weeks, or months).

Up every night for weeks, the Gabrielles' relationship with their older son began to deteriorate. None of their large, supportive family could provide real respite because Johnny was so medically fragile and required so much nursing care. Even during hospitalizations, the Gabrielles were always present and responding to nurses' questions about strategies that seemed to help Johnny. The same was true for visiting nurses at home; even when they didn't ask for help, Laura could still hear Johnny crying in his room. Recognizing the Gabrielles' exhaustion, the health care team looked for formal respite care for Johnny, but they never identified an appropriate setting. He was not sick enough for an acute care setting but was too medically complex for the available medical foster care homes.

All involved felt helpless and frustrated. This pattern persisted for approximately four months. One night, when Johnny didn't awaken at the expected one to two hours after going to sleep, his mother went to check. Johnny was dead. The cause was later determined to be aspiration. At the wake, while being consoled by a huge cadre of friends and family, the Gabrielles told themselves that at least now, "Johnny was finally sleeping" and no longer in pain. They appreciated the presence of some of Johnny's main doctors and nurses. They did not seek outside bereavement support but felt ready to face the future.

Summary

Consistent with the experiences of real children and families, these vignettes include examples of good care as well as examples of care that falls considerably short of meeting child and family needs. Bereavement care is particularly limited. Measured against the criteria for a "good or decent" death as defined in Chapter 1, some of the care described is insensitive and some leads to avoidable physical or emotional suffering for the child, the family, or both. No vignette describes a real "horror" story of care that violates norms of decency, although such cases do exist.

The vignettes also suggest that some of the dilemmas facing parents, children, and clinicians may not have a clear or successful answer—even with everyone trying his or her best. This is a particular dilemma when a child suffers from a rare condition that has few cases documented in the literature and no condition-specific research to guide physician's decisions about curative, life-prolonging, or palliative care.

No small collection of stories can adequately portray the struggles that families with a seriously ill child often experience in trying to coordinate care that may involve multiple sites (e.g., specialized referral center, outpatient clinic, community hospital, home), a large and frequently changing array of health care professionals (e.g., generalist and specialist pediatricians, nurses, social workers, child-life specialists, case managers), and differing criteria for insurance coverage of different services (e.g., inpatient care, home health services, hospice, psychosocial services, respite care, outpatient drugs and equipment).

PATHWAYS OF CARE

The vignettes suggest that just as pathways to death will vary for children, the pathways of care—that is, the mix of curative or life-prolonging care and palliative care—will vary depending on the child's condition and other factors, including family circumstances and values. Even for some conditions that are invariably fatal, the timing of death may vary considerably. For different children, the same diagnosis and initial prognosis can be followed by quite different pathways that end in death for some and, depending on the condition, extended survival or cure for others.

The unpredictability of many life-threatening medical problems can make it difficult for families to decide when further efforts to save their child will only prolong the child's suffering and dying. Faced with similar facts and uncertainties, families will differ in their responses, and their values and personalities will influence their decisions about the goals of care for their child. Some families will emphasize prolonging life until death removes the choice whereas others will, as death approaches, choose care that is focused entirely on their child's comfort and quality of life. Both may be doing their best for their child, and both may live in peace—or with regrets—about their choices.

The emphasis of care may also reflect the resources—or lack of resources—available to the child and family. For example, as discussed in Chapter 6, few children's hospitals have specialized palliative care services or consulting teams, although all hospitals should be able to provide the fundamentals of such care, for example, effective assessment and management of pain. They may not, however, have clinicians who are trained to explain the child's situation fully and compassionately, to make clear the likelihood of harms as well as benefits from different treatments, and to assure the family that it will be supported in its choices.

Traditional views of patient management have often referred to a "switch" from curative (or life-prolonging) care to palliative care. This

a. From Cure to Care: Traditional Model for Cancer Care

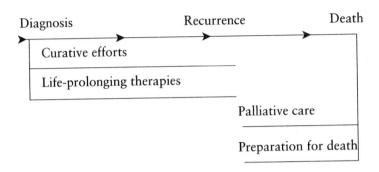

b. Integrated Care from the Time of Diagnosis Through Death into Bereavement

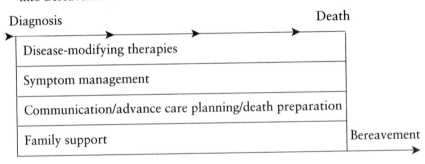

FIGURE 3.2   Sequential versus integrated models of care for advanced illness.
SOURCE: Adapted from IOM, 1997.

phrasing suggests that the two are separate worlds—even mutually exclusive—with an abrupt transition in patient care from one to the other. Figure 3.2a presents this perspective.

An alternative perspective proposes that providing some elements of palliative care closer to the time of diagnosis than happens traditionally may benefit patients and families and may coexist with and support active curative or life-prolonging treatment. For example, not only may meticulous efforts to prevent or relieve the pain and other distress that accompany certain treatments improve a child's comfort and quality of life, it may improve the child's ability to tolerate or cooperate with treatment. Just as hospice providers work with patients and families to reevaluate the goals of cure as the end stage of an illness approaches, "upstream palliative care" involves the periodic discussion of prognosis and care options and, as appropriate, the reconsideration of the goals of care during the early stages of complex chronic illnesses, for example, during "routine" visits and check ups.

Figure 3.2b illustrates the concept of integrated care in which multiple objectives are pursued concurrently after the diagnosis of life-threatening condition. The emphasis and specific elements of care may vary depending on the situation. Thus, some aspects of advance care planning (e.g., discussion of preferences for cardiopulmonary resuscitation, weighing of hospital versus home care as death approaches) are less urgent when a child's condition is possibly curable, treatments are not themselves life-threatening, and early crises such as cardiac arrest are uncommon. Likewise, if early symptoms are minimal, the emphasis may be on reassuring parents that the child's care team will do everything possible to anticipate and prevent problems and to make their child comfortable if treatments or worsening of the condition brings pain or other symptoms.

Although this report emphasizes the model of integrated care following diagnosis, situations exist in which care may indeed switch abruptly from a near total emphasis on cure or life prolongation to a total commitment to palliation, preparation for death, and support for grieving family members. For example, with some seriously injured children, physicians may initially assume—pending further evaluation—that survival is possible and work intensively and virtually exclusively toward that goal. Test results or poor response to treatment may then demonstrate irreversible damage that will lead inevitably and fairly soon to death. At that point, the emphasis of care may shift quickly to relieving any distress that the patient might be experiencing and preparing the patient (if conscious) and family members for death. When this happens, the message is never that "there is nothing we can do" but that "we must refocus on efforts" on comfort and peace and making the most of the family's remaining time together.

Similarly, for some children, the emphasis of care may always be palliative. For example, in the vignette earlier in this chapter, Sean Riley's medical condition was incompatible with extended life, but the family could have been provided active emotional support before, during, and after the birth. Physicians and nurses could have planned and prepared to manage the delivery in accord with the family's goal of having time with the baby after birth. Care would have been intensively palliative from the time of prenatal diagnosis, supporting the parents as parents before and after the baby's death and reducing their sense of powerlessness.

In yet other circumstances, the emphasis or balance of care may fluctuate over time, for example, when a child has with a progressive, fatal condition such as muscular dystrophy or certain heart conditions. In the

Gabrielle vignette in Chapter 3, the parents and other caregivers spent an increasing amount of time trying to relieve Johnny's distress. Periodically, however, Johnny was hospitalized—sometimes in attempt to relieve his apparent pain, sometimes in an intensive effort to save his life following an acute problem (e.g., an infection). The Gabrielles' physicians attempted to extend Johnny's life while doing their best to relieve his intractable distress; they explained their best understanding of Johnny's diagnosis and prognosis but did not take away his parent's hopes. To depict this as a modification of Figure 3.2b, the horizontal lines under the elements of care could increase and decrease in thickness to represent the varying emphasis on life-prolonging care or palliative care.

In sum, the ratio of palliative care compared to curative or life-prolonging care and the ratio of palliative care compared to true end-of-life care will vary for different medical conditions and at different points during the course of a fatal illness. Depending on a child's diagnosis and stage of illness as well as available resources, some palliative or end-of-life care may be delivered by specialized inpatient or home hospice teams, some by palliative care teams, and some by the primary team (e.g., oncology, cardiology, neurology) caring for the child. All will need appropriate education and training, funding, and institutional structures and processes that support the timely, coordinated provision of the right mix of care for the child and family.

The next section of this chapter reviews evidence about the adequacy of palliative, end-of-life, and bereavement care provided to children and families. Additional studies are cited in the discussions in Chapter 4 and 5 of the elements of palliative, end-of-life, and bereavement care.

WHAT DO WE KNOW ABOUT THE FOCUS AND ADEQUACY OF CARE FOR CHILDREN WHO DIE?

I had to fight with the doctors to get him on morphine. They tried fentanyl patches and other things. They did not want to send him home on morphine. I screamed and cried and got them to understand that the short time he had left must be without pain, or at a minimum of pain. He had morphine in the hospital, but didn't want it for home use. Finally, they agreed.[1]

Becky Wooten, parent, 2001

---

[1]Fentanyl, like morphine, is an opioid. The parent may or may not have known that but apparently viewed past management of the child's pain as inadequate for a child going home to die. A fentanyl patch works slowly and is appropriate for chronic and essentially unchanging pain. If the pain situation is unstable, it might be the wrong choice because once the patch is in place, clinicians cannot use additional medication to control breakthrough pain (Yaster et al., 1997; Schechter et al., 2002).

The pathway followed by a dying child and his or her family can be marked by competent, consistent, and compassionate care, by care that fails on these dimensions, or by care that falls somewhere in between these poles. In recent years, several studies and reports have attempted to document and understand more systemically the strengths and weaknesses of palliative, end-of-life care for adults (see, e.g., SUPPORT, 1995; IOM, 1997; Webb, 1997; Lynn et al., 2000; Meier et al., 2000; IOM, 2001a). They have described inadequate assessment, documentation, and management of pain and other symptoms, sometimes in combination with overtreatment, including unwanted or ineffective resuscitation and other life-support interventions. Referrals to specialists in palliative and end-of-life care have been late or altogether absent. Poor communication includes insensitive delivery of bad news, inattention to patient and family preferences, and failure to provide accurate, timely information needed by patients and families to guide decisions.

Efforts to remedy these shortfalls in palliative and end-of-life care and to increase public understanding and expectations are growing and becoming more sophisticated (see, e.g., Higginson, 1993; Doyle et al., 1998; Emanuel et al., 1999; Lynn et al., 2000; Ferrell and Coyle, 2001; AAP, 2000g).[2] The goal—still to be achieved—is to create systems that people can trust to provide competent, consistent, and compassionate care to seriously ill and dying patients and that families can count on for support and solace as they experience a loved one's grave illness or death.

What is the picture for children who die and their families? Research on palliative and end-of-life care for children and their surviving families is very sparse. Some of it focuses rather narrowly on decisions involving cardiopulmonary resuscitation, mechanical ventilation, and other life-sustaining technologies—with little investigation of the adequacy of physical, emotional, spiritual, and practical support (e.g., help in coordinating services from multiple different providers) for the children and their families. Such research as the committee did locate generally follows the pattern found for adults, reporting inadequate assessment, documentation, and management of pain and other symptoms; late consideration of the benefits of palliative or hospice care; and problems in communication.

---

[2]Useful information and links to other resources are also available on a number of Web sites, for example, those of the Center to Advance Palliative Care, Mt. Sinai School of Medicine (http://www.capcmssm.org); Project on Death in America, Open Society Institute (http://www.soros.org/death); and Last Acts, a coalition initiated by the Robert Wood Johnson Foundation (http://www.lastacts.org).

Assessment, Documentation, and
Management of Pain and Other Distress

Pain management practices and problems have been more often discussed and better documented than problems in other aspects of pediatric palliative and end-of-life care. In the past, physicians often discounted pain in children. For example, a 1960s survey of postoperative pain in children argued that they "seldom need medication for relief of pain [and] . . . tolerate pain well" (Swafford and Allan, 1967, cited in McGrath, 1998, p. 1020). Neonates were thought to lack sufficient neurophysiologic and other development to suffer pain and thus not to need pain relief during surgical procedures such as circumcision.

Both behavioral and physiological research have repudiated these arguments and clarified the existence and seriousness of pain in children (see, e.g., McGrath, 1987; Bush and Harkins, 1991; Barr, 1994; Walco et al., 1994; APS, 1995; Duke, 1997; Schechter et al., 1997, 2002; Anand et al., 1999). Nonetheless, misunderstandings and ignorance have continued. As a 1998 editorial in the *British Journal of Medicine* stated, "Current practice still falls short of the ideal of safe and effective pain relief for all children" (Zacharias, 1998, p. 1552).

Groups including the World Health Organization (WHO) and the American Academy of Pediatrics (AAP) still find it necessary to issue policy statements that remind pediatricians of their obligations to recognize and prevent or relieve children's pain and to keep abreast of research on the tools available to do so (see, e.g., WHO, 1998; AAP, 2000a, 2001a). A 1998 WHO statement on pediatric cancer pain reported that 70 percent of children with cancer suffered severe pain at some point and that such pain was often not recognized or, if recognized, not treated adequately. More recently, the AAP specifically stressed that systemic pain medications are essential to manage predictable pain associated with bone marrow aspiration and other procedures (AAP, 2001a). It likewise emphasized that reliance on sedatives or antianxiety agents alone will not only allow children to experience pain but leave them less able to communicate their distress. The AAP identified the following barriers to the appropriate recognition and treatment of pain in children including

1. myths that children, especially infants, do not feel pain the way adults do or that, if they do, there is no untoward consequence;
2. failures of physicians to assess and reassess for the presence of pain;
3. inadequate understanding of children's subjective experience of pain;
4. insufficient knowledge of strategies for assessing, preventing, and relieving pain;

5. concerns that pain management in children is too time-consuming and difficult; and

6. disproportionate fears of adverse treatment effects such as respiratory depression and addiction.

Although most pain now can be relieved (in principle if not in practice), some pain is intractable without sedation (Swarm and Cousins, 1998). Some therapies produce side effects such as nausea, itching, confusion, or sleepiness that can cause considerable distress and require shifts in pharmcologic or other interventions (McGrath, 1998). Pain may also be necessary in pursuit of certain therapeutic benefits, for example, evaluating certain injuries or judging the success of orthopedic surgery during rehabilitation. In the latter case, Walco and colleagues (1994) suggest that clinicians should ask themselves whether a less hurtful approach is possible and whether the pain inflicted on the child is the least possible needed to achieve the benefit.

Research on the adequacy of pain assessment and management in children is scarcer than that for adults, but the findings raise concern. For example, although the majority of pediatric oncologists consider themselves competent in managing pain and other symptoms (Hilden et al., 2001a), a recent study at a leading pediatric cancer center and children's hospital found that 89 percent of children dying of cancer were reported by parents in after-death interviews to have suffered substantially at the end of their lives (Wolfe et al., 2000a).[3] The most common symptoms were fatigue, pain, and shortness of breath. Half of the children suffered from three or more symptoms. The most commonly treated symptoms were pain (76 percent of cases) and shortness of breath (65 percent). Treatment was, however, reported to be successful less than 27 percent of the time for pain and 16 percent of the time for shortness of breath. Fatigue was little treated, and the study authors suggested that physicians may be unaware that some apparently effective treatments are available for this common symptom of advanced illness (or its treatments). Children with cancer who died of treatment-related complications suffered more symptoms than children who died of progressive disease.

Most studies of end-of-life care for children focus on physical symptoms rather than emotional symptoms or quality of life. In their study, Wolfe and colleagues (2000a) reported that parents of children with cancer stated that, in the last month of life, their child had little or no fun (53

---

[3]The study by Wolfe and colleagues has been replicated at another institution. Data are still being analyzed, so no findings can yet be reported.

percent), was more than a little sad (61 percent), was not calm and peaceful most of the time (63 percent), and was often afraid (21 percent). Despite the suffering experienced by their children at the end of life, 70 percent of parents described their child's death itself as "peaceful."

In the United Kingdom, several studies of children cared for by Helen House (the first pediatric hospice) documented the serious symptoms experienced by many children. One study reported that more than a third of the children who died of neurodegenerative disorders suffered from pain, most often due to muscle spasms (Hunt and Burne, 1995). More than four-fifths of all patients experienced pain in the last month of their lives (Hunt, 1990). Of 30 children with various conditions who died between 1983 and 1987, 80 percent required strong analgesics during the last month of their lives for pain, shortness of breath, or both. Children with cancer were the most likely to receive analgesics for pain, whereas children with other conditions were the most likely to receive opiates for shortness of breath (Hunt, 1990). The Helen House researchers also reported that one-third of the children who died experienced seizures, and a quarter of them suffered from excessive oral secretions (often accompanied by swallowing difficulties). In addition, they reported that the dying children were commonly described as "frightened," "grumpy," "disoriented," or "anxious and irritable" (Hunt, 1990). Even those children who could not communicate (due to age or disease progression) were described as "distressed, crying frequently" or looking "frightened."

A Canadian study of 77 children who died anticipated deaths in intensive care relied on narrative progress notes to identify how the children died (McCallum et al., 2000). Although 84 percent of the children (who had conditions such as cancer, heart disease, AIDS, organ failure, and cystic fibrosis) received opioid analgesics, only 6 percent had specific pain assessment and treatment notes recorded in their charts, and such recording was sporadic. Systematic assessment and monitoring are essential to effective, reliable pain prevention and management and to quality assurance. The study also reported that the majority of children were intubated prior to their death and that most were "comatose, sedated, or medically paralyzed," which the authors said could be interpreted as indicating "excessively invasive treatment" (McCallum et al., 2000, p. 421). Four-fifths of the patients had do-not-resuscitate (DNR) orders documented during the final hospital admission, but only 8 percent had such orders prior to that admission. The median time from recording of the DNR order to death was less than a day. In only one case did progress notes indicate that the prospect of death was specifically discussed with the child.

One study of 100 deaths in three pediatric intensive care units (PICUs) reported that nearly 90 percent of children who died had received sedatives, pain medications, or both (Burns et al., 2000). Physicians substantially increased the use of sedatives and pain medications before the withdrawal of mechanical ventilation (which was usually one of the first therapies stopped for these children). Relief of suffering (e.g., air hunger, pain) was the justification for this increase, and the only patients not receiving such care were comatose and thought not to be suffering. The researchers reported no use of paralyzing agents, the use of which they considered indefensible.

Parental and clinical assessments of children's pain and other distress may differ. For example, as shown in Table 3.1, Wolfe and colleagues (2000a) found "considerable discordance" for certain symptoms including fatigue, poor appetite, constipation, and diarrhea.

Although some observational tools have been developed to assess certain symptoms in children, clinicians or researchers often depend on parental assessments of children's pain not only in retrospective studies following a child's death but also for very young children, children with cognitive

TABLE 3.1 Discordance Between the Reports of Parents and Physicians Regarding Children's Symptoms in the Last Month of Life

Symptom	Reported by Parent but Not by Physician (N = 92) No. (%)	Reported by Physician but Not by Parent (N = 92) No. (%)	Kappa Statistic (95% CI)[a]	P Value[b]
Fatigue	44 (48)	1 (1)	−0.02 (−0.07 to 0.02)	<0.001
Pain	15 (16)	11 (12)	0.10 (−0.12 to 0.32)	0.56
Dyspnea	19 (21)	10 (11)	0.10 (−0.11 to 0.31)	0.14
Poor appetite	33 (36)	1 (1)	0.29 (0.15 to 0.43)	<0.001
Constipation	31 (34)	7 (8)	0.16 (−0.02 to 0.33)	<0.001
Nausea/vomiting	25 (27)	18 (20)	0.06 (−0.14 to 0.26)	0.36
Diarrhea	20 (22)	8 (9)	0.31 (0.12 to 0.51)	0.04

[a]Data were missing for 10 children for whom there was no documentation of clinic or hospital visits in the last month of life and for 1 child whose records were not available for review. CI denotes confidence interval.
[b]McNemar's test was used.

SOURCE: Wolfe et al., 2000a. Used with permission.

impairments, and children with very advanced disease. One review of studies comparing parental and child assessments concluded that the evidence is mixed but parents tend to underestimate their child's pain (Chambers and Craig, 1999).

A Swedish study of children being treated for cancer interviewed children and parents (Ljungman et al., 1999). It reported that "treatment-related pain was constant and dominant," that treatment- and procedure-related pain was more severe than pain due to malignancy, and that pain evaluations were unsystematic. An older study by McGrath and colleagues (1990) also reported that treatment- and procedure-related pain was common, with more than a third of the children reporting moderate to severe pain from chemotherapy and 61 and 78 percent reporting such pain from lumbar puncture and bone marrow aspiration, respectively. The study did not report on treatment strategies. A 1995 article reporting on severe pain in children dying of cancer concluded that following WHO pain guidelines was adequate for most children but that a subgroup required extraordinary measures (Collins et al., 1995). Individualized management and careful assessment of pain were essential.

Studies by Ferrell and colleagues also suggest the inadequate management of cancer pain in children (Ferrell et al., 1994; Rhiner et al., 1994). The studies assessed the impact on families of living with and trying to manage a child's pain and identified parents' feelings of helplessness and stress.

Additional studies have examined pain assessment and management for broader groups of children. A 1994 article reported on pain management practices in three Canadian neonatal intensive care units (NICUs). It concluded that procedural and disease-related pain is frequently untreated or undertreated (Fernandez and Rees, 1994).

A study by Kazak and colleagues (1996) compared distress during invasive procedures for childhood leukemia as rated by mothers and nurses. Children receiving a pharmacological-only intervention were rated as having more distress than children receiving a combined pharmacological and psychological intervention. Younger children were rated as having more distress than older children. A 1999 review of the literature on psychological interventions for disease-related pain in children identified relatively few studies, most of which had methodological problems (e.g., small sample size, no control group) (Walco et al., 1999). Taken together, the studies suggested benefits of some interventions but they were not definitive.

Unexplained variation in pain management and other practices is also a concern. One study of narcotics use for very low birth weight babies in NICUs reported a 29-fold variation in the use of opioids (Kahn et al, 1998). This kind of variation demands further investigation. Differences may relate, in part, to differences in the degree to which physicians feel legally vulnerable in administering pain medications or have misconceptions about addiction from long-term use of narcotics. Variation in methods used to assess the contribution of pain in prematurely born infants may also play a role. Pain assessment tools that have been validated in premature babies at different gestational ages and at different chronological ages should prove useful in evaluating the adequacy of neonatal intensive care, reduce unexplained variations in treatment, and reduce infants' distress (see, e.g., Krechel and Bildner, 1995).

Palliative Care Consultations and Discussions

The extent of explicit palliative care consultations is little documented for children and families. A recently published study examined all 196 deaths in an NICU between 1994 and 1997 (Pierucci et al., 2001; see also Leuthner and Pierucci, 2001). The authors reported that palliative care consultations were associated with significantly more supportive services (e.g., referrals to chaplains or social workers) for infants and families, fewer medical procedures (e.g., blood draws, radiographs, endotracheal tubes but not intravenous fluids, nutritional support, narcotics), and documentation of family emotional needs and support. Consultations prior to the child's death increased during the period studied from 5 to 38 percent. The authors could not assess whether lack of consultation reflected lack of physician or family readiness for palliative care or other factors. They did not attempt to measure the effectiveness of the supportive services provided in relieving child or family distress.

In the study by Wolfe and colleagues (2000a) cited above, earlier discussion of hospice care was associated with parental reports that their child was peaceful and calm during the last month of life. For about two-thirds of the children who died of progressive disease (rather than treatment complications), charts noted a discussion of hospice care, which occurred, on average, about 58 days before death. Further, suffering was greater in children whose parents reported that the child's physician was not involved in his or her end-of-life care. This pattern held after adjusting the analysis for cause of death, child's age at death, place of death, interval between the child's death and the parental interview, and physician clustering (Wolfe et al., 2000a).[4]

---

[4]Authors "adjusted for the possibility that the parents of patients who had the same physician may have had similar responses" and called this "physician clustering" (Wolfe et al., 2000a, p. 327).

Limitations of Life-Support and Disease-Modifying Interventions

A recent examination of the limitation of aggressive life support concluded that much attention had been paid to the question of whether and when to limit these interventions and argued that more research should focus on how to assess and improve the quality of care for patients once the decision has been made (Rubenfeld and Curtis, 2000). Studies of pediatric deaths in intensive care have found that deaths are often preceded by limitations of life support interventions—more than half of the deaths in one recent study (Keenan et al., 2000), more than one-third to one-half in an earlier study (Vernon et al., 1993;[5] Levetown et al., 1994), and more than 70 percent in a neonatal intensive care unit (Wall and Partridge, 1997). The accompanying assessment and management of pain, air hunger, or other distress has been less documented as has the timing of decisions to limit life support.

Even though death is often preceded by limitations of life-support interventions, studies also suggest that during their last month of life, the majority of children who die from chronic conditions receive some form of medical treatment that is regarded as curative or life prolonging. The earlier-cited study by Wolfe and colleagues (2000a) reported that 56 percent of children with cancer received some sort of cancer-directed therapy in the last month of their lives. More than one-third (36 percent) had undergone a bone marrow transplant, and for 60 percent of these children, the transplant was their last cancer-directed treatment. Two-thirds of children in the study had DNR orders. These orders were entered, on average, 33 days before death for children who died of their disease and 1.7 days before death for children who died of treatment-related complications. An earlier study of DNR orders in one children's hospital also reported that most of these orders were written for children who were receiving "aggressive" medical therapy in intensive care units (Lantos et al., 1993, p. 52). Orders were more common for older children than for infants. Wolfe and colleagues suggest that when life-prolonging treatment is pursued to the last, more attention to concurrent palliative therapies might reduce children's suffering.

Possibly reflecting the difficulty of changing a long-term pattern of treatment, one small study suggests that children with chronic illness hospitalized in PICUs were less likely to have life-sustaining treatment withheld or withdrawn than were acutely ill patients (Keenan et al., 2000). Levetown's 1994 study, however, reported no difference between the two

---

[5]This article used the terminology "supportive care" to describe life-support interventions, whereas the term is used here and more generally to refer to care that provides comfort to patients or families.

groups on this aspect of care. Additional research on treatment patterns for acute versus chronic conditions could inform understanding of the factors influencing treatment choices. For children with serious, chronic conditions, repeated hospitalizations may be an almost routine part of life. Families may become used to seeing the ill child "bounce back" after numerous life-threatening acute events. Then, as Ann Goldman suggests, "After a lifetime of intensive treatment, it can be difficult to abandon past patterns of care" (Goldman, 1999, p. 30).

With advances in organ transplantation, patients with conditions such as cystic fibrosis (often now young adults) and their families may regard what was previously seen as the end stage of their disease as an opportunity to be listed for a transplant, thus maintaining a hope for survival rather than preparing for death. Long-term survival, while improving, varies for different kinds of conditions (see Kurland and Orenstein, 2001), and a shortage of donated organs limits the number of transplants. Of the 45 patients who died of cystic fibrosis in Canada in 1996, an analysis found that 93 percent had been considered for transplant, 7 (17 percent) had been listed, and 2 (4 percent) had received the transplant (Mitchell et al., 2000). The analysis did not report how many received a transplant and did not die.[6] Palliative care was never discussed for one-quarter of the patients and was discussed a month before death for 40 percent.

Another study, this one in the United States, evaluated records for 44 patients more than 5 years of age who died of cystic fibrosis at one institution between 1984 and 1993. The majority of these patients were over age 20. Four died after lung transplants, and four died on mechanical ventilators in the PICU awaiting transplant (Robinson et al., 1997). Three-quarters of the patients were receiving therapeutic (e.g., intravenous antibiotics, chest physical therapy) or preventive (e.g., oral vitamins) interventions in the last 12 hours of life. Compared to surgical interventions, most cancer chemotherapy, and some other drug regimens, these therapies are less invasive and produce limited side effects. All patients had do-not-resuscitate orders, and nearly all received some opiates for pain (two of six patients who did not refused for religious reasons). Of the 44 patients, one died at

---

[6]Three-year survival rates following lung or heart–lung transplantation for cystic fibrosis are generally reported (for the last decade) to be from 40 to 60 percent (see, e.g., Balfour-Lynn et al., 1997; Hosenpud et al., 1998; Mendeloff et al., 1998; Aurora et al., 1999; Vizza et al., 2000). Transplant survival rates are higher for certain other conditions and organs, most notably kidney transplantation for end-stage renal disease. Five-year survival rates above 50 percent have been reported for children with end-stage heart disease (see, e.g., Jenkins et al., 2000; Morrow et al., 2000; Williams et al; 2000). Survival rates improve with experience with the procedure and vary with medical condition (e.g., congenital anomaly, cardiomyopathy).

home under hospice care; the remainder died in the hospital with "many of the important psychological and emotional aspects of hospice" (Robinson et al., 1997, p. 208). The authors of this study noted that while the final outcome of the disease is certain, uncertainty about short-term prognosis and the waxing and waning nature of respiratory failure in cystic fibrosis make it difficult to abandon antibiotics, physical therapy, mechanical ventilation, and similar measures. Again, some of these interventions impose relatively little burden on patients.

Despite prognostic complexities, improvements in the care of patients with unpredictable life-shortening conditions are possible. The strategy of "hoping for the best while preparing for the worst" allows clinicians and families to pursue life-prolonging interventions such as transplants with conviction and, at the same time, to be attentive to symptom management, personal goals (e.g., a family vacation), and other steps to help families make the most of the time they have.

One study of the withdrawal of life support in adults reported that "forms of life support that were perceived as more artificial, scarce, or expensive were withdrawn earlier" and that "once the decision has been made to forgo life-sustaining treatment, the process remains complex and appears to target many different goals simultaneously" (Asch et al., 1999, p. 153). If anything, the complexity of the process and the existence of multiple goals of care are likely to be even more evident when decisions involve children.

Inconsistency in clinical decisions about life-support and disease-modifying interventions is a concern. One survey study of pediatricians' decisionmaking found considerable variation in management strategies about withholding or withdrawing life-support interventions for chronically ill children as described in eight clinical scenarios (Randolph et al., 1999). For six of the eight scenarios, less than half the respondents chose the same intensity of care (e.g., mechanical ventilation, dialysis, antibiotics). For three of the scenarios, at least 10 percent chose the most intensive level of management while at least 10 percent chose comfort measures only. The most important influences on choices were the probability of acute (short-term) survival and parental wishes. Those who rated parental wishes highly were more likely to choose aggressive care when parents wanted it, even when the long-term prognosis was poor. Also, those who rated themselves as more likely than their colleagues to withdraw life support were indeed more likely to make that choice. Although the authors note that decisions in actual practice needed investigation, they observed that "variability in decision-making may lead to unnecessary suffering, lack of fairness when making decisions about neurologically handicapped infants, and inappropriate use of scarce resources in futile cases" (Randolph et al.,

1999, p. e46). They recommended clearer guidelines for decisions about limitation of life support for children.

A recent study of European neonatologists also found considerable variability in how quality-of-life was weighed in decisions in the NICU (Rebagliato et al. 2000). The authors concluded that the country in which a physician practices was the most powerful predictor of choices. The researchers also found that physician attitude, seniority of position, length of experience, and working in larger NICUs were significantly correlated with a greater likelihood of a physician's choosing to limit life-sustaining medical interventions based on predicted quality of life.

In the United States, studies examining the attitudes of neonatologists report that neonatologists frequently are willing to limit treatment in severely malformed, premature, or ill babies. One study examined the actual practices of neonatologists at a university medical center as documented in medical records. It found that 73 percent of all neonatal deaths at a tertiary NICU followed the withdrawal or withholding of life-sustaining treatment (Wall and Partridge, 1997). In contrast, a similar study in 1973 reported that only 14 percent of neonatal deaths were attributed to withdrawing or withholding treatment (Duff and Campbell, 1973). In the 1997 study, death attributable to withdrawing or withholding life-sustaining treatment was more common in severely neurologically damaged babies (more than 85 percent) than in babies with major congenital anomalies (67 percent). Neonatologists most commonly noted futility of treatment as the reason for limiting or withdrawing treatment (74 percent). They noted quality-of-life issues in 51 percent of cases (more often mentioning severe disability than unnecessary suffering as the issue). Quality of life, exclusive of any reference to the futility of treatment, was mentioned as the reason for withdrawing or withholding treatment in 23 percent of the deaths. The authors of the study observe that medical records might underdocument the importance of quality-of-life considerations based on concerns about federal "Baby Doe" regulations on treatment of infants with life-threatening conditions (see Chapter 8).

Problems in Communication

Hilden and colleagues observe that physicians report anxiety about discussing an impending death with children and their parents (Hilden et al., 2001a). Anxiety and dread may interfere with a thorough assessment of a child's emotional and spiritual well being and careful evaluation of child and family circumstances (e.g., cultural values, religious beliefs). Inadequate assessment may, in turn, compromise timely efforts to identify and relieve physical and emotional distress.

Clinicians' anxiety may also contribute to poor communication about the child's situation and prognosis, which may deprive children and families of information they need to plan for the future and weigh the pain or other suffering expected from an intervention against its probability of meaningfully extending a child's life. Certainly, most pediatric specialists have less experience than similar adult specialists in communicating a grim prognosis, although both groups have little or no training in this task (see Chapters 5 and 9).

A survey of 122 experienced emergency room physicians published in 1997 reported that few of the respondents reported any training in telling parents about a child's death or any familiarity with guidelines for such notifications (Ahrens and Hart, 1997; Maruyama, 1997). Two-thirds of the respondents described communicating with parents after a child's death as the most difficult part of emergency medicine. A similar percentage said communicating with parents about a child's death was more difficult than communicating with a family about an adult's death. Even more striking in this small survey, more than two-thirds of the respondents said that they had prolonged resuscitation efforts solely to delay telling parents that their child had died.

Khaneja and colleagues (1998) surveyed residents, fellows, and attending pediatricians at one institution to describe their general attitudes toward pediatric death and dying. Of those responding, 61 percent of all attending physicians and 73 percent of attending physicians in specialties with a higher predicted patient mortality rate reported that they sometimes consider a patient's death to be a personal failure. Conversely, residents and fellows rarely felt this sense of personal failure when a patient died. Despite feelings of failure, when a patient died, older physicians not surprisingly felt more prepared to deal with issues of death and dying than younger physicians: 13 percent of residents, 56 percent of fellows, and 71 percent of attending physicians felt adequately trained to deal with end-of-life issues, but the study did not independently assess skills. However, almost all of the physicians agreed that there was a need for further support of health care workers in dealing with death and dying (100 percent of residents, 83 percent of fellows, and 90 percent of attending physicians wanted more support). Most also agreed that the existing support systems in the pediatric department of their hospital were inadequate. Many physicians expressed a desire to attend funerals of patients, for instance, but very few had actually done so. Most cited conflicting clinical duties as a reason they were unable to attend funerals.

Other researchers as well as personal stories also point to physician anxiety and confusion about communicating bad news and discussing death and dying (see, e.g., Solomon, 1993; Nuland, 1994; ABIM, 1996a,b; IOM, 1997; Christakis and Iwashyna, 1998; Bruera et al., 2000; for pediatricians specifically, see Ahrens and Hart, 1997; Vazirani et al., 2000). Although most of these studies involve adult patients and families, it seems reasonable that some of the problems they identify will apply to communication involving children with life-threatening conditions. For example, a study by Lamont and Christakis (2001) reported that clinicians may consciously withhold information or provide cancer patients and families with misleadingly optimistic assessments and that younger adult patients were more likely to receive such misleading assessments than older patients.

A recent project to improve communication about organ donation in adult neurologic and pediatric intensive care units reported on training sessions that involved conversations between health care teams and standardized patient families. As reported in a conference poster session (Williams et al., 2001b), the researchers found that physicians were reluctant to use the "d" words (death, dying), that euphemisms confused family members, and that teamwork among team members (physicians, nurses, transplant coordinators, and clergy) contributed to effective communication. (Following training, organ donation rates increased on the study units.)

One small study of residents' competence in delivering bad news (a diagnosis of lung cancer) to adults concluded that they were not very good at it (Eggly et al., 1997). Using a 16-item instrument, the authors rated residents' skills as displayed during taped interviews with simulated patients. Residents were rated weakest in eliciting the patient's perspective. The authors concluded that the residency program was not doing an adequate job of teaching residents to use a patient-centered approach to discussions with patients. Another small study also used simulated parents as part of the process of assessing the parent counseling and information-giving skills of pediatric residents and emergency department fellows, providing feedback, and assessing improvement in subsequent discussions (Greenberg et al., 1999). The investigators reported improvements in two areas: reducing parents' feelings of dependence and improving feelings of trust. A third small study of pediatric critical care fellows using a somewhat different methodology also showed improvements following feedback by the simulated parents (Vaidya et al., 1999). Other studies have concluded (through self-reports and clinician assessments) that communications training for medical students and residents can improve their self-confidence, comfort, or skills in breaking bad news (Cushing and Jones, 1995: Garg et al., 1997; Vetto et al., 1999).

If physicians cannot face fully a child's poor prognosis and then appropriately communicate their assessment to families, timely reexamination of the goals of care and corresponding adjustments in care plans may be delayed. One retrospective study of parent and physician perceptions of the end-of-life care of 103 child cancer patients found a significant disparity between the time the physician first documented that the child was entering the end-of-life phase of his or her illness and the time the parents reported recognizing that there was no realistic chance for cure (mean difference of 101 days) (Wolfe et al., 2000b). The differences in physician and parent understanding of prognosis were not statistically significantly associated with differences in the care outcomes studied. However, when the physician's and parents' understanding of prognosis correlated more closely early on, the goals of care were more likely to be directed at lessening the child's suffering. Hospice was introduced earlier. Parents also were more satisfied with home care during the end-of-life period. When a psychologist or social worker was involved in the child's care, agreement between physician and parent assessments was more likely.

IMPLICATIONS

Children who die vary in the paths they follow, and some children with grave medical problems survive. Thus, pediatric palliative care—and if death occurs, end-of-life and bereavement care—must be flexible to meet the highly variable, changing, and sometimes difficult-to-predict needs and circumstances of children and families.

Evidence about the adequacy of current care for children with fatal or potentially fatal medical problems is limited but generally consistent with that found for adults in pointing to shortfalls in many dimensions of care. Specifically, pain and other symptoms are inadequately and variably assessed and treated, despite the availability of treatments that are effective, especially for pain. Palliative care consultations appear to increase the use of supportive services, but late or absent consideration of the benefits of palliative or hospice care is a problem. This puts children at risk of needless suffering from invasive and uncomfortable procedures that promise little or no benefit. Routine discussion and re-evaluation of the goals of care, which assists parents in making medical and other decisions, does not appear to be a part of "normal" health care for children with complex medical conditions.

More children with fatal conditions are dying after the limitation of life-support interventions, but the adequacy of care to manage any distress associated with stopping or not starting such interventions is little studied. Little research is likewise available on the prevalence, intensity, and management of symptoms other than pain and of psychological distress in children with fatal or potentially fatal conditions. Different studies point to problems in the communication of information to help families understand what may lie ahead and to make decisions about different courses of care. Barriers to these "just in case" conversations include physicians' discomfort in discussing bad news, fragmentation of care, and financial disincentives.

The literature reviewed in this chapter as well as illustrative vignettes suggest several directions for improving the effectiveness and consistency of pediatric palliative and end-of-life care. These directions include better understanding of the dimensions of pediatric palliative and end-of-life care and better understanding and application of existing knowledge and resources. Other directions include changes in the organization of care that may increase the effectiveness and reliability of such care, better training of health professionals in the principles and techniques of palliative and end-of-life care (including accurate but sensitive communication), and more research on almost every dimension of such care and the medical and other criteria for identifying children and families who might benefit from it. The next several chapters expand on these topics and also review the financing, legal, and ethical context of care for children with fatal or potentially fatal medical conditions.

CHAPTER 4

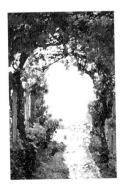

COMMUNICATION, GOAL SETTING, AND CARE PLANNING

It was terribly important for us to do exactly what was right and necessary to help our daughter. . . . Our nurse and social worker made us feel that we WERE, in fact, doing everything in our power to take care of our daughter.
Kathleen and James Bula, parents, 2001

When you first get sick, you have to live.
Katherine, 19-year-old with cancer (Sourkes, 1982, p. 112)

Except when death comes suddenly and without forewarning, physicians, nurses, social workers and other health care personnel—as well as hospitals and other health care institutions—play a central, even overwhelming, role in the lives of children with fatal or potentially fatal conditions and their families. When a child dies without forewarning, a family's encounter with medical personnel may be relatively brief but still have a profound and enduring impact.

As noted in Chapter 1, these professionals can at best help all involved to feel that they did everything they could to help, and that preventable suffering was indeed prevented. Other times, however, families' encounters with the health care system will leave them with painful memories of their child's unnecessary suffering, bitter recollections of careless and wounding words, and lifelong regrets about their own choices. In between these poles of medicine, families will often experience both excellent care and incompetence, attentiveness and neglect, and inconsistent communication of essential information.

Moving the typical experience of children and families toward the best care and entirely eliminating the worst care is an achievable goal. It is a goal that will depend on shifts in attitudes, policies, and practices involving not only health care professionals but also those who manage, finance, and regulate health care. That is, it will require system changes not just individual changes.

Child- and family-centered palliative and end-of-life care has many dimensions. One way to understand these dimensions is to view them, in a sense, as responses to families' fundamental questions and concerns following the diagnosis of child's life-threatening medical condition.

- "What is happening to me?" "What is happening with my child?" Good palliative, end-of-life, and bereavement care supports children and families with accurate, clear, and timely information about the child's condition and prognosis from the time of diagnosis through death and into bereavement—if death is the outcome.

- "What are our choices? How can we be good parents?" Following diagnosis, child- and family-centered care provides full, understandable, and timely information about curative, life-prolonging, and palliative treatment options that includes descriptions of potential harms or burdens as well as potential benefits of treatments. A central goal is to help the child and family to develop and adjust medical and personal goals based on their values and preferences as well as on medical and other circumstances.

- "How will you help us?" Appropriate palliative and end-of-life care offers a plan of physical, psychological, spiritual, and practical support that is adapted to the goals, values, and circumstances of each child and family. It is always appropriate for a child's plan of care to include such support while curative or life-prolonging therapies are pursued.

The rest of this chapter is organized primarily around these questions. The chapter tends to emphasize the role of the physician as diagnostician and communicator and as the ultimate locus of professional accountability for a child's care, particularly in the hospital. The discussion in Chapters 5 and 6 should, however, make clear that all members of the health care team—nurses, social workers, psychologists, child-life specialists, hospice personnel, and others—have specialized skills that are essential to comprehensive palliative, end-of-life, and bereavement care, including effective communication.

Such communication is especially important because parents may simultaneously hold multiple, possibly conflicting, goals that complicate decisionmaking. On the one hand, they may be profoundly reluctant to accept that their child will die, may need to feel that they have tried every option that might save their child, and may resist or resent certain offers of support (e.g., referral to hospice). One the other hand, parents naturally want to protect their child from pain and other suffering. Empathetic listening by members of the child's care team may help all involved to clarify their understanding of the child's medical situation, assess the goals of care, and fashion a care plan that reflects both medical realities and family priorities.

WHAT IS HAPPENING?
DETERMINING AND COMMUNICATING
DIAGNOSIS AND PROGNOSIS

"What is happening to me? How bad is it?" "What is happening to my child? Could she die?" General pediatricians and family practitioners may face such questions from children and families, but only infrequently are they the ones who bring the definitive word that a child has a fatal or potentially fatal condition.

In contrast, many pediatric specialists, including emergency medicine physicians, neonatologists, intensivists, oncologists, and neurologists, among others, must frequently, if not daily, inform families of a child's life-threatening condition. They may nonetheless be inadequately prepared to tell families honestly but compassionately what they need to know to make decisions and plan for the future. As described in Chapter 3, they may also so dread the delivery of such information that they fail to provide families with a complete, accurate, and timely picture of a child's diagnosis and prognosis. In addition, despite their considerable experience, they may not appreciate sufficiently the limits on how much bad news and how much complicated information people can absorb at one time.

Determining diagnosis and prognosis and then fully and sensitively informing patients and families require not only technical and intellectual skills but also empathy, education, experience, teamwork, time, and reflection. To be done consistently, it also requires supportive administrative systems (e.g., protocols, checklists, model conversation guides) and financing policies that appropriately value careful communication.

Diagnosing Life-Threatening and Fatal Conditions in Children

Aspects of Diagnosis in Children

Often, parents are the first to realize that something is not quite right with their child. For infants, the parents may recognize that their son or daughter is not achieving the expected developmental milestones—for example, raising his or her head, turning over, "cooing," or sitting. For older children, persistent reports or signs of fatigue may prompt a trip with worried parents to the pediatrician or family practitioner. This initial visit may then escalate into a nerve-wracking and protracted series of specialist consultations and tests to establish diagnosis and prognosis.

Sometimes, a critical problem is quite evident from the start, for example, when a child is badly injured as described in the vignette about "Jimmy Marshall" in Chapter 3. In such situations, a rapid series of assessments may begin with the first-response emergency personnel and continue into the emergency department, operating room, and intensive care unit. Family members may also be seriously injured or not yet located. The unavailability of a parent sometimes complicates diagnosis, for example, if a child seems to be suffering an allergic reaction to an unknown substance and is unconscious or too young to provide relevant medical history.

The technical aspects of establishing a diagnosis of cancer or heart disease may be similar in many respects for adults and children. Young children, however, present special challenges to the extent that they cannot report symptoms reliably or follow instructions (e.g., to swallow or stay still at a particular point) during diagnostic procedures. Cognitively impaired individuals of any age may present similar difficulties. In addition, diagnosing or ruling out a serious illness frequently involves painful or frightening procedures such as surgical biopsies and certain radiological examinations. Although older children and adults may also be unnerved by medical settings, young children are more likely to be upset by strange surroundings and large numbers of unfamiliar people. Child-friendly environments and special pediatric protocols, equipment, and personnel should help prevent or minimize children's pain and fear, but a young child's cooperation with diagnostic procedures may still be unpredictable.

Relatively recent technological developments that allow many fatal conditions to be diagnosed prenatally have extended the point of diagnosis sometimes months before birth. When a potentially fatal problem is identified by ultrasound, amniocentesis, or other means, an obstetrician has the difficult task of informing the parents and helping them to consider their choices. As described in the vignette about the "Rileys" in Chapter 3, perinatal hospice care is an option in some locales for parents who wish to continue the pregnancy. Whether identified before or after birth, certain diagnoses will also raise genetic concerns and should usually prompt a referral to a genetic counselor who can assist families in understanding and evaluating their situation.

Support for Children and Families While a Diagnosis Is Being Established

Frequently, parents and child patients must wait through a period of frustrating uncertainty—a diagnostic limbo—that is filled with great anxiety, hope, fear, and even grief as they anticipate the possible loss of cherished expectations for the future. Even when the basic message is "we don't yet know what's wrong," emotional support and careful and compassionate communication with parents and children are important. Parents may craft terrifying images of future possibilities until the facts are available. To support parents, clinicians may also have to manage their own frustration when a diagnosis is uncertain.

A relatively large number of rare and often or always fatal childhood disorders first reveal themselves—particularly in infants—with nonspecific signs and symptoms. Only as the child develops or the illness progresses does clearer evidence of a particular disorder become apparent. This can be frustrating for parents, who may feel that their concerns are being downplayed or ignored (NORD, 2001). Specifically identifying rare conditions can require extensive testing and may take years. According to a 1989 report to Congress, establishing a firm diagnosis took more than six years in 15 percent of individuals with rare conditions, and for almost one-third, it took more than a year (NCOD, 1989).

Sometimes a child's exact diagnosis remains in doubt, for example, if too little information from family history or from other reported cases is available to establish the significance of a diagnostic finding, such as a genetic mutation. This can cause parents even greater anxiety, especially if they would like to have more children.

Diagnostic uncertainty does not, however, necessarily affect medical management. Pursuing diagnostic clarity for its own sake may be costly, inappropriately expose children to testing risks, and subject parents to needless stress.

In addition to information and emotional support, families seeking a diagnosis for their child's problem usually can use extra assistance in navigating the health care system. Even within relatively integrated health systems, processes for coordinating multiple specialists and diagnostic procedures and their subsequent reports can be complex and imperfect. Delays and mix-ups can add considerably to the strain on children and parents, especially when the child and family have traveled far from home and their normal sources of emotional and practical support. Social workers can be helpful but typically become most involved only after a child is diagnosed.

Information Resources Beyond the Health Care Team

This chapter emphasizes information provided by the child's health care team. In reality, once they learn a child's diagnosis, many families engage in an intensive search for additional information from other sources including relatives, friends, advocacy groups, newspapers, books, magazines, and the Internet. Although not a substitute for information from clinicians, these resources do help many parents better understand their child's condition, their options, the questions they should ask, and the kind of responses they should expect.

Unfortunately, information from these other sources may be inaccurate or misleading. For example, press releases and media coverage of research developments may overstate preliminary findings and more generally create unrealistic hopes of cure or life prolongation. Such overstatements may, in turn, contribute to resistance by parents to some forms of palliative care or lead to requests for ineffective and even harmful treatments that adults might reject for themselves. To identify misunderstandings and misinformation (whatever the explanation), physicians may find it useful to ask parents what they understand of their child's situation.

One increasingly important source of information for parents, indeed all those with medical questions and concerns, is the Internet. The Internet also provides an electronic social support network for many patients and families facing serious medical problems. For example, several sites offer parent-to-parent support for families who have experienced a fetal death (stillbirth) or an infant's death from extreme prematurity or severe congenital anomalies. Sites that provide support and information for families whose child has or had a rare disorder may be especially welcome.

Little research charts how parents (or ill children or their siblings) locate or use Internet-based information, how their use varies during the course of a child's illness, or how the information influences their knowledge, attitudes, or actions. A recent survey found that 62 percent of those who used the Internet reported using it to locate health information, and over 90 percent of that group reported searching for information about a specific illness or condition, often someone else's (Fox and Rainie, 2002). The survey also found that most such users (about three-quarters) did not follow strategies that experts advise for checking a health site's sponsor, noting the date of the information, and taking sufficient time with their information search.

Other studies suggest that what consumers find on the Internet (and in books and other traditional sources) is of widely varying quality and value (see, e.g., Jadad and Gagliardi, 1998; McLeod, 1998; Eysenbach and Diepgen, 1999; Peroutka, 2000; APHA, 2001; Dyer, 2001; Li et al., 2001). Some well-managed sites include much carefully reviewed and thoughtfully presented information. Other sites provide information that is inadequately screened, misleading, inaccurate, incomplete, difficult to locate, poorly organized, outdated, or produced by groups with economic interests that could compromise the information provided. Physicians, social workers, and others advising families should review sites for clinical content and emotional tone before recommending sites, especially sites not associated with reputable governmental, professional, or other organizations.

Economic and educational disparities limit the reach of the Internet and other information resources to many patients and families. Health information, in general, tends to require high-level reading skills, even when it is intended for patients or consumers rather than health professionals (Berland et al., 2001). In addition, both before and after diagnosis, parents may find the information on the Internet overwhelming in both its volume and its content. Material intended for clinicians but available to everyone may be not only highly technical but also alarming in its specifics. Personal stories and photographs may likewise be frightening in their individual details and in their number and diversity. For example, after the birth of a very premature infant, one mother featured in an article in a major medical journal said she found the "horror stories" on the Internet so difficult that she promised herself not to read any more and to rely "more or less" on her baby's doctors and nurses for information (Richardson, 2001, p. 1504). Again, a child's care team may help guide parents to good sites.

The Internet can be more than a resource for general information and for parent-to-parent support. It is also being incorporated in telemedicine applications that support home health care for patients with life-threatening medical problems (see, e.g., Gray et al., 2000; Hersh et al., 2001; Starren et al., 2002). Chapter 6 briefly discusses some uses of telemedicine.

Prognosis: What to Expect Given the Diagnosis of a Potentially Fatal Medical Condition

Sometimes expectations for a child are clear at the time of the initial diagnosis. Certain kinds of congenital anomalies such as anencephaly are invariably fatal, although some infants may survive substantially longer than usual—dying after months rather than weeks or days. For other conditions, once an initial diagnosis is made, additional tests or waiting periods may be necessary to assess the condition's severity, the child's prospects for survival, and the implications for the child's and the family's quality of life.

Unless death comes quickly, for example, following severe injuries in a motor vehicle crash, assessment of prognosis is usually not a one-time event but a process of periodic reevaluation and discussion as time passes, as further testing occurs, and as curative or life-prolonging treatments are tried. For example, children whose leukemia recurs while they are on therapy have a less favorable prognosis than those with recurrence after treatment has ended.

Importance of Prognostic Information

When a child is diagnosed with a potentially fatal medical condition, families need information about the probable course of the condition—

including possible life expectancy and physical or mental consequences and the expected effects of treatments. The uncertainty associated with the information also should be acknowledged.

Full diagnostic and prognostic information may influence not only medical decisions but also other choices (Miller et al., 1998). For example, parents given accurate information about their child's fatal or potentially fatal medical condition may decide that it is prudent to put off the purchase of a new house or rethink a job change that would reduce family income, jeopardize health insurance, or require extensive travel. Others, if finances and the child's condition allow, may decide to take a family "dream" vacation sooner rather than later based on what they have learned. If they have a timely and full explanation of what to expect, parents may act earlier to enlist support from other family members and friends, work with teachers to create a supportive environment for the ill child and any siblings, marshal spiritual resources, and otherwise seek help to sustain them in the difficult times ahead. Likewise, if responses to therapy and the passage of time shift expectations for a child's survival and quality of life from favorable to grim, parents who are given sensitive but full information and counseling can be helped to prepare for their child's death, even if they also choose to continue experimental or other therapies. Conversely, overly optimistic assessments by physicians can deny patients and families opportunities to prepare for death and say their good-byes. It can also contribute to avoidable suffering if inadequately informed families choose burdensome treatments that will not benefit their child.

Chapter 3 reviewed some research suggesting discrepancies in physician and family assessments of prognosis. More research is needed on the causes and consequences of such differences. Possible causes include individual characteristics (e.g., styles of communication related to education or cultural background) and organizational or system factors (e.g., lack of protocols for communicating with families, poor training of health professionals).

Prognostic Uncertainty

As noted in Chapter 1, determination of prognosis is not a precise science. A number of analyses have described the limitations of quantitative and qualitative prognostic determinations for adult patients (see, e.g., Thibault, 1994, 1997; Lemeshow et al., 1995; Lynn et al., 1995; SUPPORT, 1995; Sherck and Shatney, 1996; Lynn et al., 1997; Christakis and Iwashyna, 1998; see also Appendix B). Determining prognosis for children can be even more difficult because the number of deaths is much smaller and because children's deaths from illness are somewhat less concentrated than adults in a few major diagnoses (see Chapter 2). As a result, large databases for reliable statistical analysis of survival patterns are less available and more expensive to accumulate.

For very rare conditions, even qualitative accounts of clinical experience are limited. For instance, certain neurological and metabolic disorders are so uncommon that pediatricians and family practitioners have little experience or information to use in advising families about the future course of the disease or life expectancy. They must rely on their clinical judgment and careful monitoring of a child's development, responses to treatment, and complications to provide parents with their best sense of the child's condition and future course.

Many progressive conditions have a highly variable course in children, but the reasons for this variability are not well understood. For example, research has only partly documented genetic and other factors (e.g., seizures, age at diagnosis) that put children with neurological disorders at higher risk of serious physical disability or early mortality. Similarly, researchers have undoubtedly identified only a small subset of genetic features that affect the likelihood of treatment success for various childhood cancers. Relapsed cancers are clearly harder to cure, but at the time that a relapse is diagnosed, it is not now possible to identify the children likely to be in the small group of survivors. This adds to the impetus to continue curative efforts.

Further, the same condition may follow a different course in children and adults, and a treatment may vary in effectiveness and unwanted side effects depending on the patient's age. For example, the National Cancer Institute presents advice separately for adult and childhood acute lymphoblastic leukemia (NCI, 2001a). To cite just one of many other examples, although tacrolimus has proved a generally effective immunosuppressive drug for adults who have undergone transplantation, some research suggests that children may respond less favorably (MacFarlane et al., 2001). Such differences underscore the importance of drug testing to establish pediatric dosing information (see Chapter 10).

Prognostic uncertainty may have limited practical consequences in some situations. Other times, however, it can be very consequential. As discussed in Chapter 6, for a patient covered by Medicaid or Medicare, eligibility for hospice benefits is contingent on certification by a patient's doctor and the hospice medical director that the person is terminally ill and has a life expectancy of six months or less if the disease has a "normal" course. Patients (or their surrogate decisionmakers) are also required to consent to forgo curative or life-prolonging treatments. These rules limit the ability of hospices to serve substantial numbers of adult Medicaid patients who have conditions such as congestive heart failure for which prediction of remaining life expectancy is particularly difficult and for which medical interventions during crises can add months or even years of life (Lynn and O'Mara,

2001). To the extent that determining prognosis is more difficult and uncertain in children, the rules put Medicaid-covered children and their families at a particular disadvantage if they desire assistance from a hospice.

As discussed in Appendix B, researchers have developed statistical models to assess illness or condition severity for critically ill children and to estimate their risk of death or other outcomes. The value and limitations of these models continue to be evaluated. For example, one recent study of prognosis in a neonatal intensive care unit concluded that—contrary to expectations—accuracy in predicting survival using either a statistical tool or clinical intuition did not improve with time. Instead, "most infants who die after the first few days . . . . seem to 'cloak themselves;' their ultimate demise becoming less apparent with each succeeding NICU day" (Meadow et al., 2002, p. 884). In general, prognostic models and tools tend to be more useful for some purposes such as health services management, quality assessment, and research but less so for other purposes such as guiding decisions about life-sustaining medical interventions for individual patients.

Communicating Bad News

Every word that was said the day Becky died is indelibly etched in my mind. I have replayed the words in my mind a million times. It's a never-ending tape.

Pam Borchart, parent (Maruyama, 1997)

Physicians usually will have the difficult task of telling parents what they cannot bear to hear—that their child's life is in jeopardy or that their child has died. Sometimes, as in the emergency department, physicians will be informing people they have never met before. Likewise, with a dying newborn, the neonatologist and the family may be strangers. At other times, for example, when tests show that a child's cancer has returned, physicians will be informing families they have known for the months or years of the child's illness. In some instances, the news of a child's death may come from an inexperienced resident who happens to be on duty in the intensive care unit but who has had no relationship with the family.

When a child has been injured away from home and taken to a hospital emergency department, a social worker usually serves as the communication and interpretive link between the parent and the team or teams working to save the child. Physicians may make briefer appearances to discuss tests, treatments, prognosis, and decisions. (See the vignette about the Marshall family in Chapter 3.) Nurses rarely take the lead in presenting bad news in either emergency or other situations, but they may help identify situations in which there is a mismatch between a child's condition and a parent's understanding of that condition. When there has been an emergency outside the hospital, parents may seek information from paramedics or police officers at the scene. In certain jurisdictions, death cannot be declared outside a hospital or other medical facility, and paramedics may not be permitted—or prepared—to inform parents of their child's status (Iverson, 1999). These limits do not, however, make good communication skills and sensitivity irrelevant. Communication guidelines or protocols for emergency personnel should cover situations involving both the provision and the withholding of information, including when circumstances may require a police investigation.

Although it seems reasonable that training and experience should improve clinicians' comfort and facility in communicating about life-threatening medical problems and about death, research is limited. Vazirani and colleagues (2000) concluded from a longitudinal study at one institution that pediatric residents became more comfortable with issues of death and dying over the course of their residency. At the same time, they became less comfortable with pain management out of concern that it might hasten death. As discussed further in Chapter 8, education about this and other dimensions of palliative, end-of-life, and bereavement care is limited at all levels of pediatrics training.

Most discussions about breaking bad news focus on adult patients and on families of adult or child patients. The following sections consider conversations with parents and with ill children themselves. One theme is that it is important—from the outset—to consider what, when, and how to communicate with the child patient. Depending on a child's cognitive and emotional development and preferences, the child may or may not be included in the initial discussion.

Talking with Parents

> *Things that are said at that time you remember forever.*
> Maruyama, 1997

Parents have tried to describe the impact of learning that that their child's life was in jeopardy. "Nothing in this new world makes sense. . . . In such insanity, you are dumbstruck." (as quoted in Finkbeiner, 1998, p. 5). "I don't think you understand anything until a few months go by. Maybe more than a few months" (as quoted in Finkbeiner, 1998, p.2).

Even sensitive and otherwise capable clinicians may not realize how difficult it can be for a shocked, fearful parent to absorb information. Incorrect assumptions about what parents understand, especially during a single conversation, can create confusion and distress later. If news is presented poorly, parents may recall the additional pain and, often, anger for years afterward. Personal accounts and some research suggest that physicians, whether experienced or not, will often face the telling of bad news with apprehension and inadequate formal training (see, e.g., Nuland, 1994; ABIM, 1996a,b; Christakis and Iwashyna, 1998).

Although many parents "only need to be told once that their child is dying," some may not initially accept or understand the message. For example, in one of a series of interviews about clinician experiences with families, one physician described situations in which "you can say, 'She's getting maximal therapy. She's not getting any better. That really isn't looking well [sic] and we are going to have to start to think about what if she doesn't get better . . . ' [and the parent's response is] 'So, is she going to be healthy when she goes home?' " (Bartel et al., 2000, p. 1128).

If other members of the child's care team are present during discussions with parents, they may sometimes be able to help when communication is not working. They also may participate in a timely "debriefing" to discuss how the conversation with a family went and what might be done differently and better in the future. Unfortunately, when physicians must break bad news during the evening or night, support from social workers, child-life specialists, and others may be limited because these professionals usually do not work those shifts, except for emergency departments.

Most literature on communicating bad news takes the perspective of those who must deliver the news (Girgis and Sanson-Fischer, 1995). Some studies have also sought perspectives from patients or families about what was important to them (Peteet et al., 1991; Krahn et al., 1993; Sell et al., 1993; Ahmann, 1998; Hart and Ahrens, 1998; Jurkovich et al., 2000). For example, one small survey study of 54 surviving family members of patients who had died of trauma reported that the most important aspects of delivering bad news were the attitude of the person delivering the news, the clarity of the information, privacy, and the person's knowledge or ability to answer questions (Jurkovich et al., 2000).

The literature on communicating bad news often includes guidance about how to prepare for and structure the conversation (see, e.g., Girgis and Sanson-Fisher, 1995; Ptacek and Eberhardt, 1996; Chisholm et al., 1997; Ptacek et al., 1999; Baile et al., 2000; Ambuel and Mazzone, 2001; ChIPPS, 2001; Levetown, 2001; Von Gunten, 2001). Again, little research documents whether following this guidance makes a positive difference for patients, families, or physicians (Walsh et al., 1998). As Ptacek and Eberhardt (1996, p. 496) observe, it is not clear "what of the personal, interpersonal, news-specific, situation-specific, and transmission-specific variables are important predictors of giver or receiver reactions." In general, studies suggest that considerable agreement exists between physicians and families or patients about how news should be conveyed (see, e.g., Ptacek and Eberhardt, 1996; Baile et al., 1999; Parker et al., 2001).

Box 4.1 summarizes several general principles for communicating clini-

BOX 4.1
Presenting Bad News to Families

Preparation

• Understand that respectful and clear communication is an essential professional obligation.

• Plan with members of the care team for the delivery of bad news, including the words, the tone, the time, and the place. Have information that is as complete as possible.

• Anticipate that reactions will vary, but be prepared to deal with shock, grief, anger, panic, and other strong emotions.

• Have someone trained to respond to the family's emotional and practical needs who is ready to stay with the family.

• Try to have both parents present, if clinical and family circumstances permit, and ask if they would like their child or others to be present. If the answer is yes, plan for someone to accompany the child if he or she chooses to leave.

• Find a private, quiet place where everyone can be seated comfortably and you can make eye contact with the family members and touch them if that seems supportive.

• Have a trained translator present if necessary.

• Consider taping the conversation and providing the tape to the family.

Conversation

• Indicate at the start that the news is not good.

• Show your concern, empathy, and respect for the child and family.

• Listen carefully.

• Try to get an early sense of the family, including what they already know and how they express themselves. Adjust the style and content of communication—including the use of physical contact—accordingly.

cal information and, more specifically, conveying bad news to parents about their child's medical problem. It assumes that a physician is presenting the news. Other members of the health care team bring additional skills and perspectives to bear on the complex process of presenting information effectively and compassionately. Discussions with ill children themselves are considered separately below, but many of the same points will still apply. Box 4.1 should not be interpreted as a communication protocol. (Chapter 6 includes recommendations for developing such protocols.)

Although many clinicians appear comfortable with communication guidelines and report using them, they also identify obstacles to implementing them (Campbell and Sanson-Fisher, 1998; Dosanjh et al., 2001). These obstacles include lack of time, lack of support from other professionals (especially important for residents) and from institutions, and lack of rou-

- Use the everyday language of the family rather than the everyday language of clinicians, except when clinical terms are likely to be helpful.
- Consider using sketches and diagrams to support explanations of the diagnosis and prognosis.
- Seek guidance from families about the amount and specificity of information they want, and let them control the pace and flow of information insofar as possible.
- Allow time for families to absorb and process information.
- Assess (if the child's condition permits) whether discussion of options, goals, and plans should be initiated or postponed to a defined later time.
- Check family members' understanding of what they have heard and assess what needs to be repeated or reinforced during this or later conversations.
- Reassure families that it is normal to be emotional, confused, or overwhelmed.
- Provide written information and suggest other information resources.
- Offer to help parents prepare for talking with their child if the child is not present
- Encourage parents to write down questions as they arise, so that they can be discussed later.
- Respect parents' need for hope and reassurance but avoid evasions or deceits that may undermine trust and prevent emotional and other preparation for what lies ahead.

Follow-up

- Arrange for further discussions as appropriate, including with the child (if he or she was absent), siblings, and others.
- Document the conversation (in addition to documenting diagnosis and prognosis) as a guide for future discussions.
- Reflect on the conversation and what might be done better in the future.

SOURCE: Adapted from IOM, 1997.

tine processes for feedback and dealing with emotions. As discussed in Chapters 6 and 7, health plan policies that undervalue communication and preclude reimbursement for discussions when the child patient is not present are also discouraging.

Many of the same basic principles listed in Box 4.1 will apply to later discussions with parents as a child's condition changes. Conversations may become less strained when families and clinicians have established a relationship of trust and a familiar style of communicating. This is evident in one parent's description of a crucial discussion with the child's physician after surgery and many months of chemotherapy: "The tears in his eyes when he set up the meeting and then the careful way he described everything were the final message I needed to realize that we had run out of [treatment] options" (Aney, 2001).

Box 4.2 provides an example of how an actual conversation between a physician and mother might be constructed. It does not fully depict but only suggests the professional preparation and system support (e.g., availability of written materials for families, follow up procedures) for the individual conversation.

One point that is not always emphasized is that communication is an interactive process. Early on in a conversation, clinicians can ask questions about parents' understanding of their child's situation and then craft a discussion that builds on this initial information about what parents know and what language they use to describe what they know. Also, as noted earlier, communicating about diagnosis and prognosis is usually not a one-time event but a continuing process as care goals and plans are considered and reconsidered and new information becomes available. Information may also have to be repeated. It may take considerable skill to do this without

---

BOX 4.2
Example of Communicating a Grim Diagnosis

Starting

Physician: Hello, Ms. Gutierrez. This has been a tough and exhausting time for you. Thank you for meeting with us again. This is Mandy, the social worker and Ranesha, the child-life specialist. I'm glad your friend Carlos is here with you.

Continuing

I wanted to review Maria's situation and give you some additional information about what has us so concerned. First, though, can you tell me what you understand so far?

Mother: Well yes, Maria is having problems breathing.

Checking

Physician: What do you understand is causing that?

Mother: I heard someone say something about pneumonia. My father thinks it may be from the chemical plant.

Physician: You are right that pneumonia could be one cause, and we are treating Maria for that. However, we are concerned that another problem may be causing her troubles. These problems include a form of muscle weakness called muscular dystrophy. Have you ever heard of that?

Mother: No, I've never heard of it. It doesn't sound good.

making some parents feel as if they are being bludgeoned with the message that their child will die. It may also require good communication among members of the care team so that they do not unnecessarily and insensitively go over the same issues or questions or provide conflicting perspectives.

One constraint on the use of repeated conversations to ensure comprehension of important information is that the initial news about diagnosis, prognosis, and options must often be followed quickly by treatment decisions. Parents may be asked to read and sign an "informed consent" document that describes the nature of a planned procedure and its potential benefits and risks. As described by Sourkes (1995a, p.33): "While [the consent form is] intended as a factual document, its emotional impact on the parents cannot be underestimated." To the extent that parents are shocked and only partly comprehending, their decisionmaking capacities may be impaired (Downer, 1996).

Physician: It is not good. Let me tell you more about the problem and what we can do to help. You may not understand everything in this conversation and you may forget some things. That's normal. Don't worry about writing things down. What I tell you is also in the family information notebook that we will give you. Also, that notebook has space for you to write down questions, so you should keep it with you. Then you will have a list of questions you can bring when we meet again.

Listening

Mother: I don't need to write things down.

Physician: It can very helpful. Does something bother you about it?

Mother: Oh . . . I don't write English that well.

Physician: That's okay. We can have someone who knows Spanish to help you. And in a couple of months, we should have a Spanish language version of the notebook ready.

Reassuring

Mother: I'm scared. I'm going to cry.

Physician: That's okay. It's normal to be scared. We do need to talk some right now, but then we can stop if it is too hard and set another time to talk. We will be here for you—not just me but Mandy and Ranesha and the other doctors and nurses who work specially with children like Maria. You'll meet them shortly.

After parents have learned that a child has a life-threatening medical problem, they often must then gather the emotional resources to tell others— the child, his or her siblings, their own parents, friends, teachers, and others. Physicians, social workers, child-life specialists, psychologists, and others can provide guidance and emotional support as parents undertake these difficult conversations. Time pressures, financial constraints, and other circumstances may, however, limit what they can offer.

Talking with Children

The ones who tell me are my friends.
Benjamin, child with cancer (Bluebond-Langner, 1978, p. 188)

With the advice and support of the child's care team, parents typically decide when and what to tell their child about his or her diagnosis and prognosis.[1] If parents choose not to include the child when a physician first meets with them to discuss diagnosis, they may welcome help in preparing for a later discussion with the child, perhaps even having the child's physician convey the news or at least be present. Older children may want information to come from the physician directly. Although communication clearly must be tailored to the child's developmental status and clinical status, little systematic research is available to guide parents and clinicians about the effects of different styles and amounts of communication for children of different ages and other characteristics (Stevens, 1998; Goldman, 1999).

Qualitative studies of children living with life-threatening medical conditions make clear that they are often aware at some level that they will not live to grow up or that they may die soon (Bluebond-Langner, 1978; Sourkes, 1995a). Such knowledge does not depend on explicit communication. Based on what is happening around them and to them, even young children may develop realistic apprehensions that they are going to die. Bluebond-Langner described the "five-year old boy, lying uncomfortably on his back, [who] when asked if he wanted to be turned over, said 'No, I'm practicing for my coffin'" (1978, p. 191). Another child, asked what he was going be when he grew up, replied "a ghost" (1978, p. 194).

Once it was common to try to "shield" dying children, and often adults, from knowledge of their condition. Now more agreement exists—in principle, if not in practice—that children with life-threatening medical

---

[1]The nature of the child's illness may influence parents. For example, parents of children with HIV infection or AIDS have sometimes been reluctant to inform the child of his or her status (AAP, 1999a; Gerson et al., 2001). This can harm children, especially older children who recognize that something is not right with them. With adolescents ready to experiment with sex, failure to discuss such a diagnosis can also increase the potential for harm to others.

problems should normally be informed about their condition, consistent with their intellectual and emotional maturity, medical status, and personal preferences for receiving information (Wass, 1984; Goldman, 1999). Family preferences or cultural values, which must be understood and respected, will not always be consistent with this consensus. For example, in some cultures, talking about death explicitly is seen as risky or not appropriate and in others, involvement of children in discussions about their future is not approved (see, e.g., Jecker et al., 1995; Carrese and Rhodes, 2000). In practice, the parents' values usually seem to prevail if they do not want the child told.

Although scientific research is limited, clinical experience and qualitative studies and reports suggest that failure to provide children with information and the opportunity to discuss their concerns and fears openly can lead to feelings of isolation, guilt, anxiety, and other distress (Bluebond-Langner, 1978; Sourkes, 1995a). Parents also may suffer for their evasions with their child. As one anguished father recalled, "My last words to my son were a lie" (from Goldman, 1999, p. 104). Children, however, may be very protective of their parents and siblings and may cooperate in a pattern of silence, while understanding that they are ill and may die (Bluebond-Langner, 1978). As one clinician described it, "parents want to protect their children, and children want to protect their parents . . . and you're not the parent" (Mildred Solomon, Ed.D., Education Development Center, personal communication based on interviews for the Initiative for Pediatric Palliative Care, unpublished analysis by Hardart et al., 2002).

In deciding about the content, timing, and pace of communication, parents will draw on their knowledge of their child's temperament, emotional resilience, curiosity, intellectual abilities, coping strategies, and past experiences, for example, the recent death of a grandparent (Sourkes, 1995a; AAP, 2000c). Children who have already undergone extensive testing and treatment will likely have provided clues or direct statements about what they understand or suspect and how ready they are learn more.

What is communicated will also depend, in part, on the nature of a child's medical condition and history. For example, the initial communication about the diagnosis of a usually curable cancer may emphasize that good treatments are available, that most children recover, and that the care team is committed to keeping pain and other problems to a minimum. When the diagnosis and prognosis are less favorable or when cancer has recurred, the information cannot be so positive. In these circumstances, finding ways to redefine or reframe—not remove—hope can be challenging. Once again, little research is available to guide these kinds of discussions and suggest what parents find supportive under what circumstances.

For children, cognitive development may limit what they can accurately understand about serious illness and death. A number of analyses have described the evolution of children's understanding of death (see, e.g., Wass, 1984; Stevens, 1998; Davies, 1998; Silverman, 2000). They have generally assessed developmental understanding in terms of four basic concepts: irreversibility, finality, universality, and causation. These analyses have, however, generally focused on healthy children. They may not be applicable to children who have experienced extended periods of illness and medical treatment. As parents and clinicians discuss care options for and with the ill child, they may not fully appreciate the ill child's altered sense of the world compared to well children. Further, adolescents who have lived for years with a serious condition and who may live for many additional years may continue to be treated as if they were much younger. This may interfere with their normal development toward adulthood.

In responding to a child's questions, a parent or clinician will often need to look for an underlying intent or meaning and guard against providing too little or too much information or answering the wrong question. Children's nonverbal communication—including drawings, expressions, and posture—may reveal their desires, concerns, knowledge, or suspicions more clearly than words because they lack the concepts to describe their concerns or emotions (Adams-Greenly, 1984). Stevens recounts, for example, the 5-year-old child who, on the night he died, told his parents that he did not know what to say but then sang a children's song about a rainbow (Stevens, 1998). The question of another seriously ill 5-year-old, "Doctors can't make everyone better, can they?" (Goldman, 1999, p. 96) might be both a request for reassurance and an attempt to understand more about his situation. In addition to artwork, conversations with children may be aided by the use of stuffed animals, dolls, puppets, and other toys, which may also be helpful therapeutically in helping children cope with fear, sadness, and other emotions (Sourkes, 1995a; see also Chapter 5).

For adults, detailed initial and continuing communication about diagnosis and prognosis may be driven by the patient's need to give informed consent for treatment and make financial and other plans. Children usually do not face such pressures. Unless the child needs fairly immediate preparation for surgical or other treatments, communication may be guided to some degree by his or her explicitly or implicitly indicated desire for information (Sourkes, 1995a).

Once they learn of their prognosis, children may or may not want to talk further about it with their parents. For example, one of the parents with whom the committee met felt that he and his daughter really needed to talk, but she was reluctant. Finally, she said, "Dad, okay, this is it, one time, we're going to talk. . . . [When I had] said everything I wanted to say . . . she said, 'Dad, are you finished? . . . You are getting my head all wet'" (Weil, 2001). Perhaps to spare her parents some of her anxieties, the daughter did talk more with her home-school teacher.

Later sections of this chapter consider children's participation in goal setting and treatment decisions. The discussion of decisionmaking includes the committee's recommendation that children be included in discussions and decisions consistent with their intellectual and emotional maturity, medical condition, and preferences. Chapter 8 reviews legal issues related to children's participation in decisions about their care.

Talking to Parents When Their Child Has Died Without Forewarning

My husband was called to the hospital where he tried to ask questions but received few answers.

Patricia Loder, parent, 2001

They hadn't laughed with my babies, fed them, burped them, played with them, nursed them to sleep. How could they say now that one of them was dead?

Esmeralda Williamson-Noble, parent, no date

Sometimes parents will not have to be told of their child's death because they will be there—at home or in the hospital, perhaps following a decision to forgo further life-support interventions or other planning when death is clearly approaching. Other times, physicians will have to tell parents that their child has died in the emergency department or intensive care unit. This will never be easy, even when the child has been seriously ill and treatments have been failing. The task will be particularly difficult when a child has died suddenly and without forewarning, for example, in a car crash.

Appendix F discusses some of the complexities created when a child dies suddenly and without forewarning. Such situations may involve a large cast of providers, possibly including emergency medical technicians, fire and rescue personnel, law enforcement and public safety officers, as well as hospital-based caregivers in emergency departments, on surgical teams, and in intensive care units. Each may interact with family members but under different conditions and with different constraints (including legal constraints). Each needs communication protocols and procedures tailored to these differences.

In emergency situations, some of the usual guidelines for communicating bad news may be difficult to implement, particularly if the parents or other family members have also been injured. Time for planning a conversation may be abbreviated, and time for the conversation itself may be curtailed by the need to respond to new emergencies. The expectation of a continuing relationship is usually absent, although physicians, social workers, or other designated and trained individuals can assure parents that they should call if they have questions later. They can also offer follow-up support as described below, including discussion of autopsy findings that clarify the cause of death.

Given the stressful circumstances of a child's unexpected death, the development of communication protocols and procedures and the corresponding training of emergency medical and other personnel are important but have not necessarily been a priority for health care institutions. For example, a survey of emergency department directors published in 1993 found that most hospitals did not have an organized process for informing and counseling parents whose child was dead on arrival, provided no training in how to tell parents about a child's death, and let the responsibility for doing so generally fall to the least experienced clinicians (Greenberg et al., 1993). Survey results cited in Chapter 3 suggested that emergency room physicians were poorly prepared to tell parents about a child's death and would even uselessly extend resuscitation to avoid telling them.

Recently, under contract from the federal Maternal and Child Health Bureau, the National Association of Social Workers has developed consensus bereavement guidelines for social workers in emergency departments and has received funds to train social workers in emergency services guidelines (Lipton and Coleman, 2000b; NASW, 2000). These guidelines stress the importance of preparation, including establishing protocols and procedures for communication and family support when a child dies in the emergency department; training for all department staff; designating a room to be used for private discussions with families; assigning a social worker, chaplain, nurse or other trained individual to provide support and act as a liaison between the family and emergency department personnel; and developing a plan to follow the family in bereavement. Follow-up studies should assess the implementation and results of these guidelines, which cover both the emotional or psychological dimensions and the practical aspects of working with families. In addition to these guidelines, the recent statement of the American Academy of Pediatrics and the College of Emergency Medicine on care of children calls for development, implementation, and monitoring of policies, procedures, and protocols on death in the emergency department, but the statement is not specific (AAP, 2001b).

Earlier AAP guidelines on death in the emergency department are more specific on topics that should be covered in protocols and checklists. They do not specifically discuss communication protocols but do state that departments should have a private room where family members can talk with physicians, nurses, social workers, or chaplains as well as child protection services representatives or police officers (AAP, 1994a).

When a child has died suddenly and without forewarning from injuries either before or after arriving at a hospital emergency department and the parents are not present, the general view is that a physician should notify the parents in person, for example, asking them to come to the hospital

(Levetown, 2001). Some parents may, however, make it clear in a telephone conversation that they want the news immediately. Each situation is different, and physicians, social workers, or others communicating with families should look for cues from parents or other family members about the content and pacing of discussions.

Although it may be appropriate to withhold specific information in some special situations, the committee heard that lack of information—not even a "we don't know yet" or "we are still working with [the child]"—is another burden for shocked and fearful parents. One parent, who was injured in the accident that killed her two children, told the IOM committee, "My attempts to learn the status of my children were answered only by sedative drugs, not information" (Loder, 2001, p. 4).

In its written statement to the committee, a group supporting families of murdered children highlighted the word "information" throughout the statement to emphasize its importance (NOPMC, 2001). The group also stressed that families can be obsessed with wondering what happened to their loved one and that imaginings can be worse than reality. Failures to tell the truth, even if well meaning, can be damaging, especially since families of murdered children may learn the details during police investigations or courtroom proceedings.

Among the practical matters that need to be handled competently and compassionately by social workers, chaplains, and others are (depending on the circumstances) medical examiner referrals, organ donation requests and referrals, notification of the patient's primary care physician, completion and transmission of death records, identification and notification of funeral home, and authorization for release of the body. These steps, which must be consistent with relevant state and federal laws, are necessary after most deaths, but in the crisis atmosphere of the emergency department, clear administrative protocols and procedures and associated training and monitoring are especially important. Chapter 9 includes an example of training strategies for one sensitive topic, requests for organ donation, that may be relevant for other discussions.

WHAT ARE OUR OPTIONS? ESTABLISHING GOALS

General

A child's diagnosis and prognosis will determine to some extent the kinds of goals, care options, and choices that are possible. Parents of an infant born with certain fatal congenital anomalies will have only short-term options to consider. In contrast, parents of a toddler diagnosed with a slowly progressive, fatal neurodegenerative disorder will have short-term and long-term choices to make over a period of years. The possibilities for a child just diagnosed with an often-curable cancer will differ from those for a child who has relapsed following a second or third round of chemotherapy. It would be inappropriate to emphasize options for end-of-life care during discussions with parents of the newly diagnosed child, whereas parents of the child whose treatments are failing need to learn about options for supportive end-of-life care if they are to make informed choices. In less clear-cut situations, what to tell the parents and when will necessarily be more difficult to judge. Whatever the child's status and whatever a family's goals and choices, parents should, however, be reassured that everything will be done for their child's comfort and the family's well being.

Some discussion of care goals and options will usually occur during the initial conversation about a child's diagnosis and prognosis. As already described, shock, fear, and panic may interfere with parents' abilities to absorb information and make decisions. Thus, their understanding of this initial information cannot be taken for granted. About his own experience with the very premature birth of his son (who survived), psychologist Michael Hynan wrote that some of what happens "is so horrible it must be blocked out. . . . And if you're a perinatal professional trying to explain something to me at the same time, it just doesn't register, even if I'm nodding my head. . . . I ask you [perinatal professionals] to help us when we do silly or dumb things because we are so stressed out" (Hynan, 1996, online, no page). Assessing what parents are understanding or what their reactions mean requires experience, empathy, and concentration—and the assessment may still be imperfect.

Based on their experiences and their own values, physicians and others may have expectations about what patients and families will want. They may often be correct, but one principle of patient- and family-centered care is, "Ask, don't assume" (Gerteis et al., 1993). This principle recognizes both the potential for differences in individual values and preferences and the limits on an individual's ability to absorb information. Checking understanding of diagnosis, prognosis, and treatment options (including palliative care options) should be a part of obtaining informed consent for treatment, whether or not a signed document is required. Otherwise, parents may make decisions without appreciating the expected burdens (which may sometimes be high) and the probability of benefit (which may sometimes be remote). One long-term goal should be for the parents to feel later that they did the right things and did not cause their child needless suffering.

Most parents will want to participate actively in setting goals and making decisions about their child's care. Some parents, however, may consistently defer to physicians, even when the physicians and other members of the care team actively solicit the parents' guidance in the development of care goals and plans. In contrast, in uncommon but usually very difficult situations, some parents may find themselves in conflict with their child's care team to the point that an ethics consultation or other outside mediation is needed. (See Chapter 8.)

Establishing goals and evaluating treatment options may be particularly complicated for children with very rare disorders, when physicians have little experience or literature to guide them or the child's parents. This was one of the challenges facing physicians in Chapter 3's vignette about Johnny Gabrielle and his family. As noted in that chapter, even for more common conditions, children's paths may be highly variable, more so than for adults.

A family's cultural or religious values and personal histories may shape their goals of care and preferences for information, influence their evaluation of treatment options, and affect their level of trust in a professional's advice. Research involving adults has reported differences in cultural attitudes about disclosure of information, participation in decisionmaking, use of traditional or alternative therapies, and end-of-life care (Irish et al., 1993; Blackhall et al., 1995, 1999, 2001; Hopp and Duffy, 2000; Sullivan, 2001). In addition, members of ethnic and cultural communities that have long suffered discrimination and deprivation may interpret a discussion of forgoing resuscitation or other interventions as an attempt to deny beneficial care. Some studies have reported differences in utilization of or preferences for life support and advance care planning among African Americans compared to Caucasians (Garrett et al., 1993; Gramelspacher et al., 1997; Shepardson et al., 1999; Crawley et al., 2000).

Sensitivity to cultural, religious, and other values can help members of the child's care team establish a respectful and constructive relationship with families whose backgrounds differ from their own. Profound cultural misunderstandings can be difficult to overcome, however, as devastatingly portrayed in Anne Fadiman's (1997) *The Spirit Catches You and You Fall Down: A Hmong Child, Her American Doctors, and the Collision of Two Cultures*. Discussing the relationships between the family and physicians caring for a child with epilepsy, the author writes, "It was as if, by a process of reverse alchemy, each party in this doomed relationship had managed to convert the other's gold into dross" (Fadiman, 1997, p. 223). Appendix D discusses cultural considerations in end-of-life care for children in more detail.

Integrating Palliative Care Perspectives from the Time of Diagnosis

Understandably, for parents whose child has a life-threatening medical problem, the overwhelming initial goal or desire will usually be to save their child from death. For example, the study by Wolfe and colleagues (2000b) cited earlier found that parents cited cure as their number one goal at the

TABLE 4.1   Common Goals and Examples of Supportive Care

Goal	Examples of Care
Physical comfort	Using medications and behavioral interventions to prevent or relieve a child's pain, fatigue, or other symptoms Providing physical therapy to improve function and relieve pain
Emotional comfort	Providing psychotherapy including verbal and play techniques Arranging art, music, or other expressive therapies Encouraging visits from family and friends
Normal life	Informing the child and involving him or her in decisions (consistent with intellectual and emotional maturity) Planning with teachers and administrators for a child's return to school Organizing travel or camp experiences
Family functioning	Helping parents make special time for siblings Arranging respite for parents
Cultural or spiritual values	Accommodating religious rituals and traditional customs Encouraging continuation or adaptation of family holiday traditions
Preparing for death	Planning for parents, siblings, and others to be with the child at and after death Planning for remembrances or legacies of the child's life including pictures, videos, locks of hair, and handprints or handmolds

time of diagnosis. Depending on their age, medical problem, and other factors, child patients may be as much focused on cure as their parents are.

One reason for integrating palliative care perspectives with discussion of possible curative and life-prolonging interventions is to encourage families to consider and achieve additional goals related to the child's quality of life and that of the family. Table 4.1 lists a range of such goals, some of which will be most relevant when the child's life-threatening condition extends over months or years. Without explicit consideration, these goals may be neglected—to a family's later regret and sorrow. Only the last of the goals—explicit preparation for death—requires a family to accept that a child will likely die, and even this goal does not require that a family forgo continued effort to prolong the child's life. Nevertheless, some families may be unable to face preparing for their child's death.

Another reason for integrating palliative care perspectives from the time of diagnosis is to encourage sensitive but systematic revisiting of goals and plans as a child's medical condition changes. Parents may be so absorbed in the medical, financial, and practical aspects of caring for their children and surviving day to day that they may find it difficult to recognize the need to redefine goals or identify different ways of reaching them.

When appropriate, early consultations also give families an opportunity to become familiar with palliative care personnel in advance of an expected or possible crisis and to discuss issues such as continued relationships with the child's established care team. Without such preparation, families may react instinctively by feeling that they are being abandoned and by rejecting certain options, including hospice care, without understanding what is being offered.

Given the diversity of the goals, no single health care professional is likely to be fully prepared to discuss ways to fit medical care and family strategies to the goals. Depending on the situation, physicians, nurses, social workers, psychologists, child-life specialists, chaplains, and others will have roles to play. Again, for them to perform effectively, professionals will need to be adequately educated and trained to discuss goals, identify strategies, and guide families to the appropriate and available resources.

Goals and Choices at the End of Life: Advance Care Planning

I've had the experience of having to stand at the table in the emergency room and say, it's okay to let him go. And of talking to my son [Joshua] and saying, it's okay to go, if he wants to go. For the most part, the doctors are responsive to that, but they just can't stop themselves from intervening. . . . We need to teach people how to stop and respect.

Tina Heyl-Martineau, parent, 2001[2]

Much has been written about advance care planning for adults, particularly planning for a time when they are no longer be able to make decisions or communicate preferences. Ideally, this planning is less about documents—although certain documents can be important—than it is about an ongoing process of considering values, preferences, circumstances, and expectations relevant to what a person wants at the end of his or her life (see, e.g., Larson and Tobin, 2000). A variety of initiatives have helped make advance care planning more routine and more informed. Nonetheless, most adults, even older adults and adults with serious illnesses, have not considered their own values about end-of-life care, discussed their views

---

[2]Joshua Martineau died June 30, 2002.

with family members, or completed advance directives or medical power-of-attorney documents (see, e.g., SUPPORT, 1995; Grimaldo et al., 2001; Wenger et al., 2001).

In any case, recommendations and suggestions for competent adults have only limited direct relevance for children and their families for various reasons. Except for children judged to be mature or emancipated minors (see Chapter 8), parents have the legal authority to make the medical decisions for their child, including decisions about end-of-life care, although they are often unwilling to face such decisions until the child is very near death. Children may be involved in discussions about their concerns and wishes, but their preferences about treatments will prevail only if their parents agree.

As discussed in Chapter 3, many serious illnesses in childhood run an unpredictable course of relapses and remissions, with acute events that can often be reversed for a period. Modern medical technology continues to advance and therapies that were seen as heroic just a decade ago are now considered standards of practice, such as bone marrow transplantation for relapsed leukemia or cardiac transplantation for certain heart conditions. Even when the prognosis with treatment is grim, children, families, and clinicians can postpone acknowledging an approaching death as they focus on potentially life-sustaining therapies (Goldman, 1999).

Consideration of goals for life's ending and preparation for death involves much more than signing (or not signing) orders about cardiopulmonary resuscitation and other life-support measures. It also provides the opportunity for families to think about how to make the most of their remaining time together, particularly when it is clear that time will be short. Planning for this time can even provide parents some comfort as they anticipate and grieve in advance for their child's death.

Attention to goals and choices in advance of an expected death can also help families reduce the possibility of certain distressing experiences, including unwanted interventions and even legal inquiries. For example, if an ill child dies a planned death at home and the plan explicitly provides for families to manage with no call to 9-1-1 or no race to the hospital (but with the child's care team available for consultation and support), parents may be protected by having a written do-not-resuscitate (DNR) order in their possession,[3] by having alternatives arranged in case their child's physician cannot come to the home to pronounce death, and possibly—even if the child is not under hospice care—by calling the local hospice for advice about local law enforcement practices and expectations. (Although specific

---

[3]Because success rates for resuscitation in these situations are very low, DNRs are sometimes called DNAR or "do not attempt resuscitation" orders or AND "allow natural death" orders (see, e.g., Crimmins, 1993).

requirements vary, unexpected child deaths must generally be reported to the medical examiners office.) Misunderstandings about the circumstances of a child's death can add to a family's suffering (Rosauer, 1999; Avila, 2001).

Little has been written to advise either physicians or parents on advance care planning as it may be relevant for children with life-threatening medical conditions (Hilden et al., 2001a,b; Hilden et al., 2000c). Instead, attention has focused more on clinical and ethical aspects of withholding life-sustaining interventions for children than on the goals of care and the role of palliative measures in meeting those goals (see, e.g., Lantos, et al., 1994; AAP, 1994b, 1996; Levetown, 2001). In addition to continued discussion of ethical issues, more needs to be known about variations in parents' responses and decisions when physicians have begun discussions about DNR orders, hospice, and other end-of-life choices. Such knowledge may help guide physicians who believe that continued chemotherapy or other treatments are causing the child suffering without prospect of benefit but who feel they have not been able to communicate this effectively but compassionately to parents who want to continue such treatments. This is not to imply the parents are making "bad" choices but rather to recognize that physicians' primary obligation is to advocate for what they believe is best for their patient.

Barriers to Considering Palliative Care and Advance Care Planning

Successful integration of palliative care perspectives following diagnosis means finding sensitive ways of providing parents—whatever their values and background—with timely and appropriate information about palliative care options and then encouraging their timely consideration of these options and the goals of care. Some options, particularly those related to a child's physical or emotional comfort, may not require parents to acknowledge directly that their child is likely or certain to die. For example, members of a child's care team can encourage parents to consider how to help a seriously ill child achieve a wish or goal, for example, a trip to Disney World or completion of a school activity. Some decisions about end-of-life care must, however, be explicit, for example, deciding on DNR orders or accepting hospice services, particularly if the latter choice requires agreeing to Medicaid's requirements for hospice benefits.

Because parents are often so focused on curative or life-prolonging care, discussion of hospice or end-of-life planning for their child may seem intolerable until death is very near or until continued reliance on life-sustaining technologies is finally recognized as just prolonging suffering and dying. By that time, important opportunities may have been lost to help the child and family avoid needless physical and emotional suffering.

Although few studies have examined palliative and end-of-life care for children, the study by Wolfe and colleagues (2000a) cited earlier found that children for whom hospice care had been initiated earlier were more likely to be reported by their families as peaceful and calm during the last month of their lives.

Notwithstanding the potential benefits of palliative and hospice care, it may be very difficult for parents to accept it, even if it is not presented as an "either/or" choice between life-prolonging and palliative care. For example, a couple responding to questions about their experiences wrote that "we never realized how much we needed and benefited from hospice care. . . . [Still,] we felt that to accept hospice, we were accepting Kelley's dying. Our hospice nurse and social worker would tell us that we could always discontinue hospice if Kelley got better. . . . They had many patients who stopped hospice because they went into remission or their conditions stabilized" (Bula and Bula, 2001).

Another woman who lost her daughter to cancer later wrote a member of the inpatient palliative care team, "I must stress how much I hated having to experience palliative care," and then added ". . . but the team was so comforting and so very compassionate" (Himelstein and Hilden, 2001, no page). The psychologist on the child's care team observed that the mother "dreaded the day you would darken her door."

As indicated earlier, barriers to certain aspects of palliative care and advance care planning may sometimes be cultural. For example, values in traditional Chinese and Navajo cultures may be inconsistent with explicit discussions about death and certain ways of planning for life's end. A child's care team should, however, still have a plan of care that anticipates changes in the child's status.

Recognizing that care under the palliative or hospice care label may be difficult for families to accept, several hospices have sought to make their services more acceptable and accessible to families by developing supportive programs based in their licensed home care units and then identifying them with somewhat indirect names.[4] Unlike Medicare and Medicaid, some private insurers may cover hospice services or consultations without requir-

---

[4]Examples include Caricel (Hospice of Northern Virginia), Essential Care (Center for Hospice and Palliative Care, Buffalo, New York), Children's Bridges (Hospice of the Florida Suncoast), and Carousel (Hospice of Winston-Salem and others). In a discussion of pediatric palliative care in Britain, Ann Goldman said her team was often referred to as the symptom care team or, especially early on, as the home care team (Goldman, 2000a). "Most people don't take very long to realize exactly what we do, and occasionally we'll have families who will say, "I don't think we want your help, please. We'll call you when we want you," because of the implication to them that our involvement means that their child isn't going to get better" (Goldman, 2000a, no page).

ing that curative or life-prolonging treatments cease or that life expectancy be certified as six months or less (see Chapter 7). Still, even when both clinicians and parents are prepared to consider palliative or hospice care, lack of financial, organizational, and other resources may limit access to such care.

Although far more limited than corresponding efforts related to adult end-of-life care, some organizations mentioned here as well as others have begun community information and education programs to make options more widely known to families, health care providers, religious leaders, school personnel, and others. These efforts may encourage some parents to consider end-of-life planning earlier and may reduce avoidable distress for some children but are unlikely by themselves to make a substantial difference. More creativity and more research are needed to find strategies that encourage timely discussion of end-of-life care that will prevent needless suffering, help children and families make the most of their remaining time together, and preserve parents' need to feel they have done everything possible for their child.

Involvement of Child Patients

Agreement has been growing that children should be informed about their medical condition and that they should also be involved in discussions about the goals and plan of care, including end-of-life care, consistent with their intellectual and emotional maturity, medical condition, and desire to participate (see, e.g., Brock, 1989; Burns and Truog, 1997; Hilden et al., 2000c; Hinds et al., 2001; Nitschke et al., 2001). In many situations, even children and adolescents with serious cognitive disabilities can indicate their preferences about care. In writing about the death of his 28-year-old sister, who had Down syndrome and developed leukemia, physician Chris Feudtner wrote, "Along with my family, I had contemplated every facet of her life as long as I can remember—asking constantly what mattered to her and why—with efforts simply redoubled once she became sick, commitment deepened to abide by her rules as best we could" (Feudtner, 2000, p. 1622).

Certainly, a child's cognitive and emotional maturity and preferences for involvement must be considered in preparing for initial and subsequent discussions to inform and involve children. What is appropriate for a 6-year-old—perhaps the use of stuffed animals and other play techniques to aid in explaining and assessing understanding—will not be appropriate for a 16-year-old.

Given this country's ethnic, cultural, and religious diversity, family values about discussions of death, medical care, and children's roles must also be taken into account and respected. The child's care team must be sensitive to family values and preferences but can work with families on how to inform and involve children and how to identify and respond to their concerns and wishes. As suggested earlier, failure to inform and involve children can lead to feelings of isolation and other distress. Further, it can prevent parents and clinicians from truly appreciating a child's values, goals, and experience of his or her disease and its treatment and from using that appreciation to guide the child's plan of care.

As discussed in this chapter and in Chapter 8, parents usually have the legal authority to make decisions for their child, but this is no way precludes the child's involvement in discussions and decisions about their care. Chapter 10 notes that children's "assent" to participation in research is normally expected but not necessarily required. Ethical issues may arise if children are led to believe they have choices when, in fact, their choices will be overridden if their parents disagree.

WHAT WILL HELP MY CHILD AND MY FAMILY? FITTING CARE TO GOALS AND CIRCUMSTANCES

Designing a Palliative Care Plan as Part of an Overall Plan of Care

Not all suffering caused by life-threatening medical conditions or by the pursuit of cure or prolonged life can be prevented and not all goals of patients and families can be met. Nonetheless, if suffering or the potential for suffering is not even recognized or if the goals of care are not carefully considered, then opportunities to prevent or relieve distress and to protect quality of life for patients and families will certainly be missed. Regardless of choices about curative or life-prolonging treatments, advocates of palliative care stress—to clinicians, patients, family members, policymakers, educators, researchers, insurers, and communities—that care plans should always include steps to assess and prevent physical, emotional, and spiritual suffering. As described by the American Academy of Pediatrics in its statement on pediatric palliative care, "The goal is to add life to the child's years, not simply years to the child's life" (AAP, 2000g, p. 353).

Designing a care plan that appropriately integrates curative or life-prolonging care with palliative care and preparations for death is a sensitive and sometimes formidable task. Depending on the child's medical condition, the plan of care may include a mix of preventive measures, curative or life-prolonging interventions, rehabilitative services, and palliative care. The mix usually will change over time as a disease progresses, as the goals of care are reconsidered and adjusted, and as the benefits and burdens of therapies are reevaluated based on guidance and counseling from physicians and others.

To illustrate, for a child with an eventually fatal condition such as muscular dystrophy, appropriate care for most of the child's life may include scheduling standard childhood immunizations, treating respiratory infections, providing physical therapy to slow or adjust to declining physical function, and offering psychological counseling in response to emotional distress. As the disease progresses and symptoms intensify, a palliative care plan—whether or not it goes by that name—will increase the emphasis on physical, emotional, and spiritual comfort. The plan might include participation in a camp for children with similar medical problems, art and other therapies that help the child express his or her emotions and creativity, and special arrangements to allow the child to continue in school. Antibiotics, mechanical ventilation, enteral or parenteral nutrition, and hospitalization may be chosen, refused, or adjusted as the child, parents, and health care team assess and reassess the benefits and burdens of each therapy as the condition worsens. Clinicians will ask parents about the use of resuscitation and other life-sustaining interventions such as artificial hydration or nutrition. Their decisions may be profoundly affected by what and how they are told about the likely outcomes of such measures given their child's medical situation.

Box 4.3 summarizes some of the questions that a child's care team (or teams) should consider from the time a child is diagnosed with a life-threatening medical conditions. Again, unless a child's death comes quickly, these questions may be asked repeatedly.

The responsibility of particular health care professionals for these different assessments will vary, as will the responsibilities for implementing various elements of the care plan. Physicians will take the lead in determining diagnosis and prognosis, identifying treatment goals and options to reach these goals, and assessing and explaining their potential benefits and harms to patients and families. Physicians and nurses generally share responsibility for evaluating symptoms and symptom management effects, but physical therapists, psychologists, child-life specialists, and others may also be involved in assessing a child's physical and emotional functioning and his or her reactions to medical interventions. All members of the care team should be sensitive to the emotional and spiritual well-being of the child and family, but social workers, psychologists, child-life specialists, and chaplains will be particularly attentive to this area of assessment.

Based on the multidimensional and multidisciplinary assessments of the child and the family, the child's care team has the primary responsibility—in cooperation with the child (consistent with developmental stage) and family—for developing a care plan to meet the goals of care, and then monitoring its implementation and results and making adjustments as needed. The care plan may include directions related to nursing care, medications, physical therapy, and other interventions as well as provisions for consultations with palliative care specialists, psychologists, or others who

BOX 4.3
Assessments Needed in Devising and Revising
a Palliative Care Plan

Disease Status and Symptom Assessment

- What are the child's diagnosis and prognosis? How uncertain is the child's future course?
- Is death expected soon? Would death in a few months be a surprise?
- How is the disease likely to affect the child physically, intellectually, and emotionally?
- What symptoms are present and what symptoms are likely to emerge?

Preferences and Goals

- Has the parents' understanding of their child's medical condition and care options been carefully assessed?
- Has the child's understanding of his or her medical condition and care options and his or her competence and interest in being involved in care decisions been carefully assessed?
- Do either the child or the family need more information or assistance in understanding the information already provided about the diagnosis, prognosis, and treatment options (including palliative care and end-of-life resources)?
- Do the child's and the parents' preferences appear to diverge in significant ways?
- Have the benefits and burdens of different therapy options been carefully explained?
- Have end-of-life issues and plans been discussed as appropriate given the child's condition?
- Have documents (e.g., DNR or allow natural death orders) appropriate for the child's medical status been completed and recorded in the medical record? Are copies of relevant documents available wherever they might be needed (e.g., home, school)?

Psychosocial and Spiritual Assessment: Child (Patient)

- What does the child (taking developmental status into account) understand and feel about his or her medical situation?
- How should discussions with the child take temperament and other characteristics into account?
- What are the child's hopes and fears for the present and the future related to family, friends, school, extracurricular activities, and similar matters?
- Does the child have concerns about religious, spiritual, or existential issues? Has a psychological consult or referral to a chaplain or other spiritual counselor been suggested or arranged?
- Has the child been sufficiently assured that he or she will be cared for and will not be abandoned (assuming that reassurance can be truthfully offered)?

Psychosocial and Spiritual Assessment: Family

- How are the parents, siblings, and other close family members managing?
- How have they managed difficult situations in the past?

- What are the family's main hopes and fears for the present and the future?
- What special psychological or practical issues need attention (e.g., presence of other children in the home, other family illnesses, communication or cognitive problems, history of violence or substance abuse)?
- Has assistance from a psychological counselor or from a chaplain or other spiritual counselor been suggested or arranged?
- Have family members been sufficiently assured that they will not be abandoned as the child's condition changes (assuming that reassurance can be truthfully offered)?

Child's Functional Status

- What can the child do for him or herself?
- What kind of assistance is required at home, at school, elsewhere?
- What can family members do? What outside help is needed for the family? For teachers?

Therapy Review and Evaluation

- What surgical, radiological, pharmacological, or other interventions have been employed? What interventions are planned or under consideration? What is their purpose? What are the results to date? What is expected (good and bad)? When should interventions be reevaluated?
- Are monitoring for side effects and assessment of pain and other symptoms adequate?
- What palliative interventions are being used or should be considered? What are the results to date?
- What health care providers are involved in the child's care? Are the level and mix appropriate?
- If problems arise, is reliable assistance available 24 hours a day, 7 days a week?
- What are the benefits and burdens (for child, family, and caregivers) of the therapies being provided, and what are the alternatives?
- Are the care team's perspectives and the family's perspectives consistent? Are these perspectives consistent with those of the child?

Resource and Logistics Review and Evaluation

- What is the composition of the care team and how is it functioning?
- Are additional professional and nonprofessional personnel needed? What is the availability of such personnel in the community?
- How is care being coordinated and information being communicated? Are there problems?
- What are the child's and the family's preferences about primary location of care, including at the time when death is expected? What barriers exist to accommodating these preferences?
- Are physical facilities in the home adequate (e.g., accessible bathroom)? How do transportation, economic, and other relevant resources match child and family needs? What else can be done?
- What is the financial burden on the family? Do additional sources of assistance need to be sought? Can resources be used more effectively or efficiently?

SOURCE: Adapted from IOM, 1997.

have expertise in assessing and managing particularly difficult problems such as intractable pain, delirium, and psychological distress.

In a set of recommendations for end-of-life care in the ICU, Truog and colleagues (2001) observed that for clinicians accustomed to focusing on cure and life-prolongation, it may difficult to focus on the goals of comfort and symptom management. They suggest, particularly when the end of life is approaching and the failure of curative or life-prolonging therapies is clear, it may be useful to "completely rewrite the patient's orders and care plan, just as if the patient were being newly admitted to the ICU" and then to evaluate each test or intervention in terms of how it serves the goals of care (Truog et al., 2001, p. 2335).

Involving Children in Decisions About Palliative and End-of-Life Care

Parents (or guardians or other designated adults) will in most cases retain legal authority to make decisions about a child's medical care (see Chapter 8). That legal fact does not and should not restrict parents and clinicians from involving children in discussions and decisions about their care, consistent with their intellectual and emotional maturity. As noted earlier, excluding children can lead to feelings of isolation, anxiety, and other distress.

Recommendation: Children's hospitals, hospices, and other organizations that care for seriously ill or injured children should work with physicians, parents, child patients, psychologists, and other relevant experts and with professional organizations to create policies and procedures for involving children in discussions and decisions about their medical condition and its treatment. These policies and procedures— and their application—should be sensitive to children's intellectual and emotional maturity and preferences and families' cultural backgrounds and values.

Assessing children's competence to be involved with decisions is an individual process that considers a particular child's intellectual and emotional development and understanding of the issues, his or her medical condition, and the family's values and relationships (including patterns of communication). Assessments also should consider the specific decisions in question and the probabilities and significance of possible consequences of the decisions.

Some experts see age 10 as the usual age for meaningful involvement in decisions about serious medical problems (Hinds et al., 2001). Nitschke and colleagues concluded from their research involving 43 families with children who had cancer that children as young as 5 or 6 years of age could participate in end-of-life discussions (Nitschke et al., 1982). The researchers also concluded that, in practice, the patients themselves (aged 6 to 20 years) often made the final decision between investigational therapy or supportive care for their end-stage cancer. Of the children studied, 14 chose further chemotherapy, 28 chose palliative care only, and 1 made no decision. The majority of children who chose supportive care were able to talk with their families about their fears and actively participate in family life.

For adolescents, regardless of their legal status, parents may recognize and accept that their teenager has the evident intellectual and emotional maturity to make decisions about care at the end of life. Adolescents may, however, need particularly careful assistance in understanding the available options and their possible consequences (Stevens, 1998; Hinds et al., 2001; see also Rushton and Lynch, 1992; McCabe, 1996; McCabe, et al., 1996). Some research suggests that younger adolescents do not differ greatly from adults in their ability to understand and reason about medical alternatives (Weithorn and Campbell, 1982), but other research suggests that younger adolescents are less able than older adolescents to imagine future risks and consequences of choices (Lewis 1981). Some studies suggest that involving children in decisionmaking increases their capacity to make decisions (Lewis and Lewis, 1990; Alderson, 1993).

Implementing the Care Plan

Devising a good palliative care plan does not ensure implementation. Later chapters of this report suggest how organizational problems, financial obstacles, lack of adequately trained health professionals, and gaps in scientific knowledge can compromise care. For example, institutional policies may restrict the hours during which families can visit a seriously ill child and physical structures may limit the amount of privacy, intimacy, and physical comfort available to families.

Geography is another limiting factor. Children and families in remote rural areas will generally have less access to certain palliative care resources just as they tend to have less access to other health care resources such as advanced pediatric trauma care. Regional information and consulting resources can help (see recommendations at the end of Chapter 6) but cannot overcome all geographic problems.

Supporting the Family

Even with good support from the child's care team and involved institutions, much of the responsibility for implementing and monitoring a child's care plan will rest with family members. As Hilden and colleagues have observed, families coping with a child's extended life-threatening illness "often joke that they should receive honorary medical or nursing licenses" (Hilden et al., 2001b, p. 168). Although the comment may be somewhat tongue-in-cheek, it highlights the complex tasks facing child patients and families—understanding and evaluating great amounts of information, advocating for needed information and services, making informed choices, directly providing care, monitoring a child's status, and negotiating billing, insurance, program eligibility, and other bureaucratic processes. As one parent remarked, "It's like you suddenly have a new small business to figure out and run on top of everything else going on."

The family's role in caregiving is increasingly being recognized, and more resources are being provided by hospitals, family support organizations, and other sources to help them perform this role effectively. Most practical resources appear to focus on caregivers for adults, especially elderly adults (see, e.g., ACP, 1997a,b; Karpinski, 2000; Meyer, 1998; Schmall et al., 2000; but see also CHI, 1991; Houts, 1997; Bayer Institute, 2001), although pediatric hospice programs and state and other programs for children with special needs also consider the needs of parents or other caregivers. Studies and experience suggest that many family caregivers receive little if any explicit training for what can be very demanding physical and emotional care responsibilities (Bull and Jervis, 1997; Levine, 1998; Driscoll, 2000; Rigoglioso, 2000).

In addition to providing information as described earlier in this chapter, Internet sites may suggest questions for parents to ask about the course of particular medical conditions, symptom management, and sources of assistance. Such prompting can help parents participate more effectively and fully in developing, understanding, and implementing their child's care plan. Internet sites may also provide forums for people to seek and offer information about caregiving strategies.

Comprehensive guidance for family caregivers should cover physical and emotional problems and responses for child patients, parents, and siblings (e.g., isolation, depression, anxiety); spiritual resources; practical concerns (e.g., having advance care directives at hand when they are needed, managing health insurance, obtaining help from community agencies or volunteer groups); and bereavement. The next chapter examines the spiritual, emotional, and practical dimensions of care for the child and family.

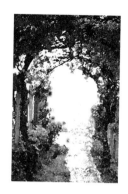

CHAPTER 5

CARE AND CARING FROM DIAGNOSIS THROUGH DEATH AND BEREAVEMENT

"I remember at the funeral the priest saying—he was trying to be comforting but [was] so far from knowing what it was really like those past months—that 'now she wasn't suffering anymore.' . . . It pissed me off . . . we had tried so hard not to make her suffer."

Susan Rheingold, physician (Himelstein and Hilden, 2001)

The prevention and relief of suffering—physical, emotional, spiritual—is a core mission of palliative care. Although not all suffering can be prevented or relieved, severe pain and other symptoms are not inevitable consequences of serious illnesses or their treatment. Continued research into the mechanisms of symptoms and palliative interventions is essential, but health care professionals and organizations can do more now to apply existing knowledge and resources to spare patients and families from physical and emotional suffering.

A broader goal of palliative care is to help children with life-threatening medical conditions and their families live as normally and as well as possible under the circumstances. Even quite sick children can often take pleasure in playing, seeing friends, continuing classes and other normal activities, and being at home in familiar surroundings. For hospitalized children, administrators and clinicians can look for ways to design physical environments, clinical routines, and special programs to minimize the obtrusiveness of intensive care units and other medical settings, encourage and welcome the presence of family and friends, and provide opportunities for play, education, and other ordinary childhood activities.

As emphasized throughout this report, palliative care is not an "either/or" proposition. Although care may sometimes focus solely on patient and family comfort, the integration of palliative care with curative or life-prolonging therapies can benefit children who survive life-threatening conditions as well as children who die and can thereby support the families of children in both groups.

This chapter examines the physical, emotional, spiritual, and practical dimensions of care for children with life-threatening conditions and their families. Although bereavement care is part of comprehensive emotional and spiritual care for family members before and after a child's death, it is—for emphasis—discussed in a separate section. Recommendations related to the discussion in this chapter are sufficiently intertwined with the discussions and recommendations about the organization and delivery of care in Chapter 6 that they are included in that rather than this chapter.

THE PHYSICAL DIMENSIONS OF CARE

General

Physical comfort should be a fundamental priority in health care for all children, but it is especially important for children who have life-threatening medical conditions and are enduring burdensome therapies. Unrelieved physical distress affects both the child and the family. It can also interfere with beneficial therapies, for example, when children in extreme pain will not cooperate with treatment.

Effective physical care for children requires a solid understanding of both the sources of distress—which can require extensive investigation—and the developmentally appropriate strategies for preventing or relieving that distress. For example, drug regimens shown to be effective in relieving a symptom in adults cannot simply be extrapolated to infants and children because developmental variations in metabolism and body composition (e.g., amount and distribution of fat, water, proteins) may affect the action of drugs. Unfortunately, many drugs have not been tested and labeled for use with children, and understanding of the underlying mechanisms of symptoms and symptom management techniques in children is underdeveloped. Federal regulations and legislation adopted in recent years provide incentives and requirements for pediatric research, including studies by pharmaceutical companies to test drugs in children and develop pediatric drug dosing information (USGAO, 2001b). Chapter 10 discusses these incentives and, more generally, the challenges—practical, methodological, organizational, legal, and ethical—of expanding the knowledge base for pediatric palliative care. It also discusses directions for future research to improve all dimensions of palliative and end-of-life care.

Particularly for younger children, family observations and reports will often be essential in determining the presence, severity, and characteristics of a child's physical distress and in evaluating the success of efforts to relieve it. In addition to providing information and observations necessary for care planning and evaluation, parents and other family members will often provide much physical and other care for their child, particularly when the child is at home. Even in hospitals, however, families may feel comforted by providing some physical care themselves. Moreover, staffing shortages or reductions may prompt them to provide care that might otherwise be provided by nurses or nurses' aides.

Depending on the expected caregiving role of family members, physicians and other members of the child's care team should assess the need of family members for training in both technical tasks (e.g., operating medical equipment or changing dressings) and mundane but possibly risky tasks (e.g., bathing or moving someone with serious medical problems). The team may also have to prepare school nurses and other personnel to help with physical care when a seriously ill child returns to school.

The focus in this section is on physical care for the child, but a comment on care for family members is also warranted. Pediatricians do not serve as personal physicians for parents, although family practitioners often do, and both may care for the siblings of ill children. In any case, if the unit of care is truly the child and the family, then generalist and specialist pediatricians, family practitioners, nurses, hospice personnel, and others should be attentive to the physical and emotional toll that a child's serious illness or death may take on family members. This attention may take various forms, including questions about possible signs of illness or stress, reminders that parents need to take care of themselves and their other children, and suggestions that a formal evaluation be sought for a family member exhibiting signs of possible medical problems. With a parent's permission, someone from the child's team might contact the parent's or sibling's personal physician to include her or him in the family support network and ensure that the parent or sibling gets additional evaluation and support during a very difficult time.

Care for Pain and Other Physical Symptoms

One goal of excellent symptom management is to prevent both disease-related symptoms and treatment-related distress to the extent possible. When symptoms do develop, the goal then is to identify and relieve them as quickly and fully as possible, while minimizing unwanted side effects, for example, the sedation associated with certain pain medications.

Achieving these goals typically involves a mix of pharmacological, behavioral, and other therapies as well as good communication with all members of the child's care team, including the parents and the child (consistent with developmental stage). Careful attention to nutrition, hygiene, posture, mobility, skin care, self-image, and other physical factors also contributes to a patient's comfort and quality of life.

Box 5.1 lists some of the most common physical symptoms experienced by seriously ill or injured children. Compared to adults, the prevalence, distribution, and pathophysiology of pain and other symptoms are poorly mapped for children living with and dying of life-threatening medical problems (Goldman, 1999). This may in part reflect the greater difficulties in communicating with and ascertaining symptoms in infants, other preverbal children, and older children with communication deficits. In addition, it almost certainly reflects a more intense focus on curative care that does not yet include adequate attention to patient comfort.

Symptoms such as pain or nausea may be related to the child's underlying medical problems, treatment for these problems, or both. Some studies of cancer pain in children suggest that diagnostic and treatment procedures may often be more immediately distressing than the disease, especially if the child is too young to understand the implications of the disease and the explanations for painful procedures (Cornaglia et al., 1984; Miser et al., 1987; McGrath et al., 1990; Ljungman et al., 2000). Also, some research suggests that children who receive inadequate pain management during an initial procedure may experience more pain during subsequent procedures than children who have been appropriately managed (Weisman et al., 1998). Given the pain and other burdens imposed by some potentially curative or life-prolonging treatments (e.g., surgical procedures, chemotherapy or radiotherapy regimens), many parents and child patients with advanced disease face emotionally difficult decisions about when the likely burdens of such treatments exceed their likely benefits.

Whatever the choices of families, those caring for children need both to better understand the pain and other distress caused by common procedures (e.g., intramuscular, intravenous, and subcutaneous administration of drugs, including pain medications) and to consider less burdensome alternatives. These alternatives may include reevaluation of the necessity for certain painful diagnostic and other procedures, the use of innovative pharmacological strategies (e.g., disks that numb the skin before injections or other procedures, pleasant-tasting oral formulations of drugs), and the application of nonpharmacologic approaches such as relaxation, imagery, distraction, hypnotic suggestion, massage, and acupuncture. In addition, child- and family-friendly physical surroundings and procedures and the presence of child-life specialists and other personnel trained to work with children may help reduce emotional distress, which, in turn, may reduce physical distress.

Although certain diagnoses tend to be associated with certain symptoms (e.g., bone pain with certain metastatic cancers, seizures with certain degenerative brain disorders, shortness of breath with certain end-stage heart conditions), children with the same initial diagnosis can differ considerably in their experience of disease-related symptoms. Likewise, although certain treatments tend to produce certain symptoms (e.g., vomiting with some forms of chemotherapy, mouth sores with some radiotherapies), children with the same diagnosis and same treatment may vary in their responses, including their experience of treatment-related symptoms. For children with advanced medical problems, the type and intensity of palliative physical care needed may be determined less by the medical diagnosis than by symptoms and other manifestations of the underlying medical condition or its treatment.

Given such individual variability, each child requires an individual assessment of symptoms and the development of a responsive care plan (McGrath, 1998; Goldman, 1999; see also Schechter et al., 1993, 1997). In addition to considering the child's diagnosis and reports of symptoms by the child or parents, clinicians should consider other characteristics of the child (e.g., cognitive capacity, personality, past medical experiences) and the family (e.g., coping behaviors, cultural values and practices). Characteristics of the health care environment may also be relevant to the development and implementation of symptom management strategies (e.g., restrictions on parents' presence during painful procedures involving children, availability of clinicians skilled in treating small patients and managing difficult symptoms, insurance coverage of certain medications or other interventions).

Studies reviewed in Chapter 3 suggest shortfalls in symptom assessment and management and point to numerous opportunities for improvement in the care of children with life-threatening medical conditions. Particularly in the area of cancer pain, one response has been initiatives to develop and implement evidence-based assessment and management protocols that stress the timely and adequate use of appropriate medications and behavioral interventions (e.g., distraction therapies) to prevent and relieve pain in children (see, e.g., WHO, 1998). Chapter 6 discusses the role of such protocols and recommends their broader development and application.

Parents as Experts on Their Child's Comfort

Once while explaining Bellini's desire for a certain positioning to a new nurse, I was told by someone watching, "Oh, you're so fussy!" Am I? Am I going overboard to want my son, who has so few options for comfort, to be comfortable, especially when I happen to know what makes him comfortable?

Susan Hostetler-Lelaulu, parent, 1999

BOX 5.1
Major Physical Symptoms That May Be Experienced by Children with Life-Threatening Medical Conditions

Pain

Key dimensions of pain include intensity, duration, and burden felt by the child. Pain is categorized as somatic, visceral, or neuropathic depending on its apparent origin. Uncontrolled pain significantly interferes with a child's functioning and well being. It can contribute to depression, irritability, and anxiety and can disrupt social relationships.

Nausea and Vomiting

Nausea (feeling that one may vomit) and vomiting are common symptoms for children with certain kinds of advanced cancer and also may be side effects of treatments such as chemotherapy. The neurophysiology of nausea and vomiting in children is not well understood. They may be prompted by a variety of stimuli (e.g., movement, odors, anxiety, medications, past experiences). Underlying causes may include gastric irritation, constipation, elevated intracranial pressure, and disturbances of metabolism.

Bowel Problems: Constipation, Diarrhea

Constipation may be caused by medications (including opioids), emotional stress, reduced intake of food and liquid, abdominal tumors or adhesions, or decreased activity. It can be extremely uncomfortable and, if unrelieved, life-threatening. Children may be somewhat less susceptible than adults, especially older adults who tend to have weak muscle tone and other problems. Diarrhea is less common than constipation in cancer patients. It is often a feature of advanced neuromuscular disorders and extreme mental retardation. Bowel incontinence is, of course, expected in infants.

Seizures or Convulsions

Seizures result from sudden, uncontrolled bursts of electrical activity in the brain. They may involve one or more of the following: a total or partial loss of consciousness; abnormal physical movement; sensory disturbances; and pain or other unpleasant sensations. Seizures can be frightening and disturbing to family members who witness them. Some fatal medical problems (e.g., certain inborn errors of metabolism) are characterized by seizures throughout their course, whereas seizures develop only in the late stages of certain other disorders (e.g., some brain tumors) or they may result from an acute problem (e.g., meningitis). Some children with fatal medical problems may independently have epilepsy or other conditions that cause seizures.

Anorexia–Cachexia Syndrome

This syndrome involves decreased appetite (anorexia) and wasting of soft tissue and muscle mass (cachexia). Severe wasting appears to be less common in children with cancer and AIDS than in adults with these diseases. Loss of appetite occurs in the late stages of many diseases. Some causes are reversible, at least for a time, but anorexia and cachexia may be an intrinsic part of the dying process for certain conditions.

Mouth Problems

Children with advanced illness may be troubled by various mouth problems, including dry mouth, sores, dental problems, and infections related to their medical condition or its treatment. Oral problems can make eating, drinking, and taking of medication unpleasant if not impossible, thereby increasing the risk of dehydration and malnutrition. Meticulous oral hygiene can help prevent such suffering in a child nearing death.

Fatigue

Fatigue may lead to sleepiness, weakness, depression, anxiety, difficulty concentrating, and other problems. It may be caused by both diseases (especially cancers) and their treatment. Extreme tiredness may interfere with a child's ability to move, bathe, or go to the toilet. The mechanisms of pathological fatigue and its treatment are poorly understood.

Dyspnea and Cough

Dyspnea (feeling short of breath) may result from a number of pulmonary, cardiac, neuromuscular, and psychological conditions. Cough can be caused by irritation; excessive mucus and other fluids; and inhalation, certain drugs, and other mechanisms.

Dysphagia

Dysphagia is difficulty in swallowing food or liquids. Developmental immaturity, brain malformations, trauma, infection, cancer, and neuromuscular diseases are common causes of this problem among children. Inability to swallow affects hydration, nutrition, and taking of medication.

Skin Problems

Skin problems that cause distress may arise from the underlying disease or its treatment or both. Problems may include itching, dryness, chapping, acne, sweating, hair loss, and extreme sensitivity to touch. Some problems, such as pressure ulcers, are less common in children than adults. In addition to causing physical discomfort, skin problems may be perceived by patients as indignities to be hidden from others.

SOURCE: Adapted from IOM, 1997, with additional information from Doyle et al., 1998; Behrman et al., 2000; and Goldman, 1999.

Parents of children with severe chronic medical conditions usually come to know their child's physical condition intimately and may become quite expert at recognizing subtle changes and other cues that suggest discomfort. Likewise, their past experience with procedures or actions that have distressed or comforted their child may help them predict how their child will respond to future procedures, which may then be considered in developing a care plan.

Although they may need the physician to interpret medically what they see, parents often act as the "eyes and ears" of the physician, especially when the child is at home. In the vignette about "Johnny Gabrielle" in Chapter 3, physicians, nurses, and others recognized and depended on the mother's expertise, even as they tried with little success to find effective ways to relieve the child's distress and reduce the mother's burden. The committee located no research investigating this topic, but it seems prudent for clinicians caring for a distressed child to inquire about what parents have found increases or reduces the child's distress—just as they inquire about other aspects of a child's medical history.

Physical Care When Death Is Imminent

Reevaluation of Symptoms and Symptom Management

Whether a child is at home or in intensive care, as death nears, certain care that has extended life or maintained comfort may become more burdensome than beneficial. For example, although dehydration is normally treated with intravenous fluids, the use of such artificial hydration for a patient nearing death may not increase patient comfort but may instead cause excessive secretions that, in turn, promote vomiting, coughing, choking, and other problems. If a patient feels thirsty or complains of a dry mouth, ice chips or small amounts of liquid combined with good mouth hygiene may be soothing (see, e.g., Twycross and Lichter, 1998). Although many hospice and palliative care experts are convinced by their experience of the merits of this approach, recommendations and decisions to avoid artificial hydration at the end of life are controversial. Little rigorous research is available to resolve disputes (Twycross and Lichter, 1998; Kedziera, 2001; but see also Finucane et al., 1999).

Depending on a child's medical condition and its progression, control of pain and other symptoms may become an increasing challenge for the care team as, for example, tumors invade vital areas, lung or kidney function deteriorates, seizures multiply, or bleeding becomes more difficult to control. Although all clinicians who care for patients should have good skills in symptom assessment and management, the expertise of a palliative care specialist may be required for difficult or refractory symptoms of advanced disease or severe injury. Families that have been able to manage their child's care at home may now need assistance from hospice or specially trained home care personnel.

Some choices in physical care and symptom management when death is imminent may cause considerable stress for clinicians and families. (Ethical and other issues in making end-of-life decisions are discussed in Chapter 8.) Pain and other symptoms can usually, but not always, be managed without sedation. When symptoms at the end of life remain uncontrolled after other alternatives are tried, one legal and generally—but not universally—accepted option is "terminal sedation," which might more appropriately be labeled "palliative sedation" (Kingsbury, 2001). The practice involves the careful increase in analgesic or sedative doses to achieve deep unconsciousness that relieves a dying patient's otherwise intractable pain, shortness of breath, seizures, hallucinations, or other severe symptoms (see, e.g., Cherny and Portenoy, 1994; Kenny and Frager, 1996; Quill et al., 1997).

Research has not shown a clear association between deep sedation and the timing of death (see, e.g., Stone et al., 1997; Galloway and Yaster, 2000; Thorns and Sykes, 2000). Nevertheless, one uncommon and unintended result of such sedation may be to hasten an impending death. Although death is not the objective, clinicians (including those who engage in palliative sedation or choose it for their family members) and others may incorrectly characterize deep sedation as assisted suicide or euthanasia (which has death as the intended means of relieving suffering) (see, e.g., Asch, 1995). Clearer and more careful education of staff and consultation with families should reduce such misunderstandings and minimize unwarranted anxieties or guilt feelings. Again, a physician should pursue deep sedation only after careful determination that other options are failing the patient and after consultation with and agreement from the parents and the child, depending on his or her condition and maturity (Kenny and Frager, 1996; Burns et al., 2000; Levetown, 2001). Clinical protocols for sedation should be established and meticulously followed.

Life Support Technologies

Just as symptom management strategies may be reevaluated and adjusted as death approaches, so the conventional use of advanced life support technologies (e.g., cardiopulmonary resuscitation, mechanical ventilation, renal dialysis) may be reconsidered and withheld or withdrawn when the physician(s), parents, and possibly the child agree that their use will only prolong dying and increase suffering. These situations are not, as sometimes described, times when "nothing more can be done." Rather, good clinical care and interpersonal skills can help prevent or minimize suffering on the part of the patient, the family, and the health care team itself.

Recent guidelines for end-of-life care in the intensive care unit urge intensivists to become "as skilled and knowledgeable at forgoing life-sustaining treatments as they are at delivering care aimed at survival and cure" (Truog et al., 2001, p. 2332; see also Rubenfeld and Curtis, 2000). Although the guidelines are not specific to children and certain details of care may differ, the general principles and perspective should provide useful guidance for pediatric intensivists. Whatever the decisions and strategies, careful communication with parents and respect for family preferences are essential to good outcomes for all involved (Kirschbaum, 1996) (see Chapter 8).

In some cases, parents may request the removal of mechanical ventilation (extubation) when death is near to allow one last opportunity for unobstructed physical contact (see Levetown, 2001; Sine et al., 2001). Procedures for discontinuing mechanical ventilation at the end of life with minimal patient and family suffering are the subject of some disagreement. Issues involve the intensity of sedation, the use of paralyzing agents, and the removal of the breathing tube (extubation) without prior steps to "wean" the patient by reducing oxygen level and pressure (see, e.g., Faber-Langendoen, 1996; Gilligan and Raffin, 1996; Truog et al., 2000; Levetown, 2001).[1]

Because some children undergo mechanical ventilation at home and children and families may prefer that removal of the equipment occur at home, protocols for discontinuing mechanical ventilation must consider home as well as hospital procedures and supports for both the child and the family. As with any other intervention, parents and other family members who will or may be present should be carefully informed about exactly what will happen as part of removing the equipment, what may happen afterward, and what can be done (e.g., administration of medications, presence of family) to keep the child comfortable.

Continued study of decisions about withholding life-sustaining interventions, the rationales for such decisions, and the associated processes of care, including comfort measures for the patient and family, would help inform the debate over compassionate and ethical end-of-life care. Better descriptive information should also help in identifying administrative, edu-

---

[1]Truog and colleagues (2001) have emphasized that use of paralyzing agents alone blocks the ability to communicate distress (e.g., feelings of pain or suffocation) without relieving it and that, even in combination with sedatives and analgesics, the agents make it impossible to determine whether these medications are working effectively. They argue that no patient should have a breathing tube removed while under the influence of a paralyzing agent unless death is expected quickly and waiting for the agent to wear off would be more burdensome than beneficial.

cational, and research strategies to improve decisions, processes of care, and outcomes. As recommended in Chapter 6, a broad-based process to develop scientifically and ethically informed pediatric guidelines for making and implementing decisions about limitations of care (including appropriate clinical procedures and comfort measures, whether life support is continued or limited) might help reduce inappropriate variability in decisionmaking, limit preventable suffering, and increase fairness.

Another issue that has sparked controversy is the presence of family members during resuscitation efforts. A comprehensive, evidence-based statement on various aspects of cardiopulmonary resuscitation recently recommended that health care providers should offer family members the opportunity to be present during resuscitation whenever possible, especially if the patient is an infant or child (AHA et al., 2000a). From their review of research, the authors of the statement concluded that family members generally do want to be present during resuscitation and that those who have been present tend to have less depression, anxiety, and other problems during bereavement than those who have not (see also Bauchner et al., 1991; Eichhorn et al., 1996 Sacchetti et al., 1996; Timmermans, 1997; Robinson et al., 1998; Boyd, 2000; Tsai, 2002).

Many clinicians have, however, feared that uncontrolled reactions by family members could interfere with patient care (as well as require responses by staff in their own right). Even their simple presence could be distracting, and support could require the diversion of scarce resources. The new recommendations specify that a staff person should be designated to be with the parents during a resuscitation attempt to explain what to expect, answer questions, and otherwise provide support.

Physical Care After the Child's Death

Physical care does not stop with death. Care of the child's body after death can be very important to families, who may be comforted by touching, cuddling, rocking, bathing, or dressing their child. Cultural and religious values may also direct such involvement—or discourage, if not forbid, it.

The consensus today among pediatric and palliative care experts is that family members should be offered the opportunity to be with their child after death and that families who lack such an opportunity (or reject it) may later regret the loss of this last time together (Sexton and Stephen, 1991; Goldman, 1999; Iverson, 1999; CPS, 2001; Levetown, 2001). Such accommodation of families is generally easier when the child dies at home rather than in an intensive care unit or other inpatient setting. If it is a priority, however, most hospitals can provide the requisite space, time, and other support. As described in Chapter 6, some hospitals have arranged a well-equipped, comfortable room that is expressly intended as a private area for families to be with their child during and after death.

Physical care after a child's death will be affected by the circumstances of death. For the child who dies quickly from severe injuries, legal requirements and other circumstances may limit care of the body immediately after death, for example, removing resuscitation tubes used in the emergency department. Parents can, however, usually be provided some private time with their child. If, however, a child has been taken to the medical examiner's office before the family arrives, family members may have to identify the child from a photograph and may be forbidden to see the child's body directly (O'Brien et al., 2001). In either situation, emergency department personnel or staff in the medical examiner's office may support families by cleaning away blood, arranging the body, and covering (insofar as possible) disfiguring injuries or wounds with clean sheets. Guidance for these personnel is based primarily on professional judgment and experience with bereaved families (Iverson, 1999; Levetown, 2001).

Stillborn infants may be presented to their parents with much the same cleansing and similar physical care that are provided to infants born alive. More preparation may be considered in other situations, for example, when the fetus has suffered substantial tissue damage (maceration or bruising) due to after-death exposure to amniotic fluid or to induced or spontaneous labor. Nonetheless, physical signs and severe deformities that might normally be shocking may be irrelevant for grieving parents (some forewarned through prenatal diagnosis) who will have only a brief opportunity for physical contact before they go home without a baby.

Parents expecting the birth of child with a fatal congenital problem can be very explicit about their preferences for physical care at birth, many of which can be honored even if the child is stillborn. For example, one parent reported on an Internet support group that she had requested, in advance of the birth of a child with known anencephaly, that the child "be quickly wiped, given a cap for her anomaly, wrapped in a blanket and have the nurse describe what she looks like to the parents before she is handed to her father first" (Kristina's Mom, no date, http://www.asfhelp.com/ASF_files/support_group_files/abiding_heart_files/wish.htm). One objective of perinatal hospice programs is to help families determine their wishes and have them honored during pregnancy, birth, and afterwards, whether or not the child is born alive (Sumner, 2001).

For the ill child who dies an expected death at home or in the hospital, little medically oriented physical care may be necessary afterwards.[2] At

---

[2]Sometimes medical equipment may need to be disconnected. In most cases, no legal requirements limit the removal of such equipment in these situations. As discussed in Chapter 4, families may want to have clear written plans and physician orders to minimize the potential for misunderstandings with emergency medical and law enforcement personnel.

their own pace, parents may wish to bathe or dress the child as one of their last physical acts of being the child's mother or father.

Families may wish to accompany their child's body to the morgue, and in some states, they can themselves take the body to the funeral home. Even after the child has been taken to the hospital morgue, it is not unknown for parents to ask to see the child once more or to make the request for family members who could not get to the hospital earlier. If it is expected that parents will see their child after an autopsy (e.g., to dress the child before the funeral), the child's physician, funeral home staff, or other aware personnel should prepare the family for what they will see (Cacciatore-Garard, 2001). Depending on family preferences or religious values, funeral homes may provide physical services after a child's death, for example, preparing the body for viewing before or at a funeral.

THE EMOTIONAL AND PSYCHOLOGICAL DIMENSIONS OF CARE

It's okay to be sad. It's okay to be mad. It's okay to cry. It's okay to laugh.

Ross, young cancer patient (Lewis, 1992).

Just as children with life-threatening problems need specialized medical and nursing assessments of their physical status and symptoms, they should also have a psychological evaluation in order to plan for truly comprehensive care. The broad elements of comprehensive psychological and emotional care include the following:

• evaluation of the child's psychological status and identification of psychological symptoms or disorders;
• provision of appropriate psychotherapy, psychotropic medications, or behavioral interventions as an integral part of the child's overall care;
• advice for the child's physician, parents, and others on additional strategies or steps that they can take to manage or minimize emotional distress;
• evaluation of the child's parents and siblings (and sometimes other family members) for psychological symptoms;
• referral as appropriate to support groups for ill children, healthy siblings and parents that allow them to share experiences in living with serious illness; and
• bereavement support for the family after the child's death.

As discussed in Chapter 6, child psychologists, psychiatrists, and other mental health professionals can provide unique knowledge and skills that broaden and deepen the emotional care of ill children and their siblings. They may gain special insight into the child's concerns, including concerns he or she may be reluctant to share with parents or physicians. Although these specialists bring particular expertise to a child's care, sensitivity to emotional distress is part of every caregiver's responsibility, including the child's generalist and specialist physicians, nurses, and others.

Parents and other family members are usually the mainstays of emotional care for children. To support them in this role, they may benefit from counseling about strategies for protecting their child (and themselves) from avoidable emotional suffering. Respite care, although not usually covered by health plans, may relieve and renew family caregivers. Wish granting programs such as those supported by the Starlight Children's Foundation (http://www.starlight.org) and the Make-a-Wish Foundation (http://www.wish.org) may give children and families a significant positive event to plan for and anticipate (Stevens, 1998).

When a child dies suddenly, bereavement care may be all that can be offered to parents, siblings, other relatives, and friends. Although bereavement care could logically be discussed here, it is, for emphasis, considered in a later section.

Special Elements of Emotional Care for Seriously Ill Children

I felt much better because I knew that I had somebody to talk to all the time! Every boy needs a psychologist! To see his feelings!
Six-year-old child (Sourkes, 1995a, p. 3)

Sadness and a certain amount of anxiety are normal responses to serious illness and may intensify as curative treatments fail and as death approaches. Although most psychological problems may be characterized as "adjustment" reactions, more severe psychopathology can emerge, particularly for children with preexisting vulnerabilities (e.g., a parent's earlier death or other loss) or with a personal or family history of psychiatric problems.

It is important to recognize normal distress and not overemphasize pathology in children, but minimizing or not recognizing real pathology is also risky. Clinical depression, anxiety, and traumatic stress reactions may seriously compromise the remaining quality of life for a child with advanced illness. They may cause intense emotional suffering, cause or increase physical discomfort, disrupt relationships with family and friends, and interfere with daily rhythms such as appetite and sleep.

Psychological symptoms in seriously ill children often have multiple possible sources. For example, the child's medical condition or its treatment or both may produce disturbing symptoms of delirium. Physical pain, neurological dysfunction, and psychological distress are closely linked if not, at times, inseparable. Because of this ambiguity, clinicians often proceed with psychological or psychotropic interventions as specific symptoms appear, even if they have not determined a precise psychological diagnosis. Preexisting or new stresses within the family may also contribute significantly to the child's distress and anxiety.

Therapeutic Strategies

Psychotherapy for the child or adolescent who is seriously ill or dying can provide the opportunity for the expression of profound grief and for the integration of all that he or she has lived, albeit in an abbreviated life span. Common issues include anger and grief at being ill, anxiety about medical procedures, worries about family members, depression caused by separation from friends and normal childhood activities, and fears of death (Bluebond-Langner, 1978; Sourkes, 1995a; Stevens, 1998). In addition to helping with these issues, counseling may also help children clarify their own views about how they want to live and how they want to prepare for death. This can affect treatment decisions.

Stevens (1998) has suggested several guidelines for health care professionals working with seriously ill children. They include understanding the child's perception of his or her situation, appreciating the child's symbolic language, differentiating reality from fantasy, encouraging the expression of feelings, encouraging self-esteem, and being open to children's ability to respond to their situation with creativity and dignity.

Some children find an outlet for their emotions and creativity in writing poetry, stories, journals, or notes to others (including notes to be read after death), and the child's care team can encourage this. Such writings may reach well beyond a child's family, friends, and care team. For example, 11-year-old Mattie Stepanek, who has a rare form of muscular dystrophy, has touched many with his poetry, which he began writing at a very young age and which includes the collection *Heartsongs* (Stepanek, 2001). Kelly Weil, who died of cancer in 1993 at the age of 11, wrote a story, Zink the Zebra, that has inspired school-based and other programs to teach children about tolerance of those who are different by virtue of physical, cultural, or other characteristics (see Chapter 6).

Psychotherapy with children involves an acute sensitivity not only to language but also to artistic expression, both literal and symbolic. Drawings often attest quite powerfully to emotional distress including sadness, anxiety, helplessness, loneliness, isolation, anger, and fear or terror (see, e.g., Sourkes, 1995a; Clatworthy et al., 1999).

With young children, play is a crucial vehicle of communication and is, thus, a basic clinical tool to facilitate emotional expression and alleviate a child's distress (see, e.g., Sourkes, 1995a; Kernberg et al., 1998; Scott, 1998). Shared imaginative play enables the child to confront the realities of life and death. The use of puppets, dolls, and stuffed animals allows the child to express difficult and painful emotions "through" the voices of these characters. Play techniques can also provide a less threatening way than direct discussion to inform children about their condition and treatments. Other expressive therapies, such as music and dance, are less often part of the psychotherapist's repertoire but also have a place in supportive care for seriously ill children (Cohen and Walco, 1999).

For children who are well enough to participate, camps that accommodate children with special needs can provide emotional support in a variety of ways (see Chapter 6). One common goal is to improve the self-esteem of campers whose medical problem has brought disfigurement, disability, or isolation (Warady, et. al., 1992; Briery and Rabian, 1999). Other goals include improving children's understanding of their illness and improving their competence in caring for themselves (Heim, et al., 1986). Inspired in part by the camp model, other group and individual recreational activities are being adapted to the needs of children with life-threatening medical problems.

While providing enjoyment and enrichment for the child, camps and other activities may also benefit the family by granting it a period of respite. Furthermore, many camps and recreational organizations involve healthy siblings, thus including them in the wider circle of care.

The Psychological Significance of School

For school-age children,, school is "the defining structure" of day-to-day life, providing constancy and routine (Sourkes, 1995a, p. 93). For the child whose routine has been wrested away by illness, school is a "normalizing axis of daily life," separated from the medical world of illness. Preparing teachers, students, and others at a child's school to reintegrate the child is an essential aspect of emotional care.

Many medical centers and hospices now offer education and consultation for schools on the medical and psychological aspects of a child's illness. They can answer questions and allay apprehensions of teachers, school nurses, counselors, and administrators, which are essential if this group is to provide a safety net for the child on a daily basis. Classmates also need to be prepared for a child's return to school. Straightforward explanations of what to expect may help relieve classmates' anxieties and minimize hurtful interactions. More broadly based programs, such as the Zink the Zebra program mentioned above, may benefit a wider group of children vulnerable to discrimination and isolation because they are "different."

Special Issues for Adolescents

The adolescent's psychological situation is qualitatively different from the young child's. "Normal" adolescence is characterized by a sense of open horizons and immortality and by the quest for identity. In contrast, an adolescent who is diagnosed with a life-threatening illness faces the disruption, if not the irreversible halting, of his or her negotiation of an independent existence.

Adolescents vary within and across the early, middle, and late stages of this last developmental stage of childhood. Moreover, family cultural values and practices will often shape adolescent experiences differently. Notwithstanding such variations and differences, certain issues dominate adolescent development: the wish for increasing independence and autonomy, a focus on body image and sexuality, the importance of peers, and the formation of a personal identity oriented to the future, not just the present (Kellerman and Katz, 1977; Zeltzer 1980). Recognition of the difference between young children and adolescents is reflected in the creation of adolescent medicine as a subspecialty of pediatrics.

Emotional care for adolescents who are facing life-threatening medical problems presents particular complexities (Thornes, 2001). During a period when developing "a life of one's own" is paramount, these young people may confront limitations in every sphere of development: physical, intellectual, and emotional. Further, they face life-and-death issues and decisions that most people do not face until much later in life. As experienced by one seriously ill girl, "You have to accept things that . . . [teens] don't normally have to face. I had to automatically be an adult and it was very hard" (Sourkes, 1982, p. 28).

For adolescents living with a medically dictated physical dependence on family and professional caregivers, psychological independence can be a major issue. Reactions of adolescents who are not granted some channel for autonomy (i.e., for making choices) may include depression, anxiety, anger, risk-taking behaviors, and nonadherance to medical regimens.

Although the specifics vary with the diagnosis and stage of illness, an adolescent's life-threatening illness often limits participation with peers, both in school and socially. Physical limitations, lengthy hospitalizations, fears of venturing out in the wider world, and fears of being "left behind" by healthy peers may compound the loneliness and isolation of serious illness. In addition, many adolescents, especially if some consequences of their illness are visible, grapple with the sense of being damaged and deviant in the outside world. "Everything about me is different. My hair is short and thin. I used to have long hair. I'm not tanned and I've lost a lot of weight. My side looks funny where they took out the rib. And you know how teenagers are—being different is the worst" (16-year-old adolescent,

Sourkes, 1995b). A poor body image, low self-esteem, and embarrassment about physical appearance may lead adolescents (and younger children also) to withdraw socially.

Seriously ill adolescents may be perceived by parents and professionals as asexual, and they are often deprived of the opportunity and privacy for sexual exploration. The emergence of sexuality is an integral part of adolescents' development, and those who are ill often mourn the fact that they may not live to have the experience of sexual intimacy. Alternatively, they may act out sexually in a quest for acceptance and affirmation. From both a psychological and a public health perspective, sexuality is a critical issue as infants and children infected with HIV now grow into adolescence (Stuber, 1992). For these and other adolescents, caregivers may find it difficult to face sexual issues and provide education and psychological counseling to respond to adolescent needs and anxieties (Joint Working Party, 2001).

Recognizing adolescents' concerns and emotional distress can also be difficult for family members and clinicians because adolescents may prefer to confide in a close friend rather than parents or professionals and because they may cope by denying how ill they are. They may try to hide their worries and fears to protect their parents. Although recognizing that guiding research is limited, Stevens (1998) has suggested some strategies for working with adolescents, including offering and negotiating choices about their medical care and personal matters (e.g., what to wear), recognizing small achievements, encouraging peer support including opportunities for discussion in settings such as camps, and using art and writing therapeutically.

Emotional Care for Families

> *[Michael's doctor] worked the entire way knowing that if Michael didn't make it, we were still going to have to get through it. So she treated us, as well as treated Michael.*
> Rose Conlon, parent, 2001

The profound and enduring impact on the family of a child's fatal or potentially fatal condition cannot be overestimated, even when the child survives. From the time of diagnosis, the relationship between the child and the rest of the family pivots around threatened or expected loss. Unless death is sudden, families will experience grief in anticipation of the child's death as well as the grief that follows death, if death is the outcome.

Support for the family may be garnered from many sources: the professional caregiving team, the extended family and friends, and the larger community. The team caring for the child and family must assess the family's needs and the availability of helpful resources. The team must also identify those families who may need more intense psychological or psychiatric intervention. As discussed in Chapter 4, the way physicians, nurses, social workers, and others communicate with families is crucial, beginning with the time of diagnosis and continuing throughout the child's illness and into bereavement.

The discussion below emphasizes emotional support while a seriously ill child is alive. It focuses on parents and siblings, but grandparents and other family members, especially those who have lived with and cared directly for the child, may also need support from the care team. Davies (2001) observes that research on the experience of the family as unit (including the patient) during palliative care is limited. In describing a study of families living with a dying family member, she identifies a complex, nonlinear pattern of responses that include redefining images and relationships, managing change, struggling with the paradox of living with dying, seeking meaning, living day to day, and preparing for death. She suggests emotional support strategies for nurses that focus on maintaining and redefining hope as illness progresses, involving the family in care planning and caregiving, and open communication.

As has been emphasized earlier, although general strategies can guide care for families, each child and family must be evaluated individually. In some cases, the child's care team may recognize emotional problems that warrant referral to other professionals.

Parents

For parents whose child has a fatal or potentially fatal medical condition, an emotional roller coaster of anxiety, anticipatory grief, and other turmoil begins with the recognition that something serious may be wrong with their child and intensifies greatly with the diagnosis of a life-threatening condition. Some parents endure from the outset the news that no options exist to cure or significantly prolong their child's life. Other parents live for a time with uncertainty, hoping that their child will be among those who will be cured but then facing the stress of difficult decisions about how far to pursue potentially curative or life-prolonging interventions.

A repeated theme in discussions with parents is that they want accurate, clear, and timely information, even if only a clear statement that the situation is uncertain. Evasions, half-truths, and other failures to communicate add to emotional distress. Another theme of parents is that they want to be listened to and recognized as experts about their child and that failure to listen to them also creates distress. Thus, much of the discussion in

Chapter 4 considered the emotional as well as the factual or intellectual dimensions of communication between parents and clinicians.

Professional caregivers also should be alert to the many dimensions of emotional distress in parents including, for example, the sense of guilt that parents may feel when they cannot save their child or because they are surviving when their child is not. Parents may also feel guilt that something they did (e.g., during pregnancy) somehow caused their child's medical problem. In some cases, they can be reassured that they were not responsible; in other situations when a parent has unintentionally contributed to a child's injury, reassurance is still important but more complicated. Marital stress is not surprising and should be a concern of those supporting the family, although evidence that a child's death contributes to higher overall divorce rates is inconclusive (see Appendix E).

The preceding discussion of emotional care for a seriously ill child noted that children may be concerned and upset about their appearance. Parents too may be sensitive to their child's appearance. Other adults, even family members and health care professionals, may overtly or subtly avoid the child, thereby contributing to both parents' and children's feelings of isolation.

As discussed later and in Appendix E, bereavement research suggests that mothers and fathers mourn differently. Their responses during the course of a child's fatal or potentially fatal condition may likewise vary, although the committee did not locate specific research documenting this. To the extent that fathers are more likely to be working outside the home and less likely to be with the child during medical visits, physicians, nurses, hospice personnel, and others may hear fewer questions or concerns from fathers and have fewer contacts with them. This means that those caring for the child and family may have to make a concerted effort to include the father and make him comfortable with the care team and the care planning process. As one stepgrandfather of an HIV positive child observed, "we must investigate if there is a male who wants to be involved, even if he is not normally present; an invitation to participate may be all that is necessary" (Smithson, no date).

The main sources of emotional support for parents will often be other family members and close friends, although some parents may find that before as well as after a child's death, others avoid them out of fear or confusion. Although parents should expect sensitivity and emotional support from the child's health care team, some may also seek or be referred for additional counseling and, when appropriate, treatment for clinical depression or other conditions.

Siblings

> *The time that he was sick was so confusing. . . . I hated to see my brother in pain. . . . Sometimes I got mad at my parents. I couldn't communicate with anybody. Really, it was because I felt a little neglected when he was in the hospital. It was lonely.*
> Susan Rae, sister (in Romand 1989, p. 21)

Parents with more than one child must find the strength to care for their ill child and for the well siblings, who are also vulnerable. Siblings are too often left out when a brother or sister is dying, both by parents who are overburdened with caring for the ill child and by professionals. Yet these children live the illness experience with the patient and parents and have many years of life ahead to negotiate the effects of the premature loss of a brother or sister. "I'm not sure if anybody could have helped but I think it should be recognized that Karen not only lost her sister, she lost the strength of the other adults in her life and the security of knowing mom and dad could protect her. She learned far too young that the world is a scary place" (Aney, 2001).

Some of the discussion about emotional support for ill children is relevant for their well siblings. For example, siblings can benefit from supportive school and camp programs and from play or other opportunities provided at children's hospitals. For example, one of the parents with whom the committee met described the help provided by child-life specialists for their well daughter, whose thirteenth birthday coincided with her brother's chemotherapy and whose fifteenth birthday came the day before his brain surgery. "[They] fixed up a goody bag for her that says 'I spent my birthday at Children's Hospital,' which is what they give to the patients. . . . That meant a lot to her. . . . They were definitely very accommodating" (Kittiko, 2001).

Siblings may also benefit from professional counseling. As they live with a seriously ill brother or sister or after that child's death, they may experience anger or jealousy, guilt, anticipatory grief, depression, and fear about becoming ill or dying. When parents decide that an ill child should die at home, well siblings may need particular attention in dealing with the intensity of that experience (Silverman, 2000).

Other potentially helpful strategies for siblings include checking for and correcting misunderstandings about their brother's or sister's medical condition, providing opportunities for siblings to "vent" their worries or resentments, alerting a sibling's teachers to the situation and enlisting their support, bringing siblings to the hospital so they can meet and observe the care team, giving them ways to be helpful, and providing the opportunity for them to say their good-byes to their dying brother or sister before and after death. "Children need to be involved and seen as active members of the family, as helpers, and as grievers" (Silverman, 2000, p. 151; see also Martinson and Campos, 1991). Davies (1998) notes that research indicates that living with a sibling who is chronically ill or disabled can have positive as well as negative consequences.

Other Family Members

Some children with life-threatening medical problems are cared for by grandparents, adult siblings, their parent's siblings, or foster parents because neither their mother nor their father can care for them as a result of death, physical or emotional disability, imprisonment, or other reasons. These children and family units are likely to experience many strains beyond the child's illness and to be in particular need of assessment and attention. More generally, caregivers should be alert to the distress of grandparents and other family members they encounter.

THE SPIRITUAL DIMENSIONS OF CARE

General

Spirituality, although often equated with religion, can be viewed more generally as the search for meaning and purpose in life and in death (see, e.g., Daaleman and VandeCreek, 2000; Miller et al., 2001). Discussions of end-of-life care for adults commonly recognize that the diagnosis of a possibly fatal illness and the approach of death may inspire spiritual reflection and a search for meaning or connection with others that may bring serenity and hope in place of fear and despair (see, e.g., Soderstrom and Martinson, 1987; Hay, 1989; Kaczorowski, 1989; Byock, 1997; IOM, 1997; Speck, 1998; Daaleman and VandeCreek, 2000; Sommer, 2001; Lo et al., 2002).

Religions provide frameworks, although not the only ones, for this search for meaning. Even individuals without a religious belief system may value and benefit from discussions with well-trained chaplains, carefully selected hospice volunteers, or others who have special empathy or insight into existential concerns at life's end. Thus, chaplains should be prepared to relate to diverse kinds of families, to support those of different faiths or no stated faith, and when appropriate, to suggest spiritual resources in the community. Hospitals may develop discussion guides for staff and volunteers to help them sensitively identify needs or concerns in ways that respect varying religious affiliations and beliefs. Religious affiliation or belief cannot be assumed from a person's name, language, or appearance.

Health care providers have traditionally made provision for certain religious rituals or practices at the end of life, for example, the "anointing of the sick" (traditionally called "extreme unction" or "last rites") in the Roman Catholic and Orthodox Christian faiths. Hospital chapels may be offered for memorial services. Hospice chaplains regularly officiate at services for children who have died. Religious groups also sponsor many hospitals, hospices, and other health care organizations and organize a variety of community-based supportive services—spiritual and practical—for individuals and families facing serious medical problems. When children are cared for at medical centers far from home, hospital chaplains may help link families to nearby faith communities for support.

The role of spiritual care in overall patient care is recognized in hospital accreditation standards (JCAHO, 1998)[3] and Medicare hospice requirements (HCFA/CMS, 1994). Medicare and other insurance programs do not, however, reimburse separately for religious counseling or other chaplain services, which increases their vulnerability to cutbacks when institutions are under acute fiscal pressure. The involvement of chaplains in spiritual care for dying patients and their families has been little studied in inpatient or home settings, even for adults (Bryant, 1993; Daaleman and Frey, 1998).

Although this discussion focuses on the role of chaplains, families also rely on their own ministers, rabbis, or other sources of spiritual comfort and enrichment. More broadly, "pastoral care" that involves the whole faith community, including lay persons, can expand the spiritual resources available for seriously ill and dying people and their families (Shelp, 2001).

Physicians, nurses, and others have sometimes been uncertain about their appropriate religious or spiritual role or connection with patients, for example, whether or when to offer to pray with them (see, e.g., Post et al., 2000; Feldstein, 2001). Such spiritual care can be profoundly comforting and may be welcomed by some patients (see, e.g., Daaleman and Nease, 1994; Dagi, 1995; Ehman et al., 1999). Still, spiritual support from clinicians has the potential, if offered insensitively, to be offensive and damaging. As suggested elsewhere, at a minimum, "the clinician's role is . . . to avoid obstructing spiritual explorations. Such obstruction is unlikely to be willful but instead to reflect the clinician's own discomfort with death as an existential phenomenon rather than a technical problem to be analyzed and solved" (IOM, 1997, p. 79).

The hazards of well-intentioned but insensitive involvement by clinical personnel in spiritual matters are cited in an employee handout from a religious health care system. It describes the case of a respiratory therapist

---

[3]Joint Commission on the Accreditation of Healthcare Organizations (JCAHO) Standard RI.1.3 "The hospital demonstrates respect for the following patient needs: . . . [RI.1.3.5] Pastoral care and other spiritual services" (RI = Rights and Organizational Ethics).

who baptized an infant suffering severe respiratory problems, thereby exposing the hospital to litigation and a $500,000 settlement with the parents (the husband was a local rabbi) (All Saints Healthcare System, 1998). The hospital had a dedicated neonatal chaplain and 24-hour chaplain coverage that included a cantor and a rabbi, but the therapist did not consult them before acting. Such extreme cases, although they should encourage sensitivity, should not discourage efforts to help patients and families with spiritual needs and concerns.

Spiritual Care for Children

a-byss'

> *My life*
> *Is halfway down*
> *An abyss.*
> *A deep*
> *Immeasurable space.*
> *A gulf.*
> *A cavity.*
> *A vast chasm.*
> *My life*
> *Is not how*
> *I planned it to be.*
> *Is not how*
> *I want it to be.*
> *Is not how*
> *I pray for it*
> *To be.*
> *In the darkness*
> *Of this pit,*
> *I see a small*
> *Light of hope.*
> *Is it possible for me*
> *To climb to such heights?*
> *To rebuild the bridges?*
> *To find my salvation?*
> *The song*
> *In my heart*
> *Is so quiet.*
> *Is so dark.*
> *Is so fearful.*
> *I dare not stay in*

This abyss.
Though deep
And vast,
I am only halfway
Down.
Thus, I am
Already
Halfway up?
Let such words
Fall onto my heart,
And raise me from this depth.

Matthew Stepanek, age 11
Used with permission.

Most discussions of spiritual issues in end-of-life care focus on adults and say little or nothing about children facing death. Clearly, children can engage in spiritual reflection and experience spiritual anguish or peace. The poem that accompanies this section shows the spiritual awareness and anxiety about life's end of the 11-year-old author, who has a progressive neuromuscular condition. The poem also documents his prayerful hope that the "song in my heart" can raise him from the depths of fear.

As described by Thayer, children with life-threatening conditions confront "issues of unconditional love, forgiveness, hope, safety, legacy, loneliness, and loss of wholeness" (Thayer, 2001, p. 173). Like adults, children may wonder, "Why me?" or "How could God let this happen?" or "Did I get sick because I was bad?" This questioning of God's purposes or caring (or lack thereof) is reflected in the perspective offered by a 5-year old who, in describing a drawing, observed, "God is a part of our family, every family. He's not doing anything" (Sourkes, 1995a, p. 133). Although some researchers have examined spirituality in children (see, e.g., Fowler, 1981; Kubler-Ross, 1983; Coles, 1990), little research has investigated the spiritual concerns of children with life-threatening medical problems and ways of responding to these concerns (Kenny, 1999; Davies et al., 2002).

The Pediatric Chaplains Network has developed a document outlining the competencies and ethical standards for chaplains serving sick children and their families (PCN, 1999a,b). One responsibility is to link an understanding of the faith development process in children to an understanding of children's intellectual and psychological development.

A careful assessment by a psychologist, social worker, nurse, or other professional of the psychosocial needs of a seriously ill child may also elicit spiritual or existential concerns by asking about a child's hopes, fears, and other emotions. Taking parents' religious beliefs into account, these professionals may be able to help child patients discuss these concerns. If a child raises specific religious or doctrinal questions in discussions with clinical personnel, deference to the family and their spiritual advisers is advised (Sourkes, 1995a).

Like social workers and others, chaplains may use art, music, and play to help children with matters of faith and meaning (see, e.g., Van Eys and Mohnke, 1985; Thayer, 2001). Older children and adolescents may benefit from techniques used with seriously ill adults, such as a spiritual assessment (see, e.g., Puchalski and Romer, 2000) or a "life review" that covers relationships, achievements, regrets, and similar issues (see, e.g., Haight and Burnside, 1993).

As far as the committee could discover, no spiritual assessment tools have been tested systematically with children. A subcommittee of the National Hospice and Palliative Care Organization has observed that the usually brief spiritual assessments by pediatric hospice programs tend to focus on parents (as spokespersons for the child) rather than on child patients themselves. It has proposed guidelines for exploring and discussing children's spiritual concerns and strengths (Davies et al., 2002).

Spiritual care for children involves more than adapting adult rituals and discussions, although the family's religious beliefs and traditions need to be identified and respected. Thayer has pointed out that "children want to have fun" and their spiritual care should reflect this (Thayer, 2001, p. 180). He also recommends that spiritual care should reflect children's developmental inclinations toward activities rather than abstract thinking and mainly verbal rituals. One example is the use of a "magic carpet" that can serve as a prop and inspiration for imagined trips to heaven or a land of no pain, where children can talk about their hopes, wants, and worries. The making of "spiritual bracelets" (akin to friendship bracelets, except that the colors of threads represent different spiritual values) can both prompt discussions about faith and other values and allow the child to create a gift. The construction and decoration of a "prayer or meditation pillow" not only offers opportunities for activity, creativity, and discussion but also leaves the child with a physical object that may later be helpful in meditation or prayer.

Spiritual Care for Family

Religious traditions and practices often provide families with some sense of order, community, and meaning during a time when they feel unmoored and overwhelmed (Silverman, 2000; see also Doka and Morgan, 1993; Davies, 1998; Goldman, 1998). As noted earlier, some rituals, such as the "anointing of the sick" are familiar in hospitals in many parts of the country, although, depending on the faith, some may not be considered appropriate for young children. When a family member is dying, members of the family's religious community may join them in the hospital room for prayers, chants, songs, scripture readings, or similar expressions. They may help plan spiritually comforting and personalized funerals and memorials for the child.

Because families are so central when a child is gravely ill, a spiritual assessment of parents and siblings is often appropriate. Again, the committee found no assessment tool that had been tested for this specific purpose. For adults, a relatively simple set of questions (e.g., do you belong to a spiritual community? how might we help meet your needs?) may be sufficient to identify those who would welcome further attention, including referral to a chaplain (see, e.g., Puchalski and Romer, 2000).

When it is offered with sensitivity and respect, the opportunity to talk with a chaplain or other appropriate person has the potential to help parents, siblings, and others close to a child who is dying or who has died to cope with their feelings of guilt, anger, or helplessness. Such discussion can also offer hope and comfort based on shared beliefs in life after death or other articles of faith.

Awareness of religious or spiritual concerns can also prepare health care personnel to present issues such as autopsy and organ or tissue donation without offense. In addition, chaplains may provide families with practical assistance, particularly if social work resources are limited (Sommer, 2001). Such practical help may include notifying other survivors or the family's spiritual adviser, preparing families if a visit to the medical examiner's office is necessary, identifying bereavement support groups and relevant social service organizations, and providing information necessary for families to make funeral and other arrangements (Iverson, 1999).

THE PRACTICAL DIMENSIONS OF CARE

Most children are legally, financially, and otherwise dependent on their parents, depending on them for food, clothing, shelter, and many other physical, emotional, spiritual, and practical needs. As they develop, children normally assume more and more responsibility for self-care.

Children who have certain serious, chronic disabling conditions may, however, remain or become substantially or totally dependent on others for such daily and recurring tasks as bathing, toileting, feeding, and dressing. Depending on family members' other responsibilities, physical strength, and emotional endurance, they may need and welcome paid outside assistance with these practical tasks. Such assistance is, however, often difficult for families to arrange and afford. As discussed further in Chapter 6, most private health insurance programs limit payment for such assistance, and state Medicaid and Title V programs are highly variable in what they cover or support.

Many families also face daunting practical challenges in identifying and coordinating multiple professional and other providers of care for a child with extensive medical and other needs. Some health maintenance organizations (HMOs) and integrated health systems reduce these burdens by themselves providing most or all of the needed services and personnel and by maintaining a unified information system to support record keeping, appointments, referrals, and other tasks. Whether they are employed by health plans, hospitals, or other organizations, discharge planners, case managers, and other paid personnel can assist families with some of the practical aspects of coordinating care. (These personnel also serve cost-containment goals, for example, helping to shorten hospital stays.)

As noted in the 1997 Institute of Medicine (IOM) report, the practical often overlaps with the physical, emotional, and spiritual dimensions of caring, and the three latter dimensions also mix with each other. For example, for a child experiencing hair loss or other changes in appearance related to chemotherapy, advice—particularly perhaps from someone with personal experience—about using wigs, scarves, or turbans or even about "making baldness a fashion statement" may help both emotionally and practically.

Box 5.2 provides examples of the many dimensions of practical support for children and families who are living with a child's life-threatening medical condition. A number involve the goal of helping the child and family maintain a normal life to the extent possible. Others concern the family's caregiving responsibilities, ready access to important information, and preparation for crises and for the child's death. When a child is seriously ill, outside support with such matters aids the child by aiding the parents.

Opportunities for practical support continue after a child's death. Particularly when a child has died suddenly without forewarning, the aftermath can be filled not only with emotional trauma and grief but also with bureaucratic requirements related to the hospital's release of the body, the medical examiner's jurisdiction, and other matters. Families may welcome assistance with the array of practical issues associated with funeral arrangements. When a child's death is anticipated, some practical matters can be planned in advance, but the particular circumstances of a child's death may still present unforeseen problems.

Given the diversity of child and family characteristics and circumstances, needs for practical assistance will vary enormously as will the challenges of meeting these needs. Although fundamental goals and principles may be consistent, strategies that meet the needs of affluent, well-educated, and stable families are unlikely to fit the single, barely literate, erratically employed parent with unstable family and personal relationships who lives in poverty in an unsafe neighborhood. Parents in the latter situa-

Box 5.2
Examples of Practical Dimensions of Care for Patients and Families

Normal Life

• What to provide for the child's immediate comfort, control, safety, mobility, and privacy: adapting, arranging and decorating the child's physical space (e.g., hospital room, bedroom, bathroom); modifying the family car
• How to manage personal care and appearance changes: developing routines and finding assistive devices for bathing, dressing, and other activities; fitting medical equipment (e.g., wheelchairs, oxygen) into life at home, school, and elsewhere; offering tips for coping with altered physical appearance (e.g., loss of hair, scarring, prostheses)
• How to continue schooling: planning with teachers and other school personnel for medical and emergency support; preparing schoolmates; arranging a shortened school day or home or hospital schooling
• How to provide for play activities and friends: adapting the home physical environment; preparing playmates for a child's return home; selecting or adapting toys, art materials

Family and Others Close to Patient

• What to do for parent caregivers: advising on employment issues and finances including eligibility for government assistance; arranging or providing volunteer or paid assistance with housekeeping, meal preparation, or respite from caregiving; short-term versus longer-term assistance
• What to do for siblings: babysitting; arranging assistance with homework and time for play, friends, and other normal activities

Planning and Quick Reference Information

• Whom to call: having easy-to-locate phone numbers (including after-hours numbers) for physician and other team members; pharmacy, medical equipment company, case manager, or other health care coordinator; family and friends to be notified of death, imminent death, or emergency
• What decisions have been made: having accessible documentation (at home, at school) of family and, as appropriate, child preferences for care (e.g., written orders to allow natural death)
• What to do for pain and other symptoms, problems with medical equipment: providing quick, clear reference guides for relieving symptoms, dealing with equipment problems, and getting additional help or information
• What to expect: providing information on signs of impending death and caregiver response
• What to do after death: plans for religious and other rituals (e.g., funeral, memorial service, wake), creation of mementos, notification of family members, funeral plans, arrangements for care of very young siblings
• What to do in the event of parental incapacity: identifying guardian and location of estate planning, financial, and other records

SOURCE: Adapted from IOM, 1997.

tion face greater practical and other burdens, but they—or at least their child—may qualify for Medicaid and for programs to help children with special health care needs. Despite their limitations (see Chapter 7), these programs often offer or provide supportive services beyond those usually covered by private health plans.

Most hospices are attuned to practical as well as clinical issues. In general, hospices have found their greatest acceptance among more educated, middle-class patients and families, although many have tried to reach out to disadvantaged individuals, families, and communities. In trying to "diversify" culturally to serve families from different economic, religious, and cultural backgrounds, they may identify a wider range of practical needs.

Assistance from friends, neighbors, employers, and others in the community can make an important difference in the experience of families living with a child's serious illness. For example, having a friend or neighbor offer to stay with a child's siblings can make it less complicated to visit a doctor with the ill child. Having someone baby-sit the ill child may allow parents a few hours respite to have a quiet dinner or to give other siblings special attention. Formal respite services that provide professional or supportive care at home or at a residential facility provide stressed families a greater opportunity to regroup physically and emotionally, whether this involves a short vacation or taking care of neglected household and business matters. Such services, which are central features of British child hospices (Goldman, 1999; Rushton, 2001), are limited in this country.

Employers can help parents whose child has a life-threatening medical problem by being flexible about working hours and leave (including provisions for coworkers to contribute leave). Employee assistance programs offered by many larger employers may help identify counseling and other resources for employees or family members. Employer-sponsored health insurance is critical to families, notwithstanding limits in coverage of palliative and hospice services. Employers will sometimes agree to waive limits in their health plans on benefits for children with life-threatening medical problems. (See Chapter 7.)

Teachers and other school personnel can likewise contribute by making practical and creative arrangements that help a child stay in school. Going to school maintains a dimension of normal life amidst much that is decidedly not normal.[4]

---

[4]Since the 1960s, federal legislation and court decisions have essentially established that states must provide free public education and related supportive services for children with disabilities, regardless of the severity of their disability. In 1994, more than 5 million children were receiving special education services as provided for by federal legislation. (For a summary of the relevant statutes and judicial decisions, see NICHCY, 1996.)

As noted earlier, faith communities not only can offer spiritual and emotional support but also can organize to provide more mundane—but very real—aid in the form of meals, transportation, shopping, and respite care. Although they may charge fees to cover some of their costs, volunteer and charitable organizations (Meals on Wheels, Ronald McDonald Houses) can likewise provide help with a variety of practical matters, such as finding accommodations while a child is hospitalized.

GRIEF AND BEREAVEMENT CARE

Parenting is a permanent change in the individual. A person never gets over being a parent. Parental bereavement is also a permanent condition. The bereaved parent, after a time, will cease showing the medical symptoms of grief, but the parent does not "get over" the death of the child.

Klass, 1988, p.178

One question I have since my sister died is "When does it stop hurting?" My mom said, "someday," and that helped. . . . I think it never completely stops hurting, but it doesn't hurt as much.

Martha, sister (in Romand, 1989, p. 31)

Once a child dies, care for that child ends. For the family, however, emotional, spiritual, and practical needs for support continue beyond the child's death. The death of a child is described as one of life's most devastating experiences, affecting parents, siblings, and a wider circle of relatives and friends.

Research suggests that the death of a loved one—whatever the age—puts the bereaved person's physical and emotional health at risk (see, e.g., Maddison and Viola, 1968; Clayton et al., 1972; Schaefer et al., 1995; Prigerson, 2001; Rubin and Malkinson, 2001; Stroebe et al., 2001b). Appropriate psychological, spiritual, practical, and sometimes physical care for bereaved family and friends is intended to reduce these risks.

Although this discussion focuses on research and analytic perspectives on grief and bereavement, the committee recognizes the need to hear the voices of bereaved parents, siblings, and others close to a child who is dying or has died. The statement to the committee from Compassionate Friends urged health care professionals to prepare themselves by reading articles and other writings of bereaved family members and not to limit themselves to the writings of clinicians and researchers (Loder, 2001). This report reflects the committee's effort to do so while being aware that the writings consulted will not reflect the full range of family experiences and circumstances.

The death of a child is never easy, but the circumstances of a child's death will affect the family's experience and the responses of health care professionals. When a child is diagnosed with a fatal or potentially fatal condition, families have some time to grieve an anticipated loss and, in some sense, prepare for the worst. When death comes with no forewarning, bereavement can be particularly difficult. The following discussion considers, first, grief when death follows an extended course and, then, grief when death comes suddenly and without warning. Appendix E provides a further review of literature, questions, and research needs related to bereavement following the death of a child.

When Death Follows an Extended Course

Grief in Anticipation

When a child's death follows an extended course, family members and others close to the child will likely experience some kind of "anticipatory grief," which has elements in common with the grief that accompanies the child's actual death. These elements include strong feelings of sadness, regret, loss, and possibly guilt and anger. When death is possible but not certain (e.g., as may be the case for very premature infants), anticipatory grief can help some parents and others to prepare for the worst outcome as they also mourn the loss of certain hopes (e.g., for a joyful uncomplicated birth and a healthy infant) (Hynan, 1996). Other parents may, however, resist such thoughts.

Grief in anticipation may also follow the prenatal diagnosis of a fatal condition. Some parents will choose to end the pregnancy and may then experience a complex range of emotions with little of the support that is normally offered to bereaved parents. Other parents will choose to try to continue the pregnancy to birth. These parents will at once be preparing for birth and for death. As discussed elsewhere in this report, obstetricians, pediatricians, and hospital personnel can help families with these preparations, as can new but not widely available perinatal hospice programs (Sumner, 2001).

Because the care team will tend to focus primarily on care for the ill child and because family members may suppress their grief or deny their needs, family members may not receive adequate emotional support. They may, as a consequence, experience more intense short- and long-term suffering. Unacknowledged grief in advance of a child's death may interfere with communication, decisionmaking, and preparations for death, which in turn may contribute to strong subsequent feelings of guilt and regret (see more generally, Byock, 1997).

As is also true once a child has died, parents who are living with their child's fatal or potentially fatal condition may receive emotional and spiritual comfort (as well as practical information) from other parents. This comfort may come informally through established friends and acquaintances (including those encountered at medical settings). It may also come through organized advocacy or support groups.

Preparing for Death

Notwithstanding their sorrow, families may find both immediate and lasting comfort and meaning in preparing for a child's death. In some cases, this may involve taking steps to allow the child to die at home. In other cases, it can mean planning for death in the hospital, if indicated by the child's medical problems and the family's preferences. In either situation, members of the care team can work with families to ensure that they and perhaps close friends have time alone with the child before and after death.

When prenatal diagnosis indicates a medical condition that is expected to lead to death at or soon after birth, families may work with hospital and hospice personnel to minimize intrusive and unhelpful medical interventions for both the mother and the infant so that the family may have as much time close to the infant as possible. When this brief time is missed, it is gone forever.

Parents can also be comforted by planning for religious or cultural rituals and arranging for mementos such as prints or molds from the dying or dead child's hand or clips of the child's hair. Many hospitals have protocols and supplies on hand to accommodate these plans or to offer them to family members faced with a loved one's sudden and unexpected death.

"Hoping for the best while preparing for the worst" can enable families to continue doing everything possible to help their child survive while accepting that death is likely and preparing for it. Again, not all families can tolerate such acceptance.

When Death Is Sudden and Unexpected

Take care of the wounded souls who are left to grieve their beloved children.

Patricia Loder, parent, 2001

When a child dies from sudden infant death syndrome (SIDS) or from unintentional or intentional injuries, which are leading causes of death for infants and children, bereavement care may be all that can be offered to parents, siblings, and other relatives and friends. Such care may range from immediate emotional support in the emergency department or intensive care unit to extensive grief counseling.

Research is sparse, but some studies and clinical experience suggest that people who experience the unexpected death of a loved one, especially a younger person, may suffer more long-lasting psychological distress than those who have forewarning (Parkes, 1975; Vachon, 1976; Lundin, 1984; Davies, 1998). Other circumstances—for example, death resulting from murder, a natural disaster, or a very public event—may add to the psychological burden of survivors. Moreover, sudden deaths of children often require investigation by the medical examiner's office, autopsy, and other procedures that can further intensify the stress and confusion experienced by bereaved families.

Yet another complication is that some sudden deaths of children result from parental abuse. Such deaths may cause anger and uncertainty among hospital staff. They may be unsure about how to handle the parents and other family members. Legal requirements have to be met, and the psychiatric status of the apparent abuser as well as other family members may require formal assessment. In these circumstances, it may be difficult to extend support to other family members, who may be viewed as complicit. Nonetheless, hospital personnel are caregivers not policymakers, judges, and juries. It remains their responsibility to offer assistance to those in need.

The discussion earlier in this chapter stressed the complexities and importance of providing information in emergency situations. Sometimes the family spends relatively little time with emergency department personnel when death is pronounced on arrival or within an hour or two thereafter. The family may be on its way home within three hours of arrival. This puts a premium on prompt inquiries and action, for example, to contact other family or friends and the family's spiritual adviser or the hospital chaplain, to offer information about bereavement support resources in the community, and to provide reassurance that family members can call the social worker or other designated person if they need assistance later and that someone will be in touch to see how they are doing.

As mentioned in Chapter 4, the National Association of Social Workers with support from the federal Maternal and Child Health Bureau has developed guidelines for bereavement care in the emergency department (Lipton and Coleman, 2000b). Appendix F considers other efforts to help emergency departments and emergency first responders improve their support for bereaved family members. The authors note, however, the lack of conclusive findings about how well the emergency medical system serves the families of children who die. As one area for future research, they suggest studies to clarify the relationship between posttraumatic stress disorder and bereavement following sudden death and the implications for family support.

Bereavement

Her words concerning his death and the choices I made also comfort me. She said, "You did the right thing." Such simple words—but what comfort they give me four years later!
Peg Rousar-Thompson, parent, 2001

Several earlier sections of this chapter have discussed ways in which health care professionals can support family members after a child's death. These supports extend from the compassion in the telling of a child's death to the offering of time for family members to be with a child after death to the providing of reassurance and various kinds of practical assistance.

Just as families vary in their other needs, they will vary in their needs for support in bereavement. Some will want or need little professional assistance in coping with their grief. Others may experience complicated grief or bereavement that is more intense and endures longer than normal. After reviewing the literature, Prigerson and Jacobs (2001, p. 1370) conclude that complicated grief symptoms "form a coherent cluster of symptoms distinct from bereavement-related depressive and anxiety symptom clusters' . . . endure several years for some bereaved subjects; predict substantial morbidity and adverse health behaviors over and above depressive symptoms and unlike depressive symptoms, are not effectively reduced by interpersonal psychotherapy and/or tricyclic antidepressants." As discussed in Appendix E, research indicates that mothers and fathers tend to mourn differently. Mothers typically report more intense and prolonged grief reactions than fathers.

Bereavement Interventions

Bereavement interventions are diverse (see, e.g., Parkes, 1998; Corless, 2001; Stroebe et al., 2001a; Worden and Monahan, 2001). Some are relatively short term, for example, preparation and protocols for the immediate aftermath of a child's death in the emergency department. Other interventions may cover an extended period or be relatively open-ended for as long as a bereaved individual wants to participate. Some focus on individual family members; others involve the family as a unit. Some are informal and rely on peers; others involve trained professionals including social workers, psychologists, psychiatrists, members of the clergy, and bereavement counselors.

Bereavement services may be sponsored by mental health organizations, hospices, children's hospitals, family-based organizations, and other groups. Internet-based options have multiplied—some offering peer support, others providing ways to memorialize a loved one. Given that death in childhood is so much less common than death in old age in this country, parents, siblings, and others may find few people with this shared experience. For this reason, Internet-based support options offer families potentially important resources, ones that need to be evaluated further for both positive and negative features.

Many questions remain about the effectiveness (and potential for harm) of different kinds of interventions to support bereaved parents, siblings, and others. Chapter 10 and Appendix E identify a number of directions for research. As with other areas of research, priorities include the identification of relevant outcomes, the development of outcome measures, the classification or diagnosis of grief and bereavement responses or symptoms, the relationship between grief and other psychological states (e.g., posttraumatic stress disorder, depression), the identification of risk or protective factors that predict the severity of responses, and the tailoring of interventions to circumstances.

Families Supporting Families

Before a child's expected death, in its immediate aftermath, and long after, family support groups offer parents and siblings comfort, information, and other assistance guided by the shared experience of bereavement. As one adult sibling wrote, although the community of the bereaved is not "a community that any of us wanted to join," it offers "sympathetic arms to hold us" (Scala, 2001, p. 6). Those involved in these family support groups know what the death of a child is like, including what it is like when weeks pass and the active support and concern of many friends, neighbors, classmates, and coworkers diminishes.

Compassionate Friends is perhaps the largest and most comprehensive of the groups offering support to families after the death of a child. A number of more focused groups such as M.I.S.S. (Mothers in Sympathy and Support) focus on families who have experienced a stillbirth, miscarriage, or infant death. In addition, a number of groups focused on specific medical conditions include bereavement support among a range of concerns that typically include support for research, insurance coverage and other financial assistance, and prevention programs.

Siblings

> *I was in a unique situation as a 5-year-old whose infant brother had died. . . . My brother's death was a void, to be sure. But in many ways, my grief, because he was so young, was more about the emotional death of my parents. My grief was about losing my parents at a crucial time in my childhood.*
>
> Jennifer, sister, no date
> (http://www.portlandtcf.org/NL112001_4.html)

> *The other scary feeling I have since Donald died is about myself dying. I thought since he was twelve when he died that I was going to do the same.*
>
> Susan Rae, sister (in Romand, 1989, p. 21)

Most discussions of grief and bereavement following a child's death focus on parents, but the loss of a brother or sister can have a lifelong effect on siblings—either directly from the loss of a significant relationship or indirectly as a consequence of parents' reactions. In 1984, the IOM report on bereavement, which focused on the research base for understanding and responding to bereavement, lacked a section on siblings' responses to the death of a brother or sister because such an information base was essentially missing. Although still modest, information about sibling bereavement is now more available (see review in Davies, 1998, Appendixes 1 and 2).

Clinical experience and the few studies of children who are themselves suffering from life-threatening illnesses suggest that they may have a more advanced awareness of death than other children (see, e.g., Bluebond-Langner, 1978; Sourkes, 1980, 1982, 1995a). For surviving siblings, however, the general literature on children's developmental understanding of death seems most relevant. In this literature, the evolution of children's understanding of death is generally assessed in terms of four basic concepts including irreversibility, finality, universality, and causation (see, e.g., Wass, 1984; Stevens, 1998; Silverman, 2000). Davies suggests that "age alone is not a reliable indicator of children's understanding of death, but it remains the most practical guideline" (Davies, 1998, p. 36).

Each child has an individual personality and way of dealing with life's normal events and problems, and each child who loses a brother or sister will have an individual reaction rooted in part in his or her own age, personality, and experiences, including relationship with the child who died. Reactions may also be shaped by the behavior of parents and others, including how news of the sibling's death is communicated and how parents cope with their own grief. Based on general guidelines about helping bereaved individuals, Davies (1998) advises those counseling parents about their surviving children to encourage parents to be honest about what has happened and what can be expected (taking into account the children's age and maturity) and to involve siblings in discussions and choices about their presence or participation in significant events (e.g., the wake or funeral). She also emphasizes that siblings, like parents, may be able to absorb only limited amounts of information at one time and may need to have information repeated and expanded.

Children of school age may find it unsettling or distressing to return to school after a sibling's death. One child who was 13 when her sister died wrote, "It was embarrassing to go back to school after Bethany died because everybody just sat there like 'What do we say to her?'" (Romand, 1989, p.16). Another child wrote that "at school they think just because [Donald's] dead he's not my brother no more" (Romand, 1989, p.22). In addition to supporting ill children, teachers and other school personnel can help ease the way for a child living with a seriously ill sibling or returning to school after a sibling's death.

Continuing Support from the Child's Care Team

After a child's death, friends, neighbors, grief counselors, peers, hospice personnel, and others in the local community may provide most of the bereavement and practical support for a family, although the extent and adequacy of such support and the extent to which families experience avoidance or neglect needs further investigation. Parents or siblings may also seek care from their primary care physician or a psychotherapist. Still, the child's physicians, nurses, social workers, and other caregivers who have often developed relationships with the family over a period of months or years can be an important source of support for bereaved parents and other family members. An abrupt end to contact soon after the child's death can feel like—and be—a kind of abandonment.

Members of the child's care team may attend the visitation, funeral, or memorial service. Reports from families suggest that condolence letters from members of the care team are welcomed. Care teams can create reminder systems for follow-up notes or phone calls to mark an important holiday or the date of the child's birth or death. Such a system might include a routine for copying the face sheet on the medical record (which will include names, addresses, and the child's birth date), noting the date of death, and putting in a "tickler" file that is checked regularly.

In some situations, families may be disturbed because the cause of a child's death is not be entirely clear. If an autopsy is performed, the physician can meet with the family to explain the findings and answer their questions. Even when an autopsy is not performed, the physician primarily responsible for the child's care should offer to answer a family's questions and refer them, if appropriate, for counseling.

The next chapter discusses further the role of professionals and health care organizations in providing palliative, end-of-life, and bereavement care for children and families. It considers that care within a broader framework of professional, institutional, and governmental efforts to improve the quality, coordination, and continuity of services for seriously ill or injured children. The chapter concludes with the committee's recommendations on a number of the issues covered in this and earlier chapters including communication, symptom management and other care processes, bereavement services, and coordination and continuity of care.

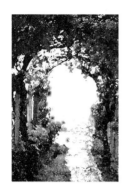

CHAPTER 6

Providing, Organizing, and Improving Care

"Was there someone in charge of your child's medical care?"
"Yes, me. Coordinating the various doctors, nurses and treatments
was the most frustrating part of the process."
Christine Aney, parent, 2001

The parents who live with the children know what is best for
that child. That was awful, the having to fight for what you knew
was best for your child.
Gary Conlon, parent, 2001

The good news . . . is that any health care organization in the
country can take immediate steps to improve how it cares for dying
patients and those who love them.
Lynn et al., 2000, p. 35

In the United States, the diagnosis of a child's life-threatening medical condition often launches child and family into a complex and confusing world of technologically sophisticated treatments, arcane terminology, and highly specialized personnel and organizations. In particular, children with a serious chronic condition will likely need both acute and chronic care involving multiple services from multiple professionals and multiple organizations at multiple sites, including the home. The coordination of such care is a difficult and frustrating burden for many parents that leaves them with less time and energy for their ill child, for other family members, and for each other. It is also a well-recognized trouble spot for health care providers.

180

This chapter begins by considering palliative, end-of-life, and bereavement care for children and their families within a broader framework of efforts to improve the quality, coordination, and continuity of care for children with serious medical conditions. In addition to strengthening accountability for care, these efforts have sought to make health care more child and family centered, to establish a locus of responsibility for the care of children with special health care needs, and more recently, to develop care coordination models for children needing care for fatal or potentially fatal medical conditions. The chapter also provides an overview of the professionals and organizations that care for children with life-threatening medical problems and their families. The final sections return to the issue of continuity and coordination with a discussion of community and regional systems of care and present the committee's recommendations.

ACCOUNTABILITY AND QUALITY

General Concepts

Although this chapter focuses on the organization and delivery of palliative and end-of-life care for children and their families, such care must be understood within the broader health care system in the United States. The deficiencies of that system in providing affordable, universal access to safe, effective, compassionate, patient- and family-centered care are long-standing. Attention often focuses on children and adults who lack insurance, but as discussed in Chapter 7, even for children and families who have health insurance, public and private health plan rules and procedures may limit professionals and organizations from offering the amounts and types of palliative, end-of-life, and bereavement care that they believe would best meet the needs of the individual child and family.

More generally, the health care system in this country is characterized by complex and often confusing organizational, financial, and regulatory arrangements that link health care professionals and institutions with each other and with governments, insurers, and other organizations. "By fragmenting the patient-physician relationship and often putting personal physicians at a distance from their dying patients, these arrangements may diminish the knowledge and intimacy that contributes to a professional's feeling of individual responsibility" (IOM, 1997, p. 122). One unintended consequence is that no health care professional is clearly responsible for seeing that patients gets needed care whatever its emphasis and whether they are at home or in the hospital. Thus, the committee believes that creating accountability for palliative, end-of-life, and bereavement care is a crucial element of any strategy to improve the quality of this care, including its coordination and continuity.

Another IOM committee has defined quality of care as "the degree to which health services for individuals and populations increase the likelihood of desired health outcomes and are consistent with current professional knowledge" (IOM, 1990a, p. 21). The literature on quality of care has traditionally distinguished three dimensions for assessment: the structure of care (e.g., information and decision support systems), the processes of care (e.g., assessing, documenting, and preventing or relieving symptoms); and the outcomes of care (e.g., avoidable hospitalizations, pain, perceptions of care). The definition of the goals of care and the development of appropriate and feasible outcome measures are essential steps in assessing and improving the quality of care and in holding professionals and institutions accountable for palliative and end-of-life care. As discussed further in Chapter 10, the development of outcome measures, whether for quality assessment or research, is a particular challenge for patients who are dying and may be sedated or otherwise not able to answer questions about their experience of care, symptoms, or quality of life in the face of death.

Solomon (2001) has noted the challenges posed by limited scientific knowledge and measurement challenges but has proposed several steps that institutions could take now to strengthen accountability and improve end-of-life care. They include establishing continuous quality improvement committees responsible for end-of-life care, collecting data as a catalyst for change, reviewing existing outcome measures and data sources and experimenting with new ones, and beginning with data collection on a small scale.

Under the rubrics of Continuous Quality Improvement (CQI) and Total Quality Management (TQM), the last decade and a half has seen an explosion of interest in the application by health care managers of formal quality improvement strategies (see, e.g., Berwick, 1989; Berwick et al., 1990; IOM, 1990b, 2001b; Horn and Hopkins, 1994; Nelson et al., 1998). Advocates have promoted principles for implementing change that include "targeting systemic defects (e.g., fragmentation and discontinuity in patient care) rather than individual mistakes; encouraging close relationships among the participants in health care transactions (e.g., physicians, patients, purchasers); using planning, control, assessment, and improvement activities that are grounded in statistical and scientific precepts and techniques; feeding statistical information back to practitioners on how their practices may differ from their peers' or depart from evidence-based standards for practice; standardizing processes to reduce the opportunity for error and link specific care processes to outcomes; and striving for continuous improvement in contrast to merely meeting established goals or criteria" (IOM, 1997, p. 126).

Once a problem area, a specific target for process improvement, and desired objectives and outcomes have been identified and investigated, a centerpiece of CQI is the "plan–do–study (or check)–act" cycle. This cycle involves four basic steps: (1) planning a change, that is, developing specific steps (e.g., data collection strategy, selection of study population) and time-table to reach the objectives; (2) doing or implementing the planned change and collecting data on outcomes and processes, including unexpected problems and results; (3) studying the change by analyzing the data, comparing results to expectations, and summarizing lessons; and (4) acting as guided by the analysis, including revising the original plan, expanding it, or identifying a new strategy. Although investments in these strategies have not necessarily been documented by controlled studies to be as successful as promised (see, e.g., Shortell et al., 1998), they have a recognized place in efforts to improve the performance of the American health care system (see, e.g., IOM, 2001b) including the delivery of consistent, effective, and compassionate palliative, end-of-life, and bereavement care (Lynn et al., 2000).

Innovative Quality Improvement Projects in Palliative and End-of-Life Care

A wealth of ideas for systematic quality improvement in end-of-life care have been generated by an initiative cosponsored by the Institute for Healthcare Improvement and the Center to Improve Care of the Dying. Leaders of the initiative subsequently discussed these ideas in *Improving Care for the End of Life: A Sourcebook for Health Care Managers and Clinicians* (Lynn et al., 2000; Web site at http://www.medicaring.org/educate/navigate/qi.html).

One chapter of the sourcebook is devoted to reports on strategies tried by a number of health care organizations to reduce fragmentation of care, improve continuity and accountability, and increase satisfaction with care. Specific, measurable objectives for these projects included reducing patient transfers (especially when death is near), providing patients and families with one or two central contact people, coordinating hospice and oncology units in a managed care system to provide a continuum of care and promote consistency in pain management, establishing reliable procedures for professionals to communicate with each other about a patient's care, and establishing and delivering on specific promises (e.g., that a known person will respond to a request for help within 30 minutes, day or night).

Some of the programs described in the sourcebook sought to coordinate care across multiple sites and providers following the model Program of All-Inclusive Care for the Elderly (PACE) that was pioneered by On-Lok Senior Health Services in California. (PACE also provided the model for the Medicaid-based pediatric palliative care demonstration projects described earlier in this report.) Other projects were focused on narrower issues, for example, developing reliable, easy ways for advance care plans to be available, recognized, and honored by providers in all settings and circumstances. The editors of the sourcebook suggested that a useful measure of continuity of care is tracking the number of health care personnel seen by a patient in a short period. They urged that patients and families should have a single point of contact but also become comfortable with several members of the care team.

Additional innovative projects and efforts to improve the quality of palliative and end-of-life care have been described elsewhere (see, e.g., Bookbinder et al., 1995; Higginson, 1993; Bookbinder, 2001; Solomon et al., 2000b, 2001b; Romer et al., 2002; see also the on-line journal *Innovations in End-of-Life Care*, http://www.edc.org/lastacts, and the Web site for Promoting Excellence in End-of-Life Care, http://www.endoflifecare.org/). These efforts do not necessarily involve the specific quality improvement approach outlined in the sourcebook. Most activities involve adult patients, but they may still offer useful direction for quality improvement efforts in pediatric care.

Practice Guidelines and Protocols for Care

Quality improvement efforts in clinical care often involve the development or adoption of formal clinical practice guidelines and administrative protocols.[1] Such guidelines and protocols are one means of providing direction and defining expectations and responsibilities for the health care professionals and organizations that care for children with fatal or potentially fatal medical conditions. As discussed in Chapter 8, they may also be useful in helping to prevent or resolve conflicts between parents and clinicians and among clinicians, for example, by clarifying the science base for medical interventions or by defining communication processes to reduce misunderstandings between clinicians and patients or families.

Insofar as possible, community institutions planning to implement guidelines or care protocols should start with up-to-date, evidence-based guidelines or recommendations that have been developed by experienced professional societies and other national groups and that, ideally, have been tested in practice settings. The rationale is to both reduce the demands on local institutions and improve the quality of the product. Unfortunately, as noted throughout this report, research findings on palliative, end-of-life, and bereavement care for children and families are limited. Even when research findings are available, they may be incomplete or in conflict. Thus, expert judgment and experience—as well as sound assessment methods and

---

[1]This discussion draws, among other sources, on IOM, 1990a, 1992, 2001b; Atkins and DiGuiseppi, 1998; Lohr et al., 1998; Woolf et al., 1999; Feder et al., 1999; Browman, 2001; Ellershaw et al., 2001; and Harris et al., 2001.

consensus development procedures—are essential in evaluating scientific evidence and in recommending courses of action in the absence of evidence. Credible and practical guidelines and protocols for palliative, end-of-life, and bereavement care should also consider the experience and perspectives of patients (when possible), family representatives, and others regularly involved in caring for patients who have fatal or potentially fatal medical conditions.

Even when methodologically sound national guidelines are available, roles also exist for local review and adaptation of such guidelines. One justification for local review and adaptation is to increase the sensitivity of care processes and procedures to specific institutional and community characteristics, including the institution's mission and priorities, the population it serves, the institution's financial and other resources, the community's resources and expectations, and state laws and regulations. Another justification is that the practical process of adapting protocols to local circumstances should promote a greater sense of local ownership and commitment to the protocols and the goals they are intended to serve. When local groups modify national guidelines, they should approach the task systematically and explain the reasons for any departures from these guidelines.

Comprehensive protocols to cover patient transfers and other events that cross institutional boundaries may require interorganizational or community-wide cooperation or agreements. Oregon provides one example of such cooperation. As part of more than a decade's work to improve end-of-life care in the state, a statewide task force has developed, implemented, and evaluated Physician Orders for Life-Sustaining Treatment (POLST)[2] as a tool to help patients have their wishes honored regardless of the site of care. This initiative has shown evidence of success (Tolle et al., 1998; Lee et al., 2000; Tolle and Tilden, 2002; see also http://www.lastacts.org/files/publications/polst0599.html).

In a few areas, interventions and care protocols are reasonably well defined and, in some cases, tested. For example, evidence-based guidelines for management of different kinds of pain, including cancer pain in children, have been developed and undergone several years of testing in the United States and elsewhere (see, e.g., AHCPR, 1994; Foley, 1994; Bookbinder et al., 1996; WHO, 1998; Du Pen et al., 1999). In addition, expectations for pain management are now articulated in accreditation standards

---

[2] The orders are presented in a bright pink document that is to be attached to the front of a patient's medical record in a hospital or nursing home. Oregon also has changed the scope of practice for emergency medical responders so that they can honor POLST provisions. In addition, the state has revised its advance directive statute and, in general, made comfort care a priority for dying patients (Tolle and Tilden, 2002).

and supporting statements devised by the Joint Commission on the Accreditation of Hospitals (JCAHO, 2001). Specific standards now state that "patients have the right to appropriate assessment and management of pain" (standard RI.1.2.8), "pain is assessed in all patients" (standard PE.1.4), and "patients are educated about pain and managing pain as part of treatment, as appropriate" (PF.3.4). Advocates have also adopted the phrase "pain: the fifth vital sign" to help increase professionals' awareness of pain and encourage the implementation of explicit pain management guidelines and protocols (APS, 1997).

The Joint Commission standards mention other aspects of palliative and end-of-life care. As noted in Chapter 5, one (RI.1.3.5) mentions pastoral care and other spiritual services (JCAHO, 1998). A broader standard (RI.1.2.7) states "the health care organization addresses care at the end of life" (JCAHO, 2001). The Commission explains the intent of the latter standard as covering

- provision of appropriate treatment for any primary and secondary symptoms, according to the wishes of the patient or the surrogate decision maker;
- aggressive and effective management of pain;
- sensitive issues such as autopsy and organ donation;
- respect for the patient's values, religion, and philosophy;
- involvement of the patient and, where appropriate, the family in every aspect of care; and
- attention to the psychological, social, emotional, spiritual, and cultural concerns of the patient and the family.

The committee believes that it is appropriate to generalize the expectation of aggressive and effective pain management to the aggressive and effective management of all serious symptoms. This would likely encourage more active efforts to develop evidence- and consensus-based guidelines for symptoms in addition to pain and to build a broader and stronger evidence base for effective symptom management (IOM, 1997; Goldman, 1999; ChIPPS, 2001; Levetown, 2001).

Unfortunately, the limited research on effective pharmacologic and other symptom management approaches for children is a concern. In some cases, symptom management and other guidelines for adult care may serve as models or starting points for pediatric guidelines, although the latter would likely have a more limited evidence base and more complex analytic task relating to children's developmental differences and other special dimensions of pediatric care. For example, as one resource, pediatric oncologists could look to the series of curriculum modules that the American Society of Clinical Oncology has developed for specific disease- and treatment-related symptoms and symptom control topics (ASCO, 2002). Notwithstanding the limited evidence base, the committee believes that practice guidelines and administrative protocols are, at a minimum, important tools for articulating institutional expectations and responsibilities and establishing a basis for evaluating processes and performance. Adoption of guidelines does not guarantee desired results. As another IOM committee warned in 1992, "guidelines for clinical practice are a promising but not a quick or sure strategy for improving and rationalizing the overall use of health care services. . . . Persistent commitment over the long term is required from both policymakers and health care professionals" (IOM, 1992, p. 4). The last decade has confirmed that assessment. Even when health care personnel agree with the basic message of a guideline (i.e., have identified, reviewed, evaluated, and accepted the guideline), formidable barriers to implementation exist, including habitual practice patterns, countervailing patient preferences, time pressures, financial disincentives, liability concerns, and lack of supporting information and administrative systems. Some barriers (e.g., inadequate information systems) can be acted on locally, at least in part, but other barriers (e.g., financial disincentives) lie largely beyond the reach of individual institutions and require system-level changes in policies and practices.

THE CHALLENGES OF COORDINATION AND CONTINUITY

Although the rationale for specialized pediatric services to serve seriously ill or injured children is persuasive, the system has some limitations. Many communities lack the population base and resources to support such services, so some children and families must travel long distances to get specialist and subspecialist care. They thus are separated from their normal sources of support including other family members, friends, and the child's usual physician. When the child and family return home, they may have to rely on professionals and providers with limited experience in caring for children with advanced illnesses or providing palliative and end-of-life care. The coordination, continuity, and quality of a child's care may suffer as a result, especially if follow-up protocols, consultation, and other support from specialist professionals and medical centers are limited.

When children can be treated in or near their home community, coordination and continuity can still be difficult and frustrating when multiple providers and services are involved. Even within a single institution, coordination and communication may fail during shift changes, discharge preparation, and other predictable transitions.

In parents' stories of their experiences with a child's life-threatening illness and death, two frequent themes are the burden of coordinating the many elements of their child's medical care in a fragmented care system and the difficulties of maintaining continuity in care and sustaining trusted relationships. Parents find themselves spending hours on the phone trying to identify, schedule, and coordinate providers and services and also struggling with health plan requirements and procedures. They may have to ensure that essential medical information and care plans (e.g., orders about life-sustaining care) accompany their child from one provider to another and still repeatedly explain the child's history and their experiences and preferences regarding the child's care.

Recognizing the financial, psychological, and other costs of poorly coordinated care, health care professionals, administrators, accreditation organizations, insurers, and regulators have created and refined a number of structures and processes for integrating diverse services and smoothing the transition of patients from one caregiver, care team, organization, or setting to another. They may fail in implementation for various reasons (e.g., poor information systems, inattentive management, inadequate resources), but the basic mechanisms are reasonably well accepted. These mechanisms, which may also serve cost control objectives, include the following:

- discharge planning procedures to ensure that patients leave hospitals, nursing homes, and other institutions when it is medically appropriate and when appropriate follow-up care has been planned and arranged;
- case management programs, which may coordinate both health and social services for patients and families, particularly patients with serious chronic problems and limited financial resources;
- disease management programs to improve the continuity, consistency, and effectiveness of care, including self-care, for individuals with specific medical problems such as diabetes or asthma;
- standardized procedures for patient transfers and follow-up among hospitals, home care agencies, hospices, and other organizations that have overlapping service areas;
- patient, family, and general community educational efforts intended to inform people of programs that may assist them in obtaining and coordinating services and of steps they need to take to navigate the care system; and
- medical information systems that follow people across settings and providers of care, so that plans of care, preferences, and records are accessible whenever needed.

These and similar arrangements have not generally been designed with the needs of dying patients and their families in mind. Most could, however, be adapted or adjusted to include objectives and procedures focused on the coordination and continuity of palliative, end-of-life, and bereavement care for adults and children.

In addition to the mechanisms identified above, a number of other coordination strategies have been developed to assist children with special health care needs and their families.[3] The "medical home"—one broad approach for these children and families—is discussed below as is a strategy to integrate and coordinate palliative care for children hospitalized with life-threatening conditions. Both can be seen as elements of larger initiatives that attempt to put the needs and preferences of children and their families at the center of health care systems.

Although many strategies focus on coordinating multiple providers and sites of care, strategies to preserve continuity of care are also important. Continuity is a complex concept that overlaps with but is not identical to coordination of care. Fletcher and colleagues (1984, p. 409) distinguished between "a thread" that ties episodes of care together (continuity) and the relationship of various components of care (coordination) but also noted that the terms may be used interchangeably. As used here, continuity implies that needed services will be provided without disruption. It also implies that a child and family are able to maintain trusted relationships and patterns of care that have been forged and tested over time, especially during the course of a child's serious illness.[4] With discontinuous relationships, it is difficult if not impossible for individual physicians and other members of the care team to promise that they will "be there" when patients and families need them (Lynn et al., 2000).

Some studies suggest that continuity increases patient and family satisfaction with care and can reduce hospitalization and, possibly, costs. For example, one recent cross-sectional study on continuity of care in a primary care clinic reported that continuity of care was associated with higher parent ratings on items about providers' respect for parents' views, careful listening, and understandable explanations (Christakis et al., 2002; see also Gill and Mainous, 1998; Gill et al., 2000; Christakis et al., 1999, 2001).

---

[3]As discussed in Chapter 2, these children "have or are at increased risk for a chronic physical, developmental, behavioral or emotional condition and . . . also require health and related services of a type or amount beyond that required by children generally" (McPherson et al., 1998, p. 138). Many of these children have conditions such as vision loss, mental retardation, autism, and serious learning disorders that are not expected to lead to death in childhood. A small percentage, however, have congenital anomalies, progressive neurodegenerative diseases, and other conditions that are often or always fatal.

[4]Sometimes continuity refers more narrowly to a "usual source of care," which could be a clinic with no guarantee of continuity with a particular caregiver. Other dimensions may include continuity of records and information. See, for example, Donaldson (2001).

Continuity is usually valued, but other considerations must also be weighed, for example, a family's desire to bring a child home rather than stay at a distant, specialized treatment center. Further, hospital or hospice rules, health plan requirements, licensure restrictions, and other policies can limit continuity, although creative and persistent families, social workers, physicians, and other team members may find ways around some restrictions in individual situations. Nonetheless, unless institutions establish systematic processes and protocols for handling special situations, arranging waivers to rules, and, more generally, making continuity planning a part of the care process, it will be difficult to sustain continuity of care and keep the focus on the child and family rather than on institutional requirements and conventions.

When primary responsibility for a child's care shifts, those who have cared for a child may still seek ways to maintain some degree of continued communication and involvement with the child and family. If a child has been appropriately referred to hospice after the failure of chemotherapy and other cancer treatment, the hospice team and the oncology team can encourage continued relationships, for example, through regular phone calls. Similarly, a child's primary care physician can call to keep in touch while a child is under a specialist's care.

Child- and Family-Centered Care

General

As described by advocates, the movement for family-centered care targets the subordination of the needs of the child and family to the needs of the health care system (see, e.g., Shelton et al., 1987; Johnson et al., 1992; Shelton and Stepanek, 1994; see also Harrison, 1993). Although the ideas championed by this movement have roots that extend back to the 1970s and before, they were given particular emphasis in the late 1980s by advocates for families whose children have special health care needs (as defined in Chapter 2).

The commonly cited elements of family-centered care for children with special health care needs do not explicitly include informing children, involving them in goal setting and care planning, and respecting their individual values and concerns. One reason may be the movement's focus on children who have cognitive limitations or serious emotional disorders. Also, parents have legal authority to make decisions for their child and are usually the child's primary caregivers.

Beyond the special needs community, proponents of patient-centered care have argued for understanding care "through the patient's eyes" (Gerteis et al, 1993). A child-adapted version of that perspective would

---

BOX 6.1
Elements of Child- and Family-Centered Health Care

• Recognizing that the family is the constant in a child's life, while the role and importance of health care and social service systems vary and the people staffing those systems change
• Understanding and accommodating the individual strengths and characteristics of the child and family, including their coping strategies and their cultural, ethnic, religious, and other values
• Sharing unbiased, timely, complete, responsive, and understandable information with families about their child's diagnosis, prognosis, and care options
• Sharing information with the child and involving the child in goal setting and care planning, consistent with the child's developmental status and preferences and the family's values
• Promoting and assisting collaboration between families and professionals at all levels (i.e., in direct patient care, organizational processes and decisions, and community- or system-wide policies and practices)
• Designing sustainable care processes and care systems that meet the differing developmental needs of infants, children, and adolescents
• Developing care processes, systems, and policies—within both institutions and communities—that respond to child and family needs for flexibility, continuity, emotional and financial support, cultural and ethnic sensitivity, and education about caregiving responsibilities
• Encouraging and assisting family support groups, peer counseling, and other lines of family-to-family communication
• Encouraging child-to-child lines of support and communication, consistent with the child's developmental status and preferences and the family's values

---

SOURCES: Adapted from Shelton et al., 1987; Johnson et al., 1992; and Shelton and Stepanek, 1994.

---

attempt to understand pediatric care "through the child's eyes." To that end, the committee recommended in Chapter 4 that children with life-threatening medical conditions be involved in care planning and decisionmaking, consistent with their intellectual and emotional maturity and with the family's background and values.

In Box 6.1, the committee has amended and supplemented the commonly cited core elements of family-centered care to add explicitly the recognition and involvement of the child whenever possible. In addition to adding child-centered elements, the list of core elements also mentions education of family caregivers. This reflects the importance of appropriately training family caregivers to provide care that is often provided by nurses or other trained health care personnel.

The Medical Home

The "medical home" is a core component of strategies to implement the elements of family-centered care for children. The concept has its fullest expression as a means of improving the continuity and coordination of care for children with special health care needs and eventually supporting the successful transition of these children to adult services. Insofar as possible, the goal is to meet all of the child's and the family's needs—medical, psychosocial, educational—in the local community.

The medical home concept has been developed and promoted by a coalition including the American Academy of Pediatrics (AAP), the federal Maternal and Child Health Bureau, Family Voices, and other groups (AAP, 1992, 1995b, 1999b). As defined by the Maternal and Child Health Bureau (MCHB, 2000a), "a medical home is the collaborative effort between primary care providers and children with special health care needs and their families to ensure that care is accessible, family-centered, continuous, comprehensive, coordinated, compassionate, and delivered in a culturally competent environment" (MCHB, 2000a). The ideal elements of the medical home, as described by the AAP, are listed in Box 6.2. Some of these elements

---

BOX 6.2
Ideal Elements of the Medical Home for Children

1. Provision of preventive care including, but not restricted to, immunizations, growth and development assessments, appropriate screening, health care supervision, and patient and parental counseling about health and psychosocial issues
2. Assurance of ambulatory and inpatient care for acute illnesses, 24 hours a day, 7 days a week; during the working day, after hours, and on weekends, 52 weeks of the year
3. Provision of care over an extended period of time to enhance continuity
4. Identification of the need for subspecialty consultation and referrals and (the ways to obtain these services); provision of medical information about the patient to the consultant; evaluation of the consultant's recommendations; implementation of recommendations that are indicated and appropriate; and interpretation of these to the family
5. Interaction with school and community agencies to be certain that special health needs of the individual child are addressed
6. Maintenance of a central record and database containing all pertinent medical information about the child, including information about hospitalizations; this record should be accessible, but confidentiality must be ensured

---

SOURCE: AAP, 1992.

193

are in place but the concept remains, for the most part, an ideal rather than a generally implemented reality.

The AAP notes that geographic barriers, personnel constraints, practice patterns, and economic and social forces make the ideal medical home unobtainable for many children. For example, many children with special health care needs are covered by Medicaid, but reimbursement for physician services and capitation rates for Medicaid managed care plans are so low that they deter pediatricians from providing that ideal (see Chapter 7).

The goals of the medical home and the goals of palliative care and end-of-life care for children are fully compatible. Efforts to implement the medical home concept for the larger population of children with special health care needs should benefit the smaller group of children who die of complex chronic conditions. These efforts may also provide models for the coordinated care of children with more acute medical problems who alternate for shorter periods between inpatient and community care before they die. In turn, even though generalist pediatricians and family practitioners will usually care for relatively few children who die, their preparation in the basic principles of pediatric palliative care can benefit the much larger population of children with serious medical conditions that are not expected to prove fatal in childhood. (Chapter 9 examines education and training in palliative and end-of-life care for generalist and specialist pediatricians and family practitioners.)

Pediatric Advanced Illness Care Coordination

One strategy for coordinating care that focuses specifically on patients with fatal or potentially fatal diagnoses emphasizes communication and decisionmaking. Following a model originally developed for adults (Tobin and Lindsey, 1998), the Pediatric Advanced Illness Care Coordination (PAICC) program is intended to integrate and standardize pediatric palliative care within the routines of medical care for children with serious medical conditions (Himelstein et al., 2002). The approach also reflects current principles of case management and disease management.

The adult program is operating in 40 institutions in the United States (Dan Tobin, M.D., The Life Institute, personal communication, March 6, 2002). The pediatric program is being introduced in a number of medical centers around the country including The Children's Hospital at The Cleveland Clinic, the Children's Hospital Wisconsin, Hackensack University Medical Center, and the University of Texas Health Sciences Center at San Antonio. The care coordination program can work in tandem with different specialty care teams and with the medical home of a child with special health care needs.

Two central features of the pediatric program are the designation of a care coordinator to work with health care teams and families and the availability of three manuals—one for the child's main physician and other caregivers, one for the care coordinator, and one for parents. The care coordinator keeps the patient and family at the center of care, with a focus on their information needs and psychosocial concerns. He or she also initiates conversations about end-of-life issues and decisions and coordinates and orchestrates care—possibly providing some care but also helping families find, obtain, and coordinate resources. The coordinator offers information and support services to parents while making clear to parents that they can call the coordinator for assistance even if they do not want to accept the services.

The manual for care coordinators is a training guide that includes modules on communicating compassionately and effectively with children and families about diagnosis and prognosis, planning and decisionmaking, helping families cope with fear, and supporting them in preparing for death. The manual for families is intended to help parents gain some control over the experience of having a child with a life-threatening condition. It urges them "not to put this manual down because you do not want to think about the worst" (Hilden and Tobin, 2002, p. 6).

Key elements of planning for PAICC include the identification of resources for palliative and end-of-life care within hospitals and in communities, the identification of sources of referrals for pediatric palliative care (e.g., oncologists, intensive care nurses, discharge planners, health plan case managers, chaplains), and the assessment of clinical services, inpatient palliative care resources, relevant administrative procedures, and potential barriers to program implementation. Other elements include initial and ongoing training of program staff, strategies for educating providers and winning their support, procedures for introducing the program to patients and families, processes and tools for documenting communication and information, and formal evaluation of processes of care and outcomes. Among the outcomes sought by the PAICC model are

- increases in (1) the frequency and timeliness of referrals to palliative care experts and (2) the interval between do-not-resuscitate (DNR) and similar orders or advance care directives and the time of death;
- improved documentation of communication about end-of-life care;
- increases in staff satisfaction with providing end-of-life care and serving children with advanced illness; and
- improvements in children's quality of life and in the satisfaction of children and families with the care and information provided.

Any strategy to improve the coordination, continuity, and effectiveness of care for seriously ill children and their families depends on the commitment, preparation, and support of an array of health care professionals. The following section first discusses individual categories of professionals. It then considers various kinds of pediatric care teams, which also are intended to serve as a means of coordinating the care needed from different categories of health professionals.

HEALTH CARE PROFESSIONALS

To evaluate and meet children's special physical, cognitive, and emotional needs as they develop from infancy to adulthood, an array of specialized health care professionals and health care organizations have evolved over the last century and more. These professionals include general and specialist pediatricians, pediatric nurse practitioners and nurses, child psychologists, child-life specialists, pediatric social workers, and others with training in various aspects of care for infants, children, and adolescents. Children's hospitals specialize in treating ill or injured children, and some home care and residential care facilities also concentrate on care for children.

In addition, children may receive care from professionals and organizations that do not specialize in pediatric services. For example, a seriously injured child may be taken to the nearest Level 1 trauma center but may then be transferred to a center specializing in pediatric emergency and intensive care. The transfer may also be from more to less specialized care, for instance, when children who have returned home after treatment at a center specializing in pediatric oncology may receive follow-up hospital care at a community hospital. This mix of specialized pediatric and other providers complicates efforts to describe, assess, and improve the provision of palliative, end-of-life, and bereavement care to children and their families.

Physicians and Nurse Practitioners

Any physician can legally care for a patient of any age, but pediatricians are uniquely educated to diagnose and treat children. In 1995, data from the American Medical Association showed 50,000 physicians in the United States who designated themselves as practicing pediatricians (board certified and non-board certified) (Randolph et al., 1997; DeAngelis et al., 2000). More than 90 percent were involved in direct patient care.

Family practitioners are also trained to provide primary care to both adults and children, more often older children and adolescents rather than infants and preschoolers (AAP, 1998b). According to data from the 1980s and earlier, family practitioners provided 15 to 25 percent of physician services received by children, possibly more in rural areas (Budetti et al., 1982; Abt Associates, 1991). In addition, about 5,800 pediatric nurse practitioners have been certified (DeAngelis et al., 2000). The amount of care provided to children by specialists and subspecialists who care mainly for adults is not documented (Gruskin et al., 2000).

Because most children are healthy and require mainly preventive and other primary care, general pediatricians and family practitioners are less likely than generalist physicians caring for adults to encounter and care for patients with fatal or potentially fatal diagnoses. When they do encounter such child patients, they typically refer them to appropriate pediatric oncologists, cardiologists, or other subspecialists. The committee identified no data on the nature or extent of generalist involvement in the care of children with life-threatening medical conditions and likewise found no information on the nature or extent of clinical guidance or consultation provided to generalist pediatricians by local or regional specialists. Although committee members were aware that some managed care organizations require that children be returned to the care of primary care physicians if it is judged that continued curative or life-prolonging treatments will be ineffective, they located no systematic information on such policies or their consequences.

Pediatric subspecialists vary considerably in the amount and kind of care and support they provide to seriously ill or injured children.[5] For example, radiologists or surgeons who treat pediatric cancer patients provide essential services but often have relatively limited ongoing involvement and do not have primary responsibility for the child's care. Pediatric emergency medicine specialists may provide very intensive services but for a relatively limited period before a seriously injured or acutely ill child dies or becomes the responsibility of a critical care specialist. In contrast, pediatric oncologists, neurologists, cardiologists, pulmonologists, and certain other specialists may have close relationships with children and families that extend for years. Neonatologists, obstetricians, and other specialists, including the nurses who staff neonatal intensive care units and delivery rooms, provide intensive care—sometimes briefly, sometimes for months—for a substantial proportion of children who die.

---

[5]The American Board of Pediatrics recognizes 13 pediatric subspecialties: adolescent medicine, cardiology, critical care medicine, developmental–behavioral pediatrics, emergency medicine, endocrinology, gastroenterology, hematology–oncology, infectious disease, neonatology–perinatology, nephrology, pulmonology, and rheumatology. Certificates are awarded in conjunction with other specialty boards in the areas of clinical laboratory immunology, medical toxicology, neurodevelopmental disabilities, and sports medicine (ABP, 2002).

Each category of specialist should be prepared to provide palliative, end-of-life, and bereavement support appropriate for the children and families they serve. In August 2000, the American Academy of Pediatrics issued a policy statement stating that "all general and subspecialty pediatricians, family physicians, pain specialists, and pediatric surgeons need to become familiar and comfortable with the provision of palliative care to children" (AAP, 2000g, p.356). Pediatric specialty groups are also beginning to recognize the importance of more systematic attention to palliative and end-of-life care for children and their families. For example, the Children's Oncology Group has organized an End-of-Life Care Subcommittee that will work to develop the evidence base for palliative care within the framework of clinical trials (COG, 2001). Chapter 9 describes other initiatives sponsored by pediatric professionals that focus on the education of clinicians.

Within the relatively new field of palliative medicine, the emphasis is overwhelmingly on care for adults, especially elderly adults who account for more than 70 percent of Americans who die each year.[6] A small cadre of pediatric palliative care specialists is, however, emerging to provide leadership and support for the larger pediatric care community.

Nurses

Both parents had to work. They were very, very poor people. . . . So the nurses just did everything. Every single bit of love those children had in their last moments came from the nurses, and you know that was a gift.

Salvador Avila, parent, 2001

For nurses as for physicians, specialized training in pediatric nursing recognizes children's unique developmental needs. Further specialization in neonatal and critical care reflects the very particular demands of caring for premature infants, infants with severe congenital anomalies, and critically ill or injured children. Other organized areas of nurse specialization include pediatric oncology and cardiology.

Nurses play a central role in providing day-to-day palliative care and home hospice care for adults. Experienced hospice nurses tend, however, to

---

[6]Palliative medicine is not a formally recognized medical specialty. Groups such as the American Academy of Hospice and Palliative Care Medicine (AHPCM) have, however, organized to build the field by promoting and providing education, research, clinical practice guidelines, public information, and advocacy. AHPCM also has developed certification standards, which do not distinguish between adult and pediatric care; the organization has certified some pediatricians as palliative care specialists.

have no training in pediatric care, and experienced pediatric nurses tend to have little training in palliative and end-of-life care.

Even experienced hospice nurses and other hospice staff may fear caring for dying children and find it very stressful, especially if they do not receive specialized training and ongoing support. Some nurses may also find it hard to separate their professional roles from their feelings as parents (Sumner, 2001).

More guidance on pediatric palliative nursing is becoming available. A comprehensive new textbook of palliative nursing (Ferrell and Coyle, 2001) includes three chapters specific to pediatric care (Hinds et al., 2001; Levetown, 2001; Sumner, 2001), and the major text on palliative medicine has from its first edition in 1993 included chapters on care of children (Doyle et al., 1998). (Other educational initiatives are described in Chapter 9.)

In the course of its work, the committee heard concerns that a nationwide shortage of nurses extends to pediatric care, especially pediatric home health care (NAPHACC, 2001). Another issue for home health care nurses is their isolation, which limits their opportunities to learn from peers as well as from the on-site training programs that may be available in hospital settings. Similarly, hospice nurses may also find that visiting patients at home, while rewarding in many respects, leaves them feeling somewhat isolated from other team members. Joint visits with other team members, team meetings, and other strategies, such as joint hospice-hospital or hospice-home care programs, may encourage learning and reduce isolation.

In its statement to the committee, the American Association of Critical Care Nurses (AACCN, 2001) noted that despite the time nurses spend with children in intensive care and with their families, nurses are not the key decisionmakers and are not always consulted in the development of a child's care plan. One result, the group suggested, is that the care plan may be based on incomplete information about the child and family. Implementation of the plan may also suffer as a result of unacknowledged differences in physician and nurse perceptions.

Even nurses who never expected to encounter seriously ill children may become involved in caring for children with life-threatening medical conditions. As discussed further below, as the number of medically fragile children enrolled in schools has increased, school officials and school nurses have been challenged to support medication regimens for these children, to prepare for cardiac arrest and other medical emergencies, and to cope with other challenges once largely unknown to school health personnel (AAP, 2000d; see also Chapter 8). The school nurse also may educate a child's teachers, other school personnel, and the child's classmates and their families about an ill child's condition and ways of easing the child's reentry and continuation in school.

Social Work and Mental Health Professionals

Child psychologists and psychiatrists, as well as social workers, may be called on to provide psychological care for seriously ill or injured children and for their families, before and after a child's death. Social workers have typically been an integral part of palliative and hospice care teams, available to families (parents especially) for help with emotional and practical concerns, including identifying community resources (e.g., home health agencies, funeral homes). In the hospital emergency department and intensive care unit, they often serve as the communication link between parents and the team caring for a seriously injured or suddenly ill child. In these stressful and often confused situations, their role is to help ensure that needed information is successfully communicated and that parents have an adequate opportunity to raise questions and concerns so that they can more effectively participate in decisionmaking about their child's care.

The entry of child psychologists and psychiatrists into the field of palliative care is a relatively recent development. Their inclusion in the care team extends the emotional care available to seriously ill children and their siblings, particularly in assessing and treating symptoms such as depression and anxiety that can substantially diminish an ill child's quality of life.

One important goal for all staff in a children's hospital is to help children maintain as much normal life as possible. Child-life specialists contribute to this goal. Based on a 1998 survey, the National Association of Children's Hospitals and Related Institutions (NACHRI) reported that 97 percent of 112 responding hospitals employed at least one child-life specialist (NACHRI, 1998). Similarly, the American Academy of Pediatrics has reported that 97 percent of children's hospitals and 82 percent of hospitals with pediatric residency training programs (in general or children's hospitals) employed child-life specialists (AAP, 2000c). Large physician groups may also use child-life specialists.

Child-life specialists do not fit neatly into usual professional categories. As experts in communicating with children, they can help "translate" between clinicians and children. They may engage children in developmentally supportive and therapeutic play and in therapies using art, music, and dance. As discussed in Chapter 5, these techniques may help children express and cope with difficult emotions and offer relief from the stress of illness and medical treatment. In addition, child-life specialists may employ distraction and other behavioral techniques to help manage pain and other symptoms. In children's hospitals, they also help provide supportive environments for siblings of sick children to play and interact with siblings of other children who are coping with similar situations. Particularly for children hospitalized repeatedly or for extended periods, child-life specialists become familiar people with whom children can safely share fears, worries, and hopes that might otherwise be unexpressed. With the child's permission, these concerns may be communicated to parents and the care team. Child-life specialists typically work "9 to 5" and, thus, are not available to support children, families, and physicians when crises arise outside those hours. Unlike psychiatrists but like nurses and, often, clinical social workers and clinical psychologists, child-life specialists cannot directly bill insurers for their services. In times of particular fiscal stress, their services are vulnerable to discontinuation.

Providers of bereavement care may come from a variety of backgrounds including social work, psychology, and nursing. Helping bereaved people may be a full-time responsibility or one aspect of the work of a chaplain, social worker, funeral director, hospice volunteer, or other interested individual.

Other Personnel

Chaplains provide spiritual care to patients and families in hospitals and other care settings. They also provide emotional support and comfort and practical assistance to families coping with the death of a child (Sommer, 2001). As discussed in Chapter 5, provisions for spiritual care are part of hospital accreditation and Medicare hospice requirements. In general, however, the extent of chaplains' involvement with dying children and their families is little documented or evaluated.

Hospital teachers provide individualized and group learning for patients well enough to leave their beds during the day. They also make rounds to help children who are confined to their rooms. Other teachers specialize in home tutoring. Hospital and home teachers can establish close relationships with children, who may feel comfortable sharing concerns with a home teacher rather than adding to their parents' worries and stress (Weil, 2001). In addition, although such links are more the exception than the rule, videoconferencing and other technologies provide opportunities to help homebound children maintain contact with children, teachers, and resources at their regular school (Bowman, 2001).

Phlebotomists, respiratory therapists, physical therapists, and others who are skilled in working with small patients can reduce the physical and emotional distress caused by diagnostic and therapeutic procedures. Ideally, they will have equipment (e.g., needles and other intravenous equipment, breathing tubes, oxygen masks) appropriate for children of different sizes, and they will also develop skills in reassuring or distracting children and otherwise reducing their fears and anxieties. General hospitals with no pediatric unit are unlikely to have such specialized personnel and equipment.

Pediatric Care Teams

Multidisciplinary care teams are a feature of much pediatric emergency, chronic, and acute care, especially for children with complex conditions that require a period of inpatient evaluation and treatment. Thus, the neonatal intensive care team concentrates on the specialized needs of fragile newborns (including premature infants and those with serious congenital anomalies) and their families. The pediatric oncology team cares for children with cancer and their families. Emergency care teams work intensively for a compressed period of time to assess and stabilize children before transferring them to other care teams. Although health services are usually not organized to encourage it, a care team or some members of the team may provide both inpatient and outpatient care (e.g., inpatient and outpatient chemotherapy).

Regardless of the site of care, the usual goals of pediatric care teams working with children with serious medical conditions are multifaceted. They include

• providing and coordinating care appropriate to all the physical, emotional, spiritual, and practical needs of the individual child and family including family needs after the death of a child;
• caring for the child and family as a unit;
• encouraging information sharing and consistency among team members and relevant others so that families do not receive conflicting or confusing messages from professional caregivers;
• integrating family members into the care team and, thus, involving them more fully in establishing the goals of care and in making decisions; and
• preparing for and coordinating transitions in the site or emphasis of care and providing continuity.

Ideally, team care is not only multidisciplinary (i.e., involves members from several disciplines) but also truly interdisciplinary (i.e., "is more than the sum of its parts"). Although the terms multidisciplinary and interdisciplinary are often used interchangeably, as used here, interdisciplinary refers to structures and processes that (1) encourage individual team members to understand and incorporate the perspectives of other disciplines into their own assessments and practices (consistent with licensure and other reasonable constraints), (2) reduce disciplinary misunderstandings, discord among team members, and gaps or discontinuities in care, and (3) forge more productive relationships and practices among individuals with different disciplinary backgrounds.

The composition of pediatric care teams will naturally vary depending on the nature of the child's medical problem and the settings and kinds of services needed. The resources, traditions, and philosophy of the employing organization may also influence team composition. In general, however, the core of an inpatient team caring for a seriously ill or injured child includes a primary subspecialist physician (e.g., pediatric oncologist or cardiologist), one or more nurse specialists, a psychologist or social worker, perhaps one or more residents or fellows, and possibly a child-life specialist. Other subpecialists (potentially, but at present rarely, including a palliative care specialist) are brought in as needed. Supporting members of the team may include pharmacists, respiratory therapists, physical therapists, genetic counselors, dieticians, and chaplains.

Team care is widely viewed as central to inpatient palliative care and home hospice programs for both adults and children and their families. To the extent that inpatient palliative care teams exist in either adult or pediatric care, they generally serve as consultants to other specialty care teams (e.g., oncology, cardiology, nephrology) that retain primary responsibility for a patient's care, especially for children who are continuing to receive curative or life-prolonging therapies. The core of an inpatient consulting team may be nurses supported by a physician who is involved as needed. If the focus of care is primarily palliative and home based and if pediatric hospice services are available in the community and accepted by the parents, a home hospice care team may assume primary responsibility for care of the child and family. Again, nurses usually play a central role in hospice care teams.

When a child goes home for care that is primarily palliative, some families may prefer that the child's oncology or other care team continue to take the lead, especially if the child and family are local. Geographic distance can, however, make this approach to home care impractical, and some families may prefer to have the child's general pediatrician or family practitioner assume primary responsibility for the care of a child at home. As noted earlier, managed care rules may require such a transfer of responsibility if the focus of care shifts from cure or life prolongation to palliation.

Despite their seeming ubiquity, little systematic research appears to have focused on the numbers, structure, or performance of different kinds of pediatric care teams.[7] Given (as reported below) the limited number of

---

[7]Team care is often a part of a multi-element intervention in which the individual elements or processes of care are not evaluated separately. Some relevant research may be categorized under "key words" that involve related concepts such as "care coordination." For example, some research has examined the contributions or acceptance of specific professionals (e.g., nurse practitioners, social workers) in different environments (see, e.g., Burl et al., 1994; Inati et al., 1994; Aquilino et al., 1999; Dechairo-Marino et al., 2001). Team care is often associated with the use of formal clinical practice guidelines and quality improvement initiatives to

inpatient and hospice palliative care programs for children, the number of specialized teams providing pediatric palliative and end-of-life care cannot be large. Increased implementation of pediatric palliative care will almost certainly involve more interactions between palliative care teams (both inpatient and home hospice based) and oncology, neonatal, and other care teams. Descriptive research to map the nature and frequency of such interactions among teams would provide useful preparation for subsequent assessments of performance (see Chapter 10).

In general, the effectiveness of care teams has been linked to conditions such as (1) appropriate composition and size of the team, (2) sufficient financial and other resources (e.g., information and communication technologies), (3) successful processes for setting goals, coordinating activities, evaluating performance (both processes of care and outcomes), and preventing or resolving conflicts; and (4) supportive professional and organizational cultures, (see, e.g., Fried and Rundall, 1996; Shortell et al., 1994; Opie, 1997; Mickan and Rodger, 2000). The fourth area—supportive professional and organizational cultures—is widely viewed as a major barrier to successful team functioning. In particular, the preparation of health care professionals to work in teams has been limited.

Although health professions education, in general, has a strong disciplinary and hierarchical character, preparation for teamwork is increasingly recognized as essential (see, e.g., O'Neil et al., 1998; Knebel et al., 2001; see also residency program requirements listed at http://www.acgme.org). Chapter 9 notes the importance of preparation for team care in undergraduate, graduate, and continuing health professions education. Chapter 10 urges more research into the dynamics of team care in different contexts (e.g., inpatient and outpatient care, primary and specialist care), its outcomes, and methods of successfully preparing professionals to function as members of teams.

ORGANIZATIONS AND SETTINGS OF CARE

As described in Chapter 2, more than 56 percent of child deaths (under age 19) in 1999 occurred in inpatient hospital settings, and another 16 percent occurred in outpatient hospital sites (primarily the emergency department). Approximately 5 percent of children were declared dead on arrival at a hospital. Children, unlike adults, rarely die in nursing homes, although some severely disabled children die in other residential care facili-

---

reduce unwanted variability in care processes and outcomes. Some studies suggest problems in the multidisciplinary care component of such initiatives, for example, staff turnover or interpersonal conflict (see, e.g., Qualls and Czirr, 1988; Weissman et al., 1997).

ties. For children with complex chronic conditions, the proportion of deaths occurring at home has been growing but is still smaller than for adults with such conditions. For both groups, most will receive inpatient care during advanced stages or exacerbations of their illness.

Inpatient Care

Because so many children die in the hospital and because inpatient curative and life-prolonging treatments so often continue for children until death is imminent, the availability and quality of inpatient palliative, end-of-life, and bereavement care are important for these children and their families. Even though increased availability and acceptance of pediatric home hospice programs may reduce the amount of hospital care provided to children with complex chronic conditions that end in death, inpatient care at the end of life is likely to remain more important for children than for adults.

Inpatient care may increase a parent's sense of security and relieve the family of complex care responsibilities, but it usually affords less privacy, intimacy, and family access and control than does home care (Chaffee, 2001). Whether a hospital specializes in pediatric care may affect these and many other dimensions of care for children with life-threatening medical conditions.

General Hospitals

We were shipped back to our local stupid hospital for the last blood transfusions. The staff was used to broken bones and healable stuff. They hadn't a clue about cancer and the finality of Eric's situation.

Becky Wooten, parent, 2001

Given the limited number and geographic distribution of specialized pediatric emergency and inpatient services, many children with life-threatening medical problems and their families must depend on general hospitals for care. In addition, children and families served by children's hospitals distant from their home community must often rely, at some point, on a local general hospital for follow-up or crisis care, and some children will die there. This makes the quality of pediatric palliative services an issue not just for children's hospitals but for any hospital that cares for children.

The pediatric services of general hospitals vary considerably, ranging from minimal in small rural and community hospitals to intensive and sophisticated in large medical centers. Clinical services provided by pediatric units in these latter centers may differ little if at all from those provided in centers with pediatric units that describe themselves as children's hospitals.

A recent Washington state study reported that 80 percent of the state's nonpediatric hospitals provided some pediatric services and that one-quarter (mostly large hospitals) had separate pediatric units (EMSCWS, 2000). Of the 64 percent of state hospitals with intensive care units (ICUs), two-thirds provided intensive care services to children. Exactly equivalent national statistics are not readily available, but data from the American Hospital Association's 1998 survey of community hospitals indicate that about half of the 4,600 responding hospitals provided some pediatric medical or surgical care (not differentiating between pediatric and nonpediatric hospitals) (American Hospital Association, 2000). About two-thirds of the responding hospitals reported providing (adult) ICU services, but only 9 and 17 percent of responding hospitals reported that they provided pediatric or neonatal intensive care services, respectively.

Children's Hospitals and Related Institutions

In 2001, NACHRI, the association of children's hospitals and related institutions had 161 members, 47 of which were self-governing, freestanding, comprehensive children's hospitals located in 24 states, the District of Columbia, and Canada (NACHRI, 2001a,b). Other member hospitals function as units of larger hospitals, most of them university based. A few members are specialty hospitals that limit services to specific conditions such as neuromuscular or orthopedic problems. A number of hospitals with significant pediatric services are not members of NACHRI, but the committee found little summary information about these institutions.

One emphasis of modern children's hospitals is the design and construction of facilities that incorporate child- and family-friendly physical elements, for example, nonfluorescent lighting, carpeting, play areas in waiting rooms, gardens, and family beds in patient rooms (Komiske, 1999). One potential advantage of freestanding children's hospitals is that they do not have to compete with adult medicine for space or attention when facilities are constructed or remodeled.

Freestanding children's hospitals, although they represent just 1 percent of all hospitals, are said to serve an estimated one-quarter of hospitalized children with congenital or chronic disease, and in combination with pediatric units of major teaching hospitals, they care for a substantial majority of these children (NACHRI, 2001a). In response to surveys, NAHCRI member hospitals have reported that 57 percent of their inpatient admissions, 68 percent of their inpatient days, and 76 percent of their inpatient charges relate to care for children with congenital or chronic conditions.

Many of these conditions are not, however, considered likely to prove fatal in childhood.

The focus of children's hospitals on children with serious medical problems is also suggested by data showing that catastrophic cases (those generating charges of more than $50,000) account for about 5.5 percent of cases in freestanding, acute care children's hospitals compared to 1.5 percent in pediatric programs of general hospitals (NACHRI, 1999). Almost half of the children cared for by children's hospitals are poor or uninsured, emphasizing the "safety-net" role played by many of these hospitals in their communities.

Care for critically ill newborns is sufficiently specialized that they are typically cared for in specialized neonatal intensive care units (NICUs) while infants, older children, and adolescents with critical medical problems are cared for in pediatric intensive care units (PICUs). Although specific figures are lacking, a substantial fraction of children who die will die in these units and will do so following decisions to limit life-support (see Chapter 4).

On average, intensive care beds account for about one-quarter of all beds in freestanding, acute care children's hospitals, compared to about one-tenth of pediatric beds in general hospitals (NACHRI, 1999). Like trauma centers, NICUs and PICUs are classified into different levels. For example, Level III NICUs are expected to serve the highest-risk neonates and to have consultation and transfer agreements with hospitals that have Level I and Level II units or no units.

For cancer and certain other serious conditions, specialized diagnostic, treatment, and research centers have developed, usually as units of major university-based children's or other hospitals. Some research suggests that specialized pediatric cancer centers are linked to better survival outcomes for children with cancer (Meadows et al., 1983; Kramer et al., 1984; Stiller, 1988; Wagner et al., 1995). The committee located no studies documenting differences in quality-of-life outcomes.

In guidelines on cancer centers, the AAP noted that safe but "resolute" use of the treatments (e.g., chemotherapy, radiation therapy) that are emphasized at these centers can have "devastating morbidity and appreciable mortality" (AAP, 1997b, p. 139). The guidelines do not, however, mention specifically the corresponding need for intensive and effective pain and other symptom management capabilities and for psychological, spiritual, and other support for children undergoing these treatments and for their families.[8] An earlier statement on pediatric cardiology centers likewise did

---

[8]The guidelines include a general reference to family support services and note the role of social workers is assisting with family fear, anxiety, and worry. They do not specifically mention grief and bereavement support.

not mention palliative care (AAP, 1991). The recent AAP policy statement on palliative care strongly endorses offering such care early in the course of illness for children with an "ultimately terminal condition" (AAP, 2000g). In addition, recent AAP (2001b) guidelines for pediatric emergency medical facilities called for explicit policies related to death in the emergency department and to DNR orders. Unlike earlier (1995) guidelines, the new guidelines do not explicitly mention support and follow-up for grieving families.

Although children's hospitals may emphasize child- and family-friendly environments, one area of concern has been the harsh nature of the traditional NICU with its bright lights, noise, frequent handling, and frequent invasive and painful procedures. Parents of premature infants have noted the lack of research justifying the traditional NICU environment and urged less invasive care and more access for parents and other family members (Harrison, 1993). Recent AAP (2000a) guidelines on the prevention and management of pain and stress in neonates mention the need to minimize noxious environmental stimuli, and an earlier statement focused specifically on noise (AAP, 1997c). Such efforts to "humanize" neonatal intensive care should benefit all fragile neonates—those who survive and those who die—and their families. They also provide an opportunity for research to assess and improve infant quality of life as well as to reduce morbidity and mortality.

The social environment of neonatal and pediatric intensive care may also be unfriendly. For example, time and space restrictions on family access to a critically ill or injured child—especially when death is imminent—may add to the family's emotional and spiritual distress and increase its suffering after the child's death. Thus, the Canadian Pediatric Society's guidelines on care for families experiencing perinatal loss recommend that "visiting policies should be around the clock, including during bedside rounds" (CPS, 2001, p. 471). The guidelines also state that families should have time and a private place to be with their baby after death.

A recent survey of children's hospitals in the United States found that over 80 percent of the respondents reported open visitation policies for parents with children in NICUs, PICUs, and general inpatient units (Susan Dull, NACHRI, personal communication, July 16, 2002, based on data from George Little and JM Harris, II). Approximately 70 percent reported policies allowing parent access to the child's medical record in the NICU or PICU; about two-thirds reported involving parents in the development of the child's care plan.

Availability of Inpatient Palliative Care and Hospice Programs

A number of children's hospitals have created inpatient palliative care or hospice programs, but they do not appear to be the norm. In preparing for its statement to the committee, NACHRI circulated a special survey to its member hospitals to obtain information about their palliative services. Of 161 member hospitals, 48 (30 percent) responded (NACHRI, 2001a). Two-thirds of those responding said they were currently not able to provide the full array of palliative services. Almost a third of respondents indicated limited or no availability of inpatient or home palliative care or hospice programs. More than half indicated that lack of such services in the community limited their ability to discharge patients appropriately. Most but not all respondents (85 percent) reported pain management services; one-quarter of this subgroup reported having a pediatric palliative care team. Three hospitals reported the use of dedicated pediatric hospice or palliative care beds. In addition to these results, the survey cited at the end of the preceding section found that 82 percent of respondents reported regular assessment of children's pain in the PICU, but the figure reported for NICUs was 69 percent.

The committee located no information on pediatric palliative care programs in other hospitals, but the number is likely to be low. For hospitals overall, survey data suggest that palliative care programs are far from common and that formal pain management programs have been slow to develop. The American Hospital Association's 1998 survey of more than 6,000 community hospitals in the United States, which had responses from more than 4,800 hospitals, found that just 15 percent of those responding reported any "end-of-life services" whereas 36 percent reported a formal pain management program (American Hospital Association, 2000; Pan et al., 2001).[9] A follow-up survey of just over 2,000 hospitals with end-of-life or pain management programs or both asked about palliative care programs (meaning an inpatient palliative care unit, a hospital-based palliative care consultation service, an outpatient palliative care service, or a hospital-based hospice unit). Of the approximately 1,100 hospitals responding to this survey, 30 percent reported having a program and 20 percent had plans to establish one (Pan et al., 2001). More than 85 percent of the patients served by the programs reported in the survey had a cancer diagnosis. The most common reason for a consultation was pain management, which accounted for almost two-thirds of consultations, with consultations about the goals of care a distant second (one-quarter of the consultations).

Overall, the two NACHRI surveys as well as other reports and committee experience suggest that the capacity to provide comprehensive, reliable palliative and end-of-life care is quite limited, even in the hospitals that

---

[9]End-of-life services were defined as "an organized service providing care and/or consultative services to dying patients and their families based on formalized protocols and guidelines" (Pan et al., 2001, p. 316). Virtually all hospitals have ethics committees and chaplains that are concerned with end-of-life issues.

specialize in treating children with life-threatening medical problems. Lack of pediatric hospice and similar care in the community further compromises the capacity of professionals in children's hospitals to meet the needs of dying children and their families by discussing and providing timely referrals to such services.

Elements of Pediatric Inpatient Palliative Care

Based on home hospice concepts, some of the basic elements of inpatient end-of-life care for children and their families were outlined as early as 1982 (Silverman, 1982; Whitfield et al., 1982). These elements included broadening the decisionmaking process to include the family and the health care team, as well as the child's physician, and providing a comfortable, private room for families of terminally ill children.

Central to most inpatient programs—whether for adults or children— is a referral and consultation service staffed by palliative care specialists, generally including physicians, nurses, social workers, and chaplains (ChIPPS, 2001; Levetown, 2001). Nurses may form the core of the team. Depending on patient and family needs and the concerns of the patient's regular care team, an inpatient palliative care consultant may

- help the patient, family, and their care team to understand and evaluate care options (e.g., starting or not starting mechanical ventilation, accepting hospice care) and determine the goals of care (e.g., prolonging life, emphasizing quality of life);
- work with the family and the care team to develop, implement, monitor, and if appropriate, revise the child's plan of care;
- assist in evaluating and managing patients with difficult symptoms and in providing emotional support to patients and family members including after a child's death;
- make referrals, as needed, to other physicians, psychologists, child-life specialists, chaplains, clinical social workers, and other relevant professionals;
- help with patient transitions between inpatient and home care and advise or otherwise assist home health care and home hospice personnel with developing and implementing the child's plan of care at home; and
- supervise the care of home hospice patients who require hospitalization for symptom management or family respite, whether or not the child and family have previously been cared for at the hospital.

A recent report on one inpatient program for neonatal intensive care portrayed service patterns that were generally consistent with the description above. Based on an analysis of care for nearly 900 infants admitted for neonatal intensive care during a 30-month period ending in June 1998, the researchers found that the primary reasons for palliative care consultations were to assist with home hospice arrangements, advise on comfort measures, support the consideration of options such as DNR orders, and provide comfort to grieving families (Leuthner and Pierucci, 2001). Approximately one-quarter of the 51 infants who died during the study period received a palliative care consultation. An earlier study, which covered all infant deaths at the same institution, reported an increase in consultations over time from 5 percent in 1994 to 38 percent in 1997 (Pierucci et al., 2001).

One objective for inpatient pediatric palliative and end-of-life care is the availability of at least one room with home-like features. Such rooms may be equipped for mechanical ventilators, monitors, and other technologies, but the focus of both services and physical environment is still on peace and comfort (Levetown, 2001). For example, two Texas hospitals (University of Texas Medical Branch at Galveston and Christus Santa Rosa in San Antonio) have created a large room or suite (referred to as "Butterfly" rooms) that provides sofa beds and comfortable chairs for family and friends, kitchenette, television, carpeting, and other similar features. If parents wish the presence and support of extended family and friends when a child's death is expected, the rooms can accommodate more than 30 people.

Box 6.3 presents a number of questions that may be useful for clinicians, hospital managers, and patient and family advocacy groups concerned about the availability, structure, effectiveness, and accountability of inpatient palliative or hospice care in a specific institution. These questions were adapted from a set that focused on adult care and take into account the discussion in Chapters 4 and 5. The committee believes that many of the basic features of inpatient palliative care services apply across the age spectrum.

The committee notes that those providing inpatient palliative or hospice services for children sometimes emphasize that their acceptance criteria do not require that the child's life expectancy be six months or less or that the child and family forgo curative care. As discussed in Chapter 7, Medicaid and some private insurers' hospice benefits include these criteria and also restrict coverage and payments for palliative or hospice care in other ways. Thus, to provide a comprehensive array of inpatient palliative care or hospice services for children and their families, hospitals and hospices will often have to rely on private fundraising and contributions. In Chapter 7, the committee recommends that coverage of pediatric palliative care be expanded and limitations on hospice coverage be eased.

Palliative and End-of-Life Care in the Home

Most home care arrangements assume that parents will provide substantial amounts of patient care, including care that involves advanced technologies such as mechanical ventilation and IV administration of powerful medications. For a child with a progressive neurological disease, such care at home may continue for years and may differ little on a day-to-day basis from care for children with severe conditions that are not expected to prove fatal. For other children, care at home may last only a short period once parents accept that curative or life-prolonging treatments have failed their child and decide that death at home rather than in the hospital will be most comforting to the child and family.

Hospices will serve some of these children and families, although, as described below, many hospices rarely if ever care for a dying child. Further, because families are often reluctant to accept the concept of home hospice care or the coverage conditions imposed by Medicaid and some private health plans, they may turn to home health care agencies for essential assistance.

General

> *The visiting nurse gave me literature on what to look for as death approached. She was the glue that held us together. . . . She came and dressed Eric and made phone calls after he died. She later told me that this was the first death she had dealt with. She was so calm and she kept me from losing it.*
>
> Becky Wooten, parent, 2001

> *We were happy with our home health care company, and things were going well. But when we got home from our spring break vacation, [our son] took a turn for the worse that required the hospice care.*
>
> Winona Kittiko, parent, 2001

Because hospice care may not be acceptable, available, or appropriate for all children and families who could benefit from palliative or end-of-life care at home, it is important to consider the role of home health providers as well as hospices in providing palliative and end-of-life care (Liben and Goldman, 1998). Providers of pediatric home health care services include children's hospitals, other hospitals, home health care agencies, hospices, and independent professionals. Some providers specialize in home health care for children (see, e.g., NAPHCC, 2001), but the committee found no comprehensive data on the pediatric caseloads for these or other home

BOX 6.3
Questions About Inpatient Palliative, End-of-Life, and Bereavement Care for Children and Their Families

Training and Preparation

- Are nurses and others who staff neonatal and pediatric intensive care units, emergency departments, and specialty services trained to recognize children and families for whom the goals of care should be reconsidered?
- Are trained staff and procedures in place for arranging care and consultations to support clinicians, children, and families in assessing and reassessing the goals of care and the ways of meeting those goals as they relate to physical, emotional, spiritual, and practical dimensions of care?
- Have hospital personnel been provided training and assistance in developing skills in communicating bad news, discerning child and family wishes and concerns, and respecting dignity through their language and other behavior?
- What training, clinical practice guidelines, symptom assessment protocols, and other supports are in place to ensure that the child's and family's needs for palliative, end-of-life, and bereavement care are routinely assessed and met?
- Have practices for limiting life-support interventions been reviewed to determine whether they should be modified to reduce distress for patients, families, and staff?
- Are resources and procedures available to help staff cope with the stresses of caring for critically ill and injured children?

Staff, Facilities, and Other Resources

- What internal or external expertise in pediatric palliative and end-of-life care is available to help clinicians and families with clinical evaluation, symptom prevention and management, decisions about life support, advance care planning, bereavement support, and other matters? How is this expertise organized and shared? Are other personnel routinely educated about the availability of this expertise and expected to use it when appropriate?
- What care options are available for dying children within the hospital, for example, a designated bed or unit that provides a home-like setting and is governed by different rules regarding visiting hours, number and age of visitors, and other matters? Are relevant personnel throughout the hospital aware of these options?
- Can hospital procedures and the physical environment be modified in ways that reduce stress and discomfort for children and families wherever care is provided within the institution?

Responsiveness

- How well are children and families informed about who is responsible for the child's care, what they can expect, and to whom they can look for information and assistance? Is continuity in relationships supported?

• How specifically are the preferences and circumstances of children and their families determined, assessed, recorded, and accommodated—throughout the child's medical course?
• Are care processes focused narrowly on written orders or more broadly on a comprehensive care plan? Are all dimensions of care addressed—physical, emotional, spiritual, and practical?
• What support is available for siblings?
• What structures and processes are in place to prevent, moderate, or mediate conflicts among clinicians, families, and children?
• What provisions are made for non-English speakers, cultural minorities, and others who may not fit routine administrative and clinical procedures?

Continuity, Coordination, and Community Resources

• What protocols and procedures are in place to promote continuity and minimize unwanted transfers and other disruptions in relationships, especially at the end of life?
• What structures and processes are in place to help children and families to identify needed resources and assist with appropriate transitions to or from the hospital and other care settings? Are procedures in place to see that care plans (including preferences about life support interventions), contact information, and prescriptions accompany the patient during transfers?
• What relationships exist with home health agencies, hospices, bereavement support groups, and other organizations that care for or assist children and their families?

Information Systems and Evaluation

• Are clinical information systems in place that reliably document and update treatment decisions (including orders about resuscitation and other life-support interventions), symptom assessments, care processes, patient responses and outcomes, and similar matters?
• Do information systems support the timely provision of information to all involved staff in all parts of the institution and at all times of the day?
• Do information systems provide clinical decision support in the form of easy access to guidelines for pediatric palliative care, prescribing protocols, reminders or alerts, and other information relevant to symptom prevention and relief for children of different ages and with different medical problems?
• What structures and processes are in place to evaluate and improve the quality of care provided to children who die and their families?

SOURCE: Adapted from IOM, 1997; see also ChIPPS, 2001; Levetown, 2001; Hilden and Tobin, 2002; and Himelstein et al., 2002.

health care organizations. The caseload of most agencies is dominated by elderly Medicare beneficiaries (HCFA, 1999). In 1996, nearly 14 percent of those age 65 or over had one home health visit compared to less than 2 percent of children under age 6 and less than 0.5 percent of those aged 6 to 17 (Kraus et al., 1999).

The frequency, duration, and type of home health care services will vary depending on the child's and family's needs, geographic location, state licensure requirements, community availability of appropriate personnel, and family insurance and other financial resources. For some children located in rural areas, home health care providers may supplement in-home care with interactive and other telemedicine technologies. The committee found no data describing the extent of such services in this country, but discussions with major vendors suggest that fewer than 200 of the nearly 20,000 home health agencies provide telemedicine services to any of their patients (Field and Grigsby, 2002).

Because families are usually expected to take major responsibility for home caregiving, the AAP guidelines for home care for children with chronic disease recommend that if possible a family should have at least two members who are trained and prepared to take care of the child at home (AAP, 1995c). The guidelines also suggest that family members should, ideally, be prepared for their caregiving role by providing as much care as possible in the hospital before the child's discharge. Further, the guidelines call for children to be included in home care training and education and to be responsible for self-care whenever possible.

Depending on the child's diagnosis and care plan and family circumstances, including the child's insurance coverage, home health care agencies may provide nurses, home health aides, physical therapists, social workers, and others to assist the child and family. Those providing pediatric home health care state that it generally requires more specialized skills and more time, thus allowing care for only two to three children during a day rather than the usual five to six adults (NAPHACC, 2001). (For a general guide to palliative care in the home, see Doyle and Jeffrey, 2000.)

Some children and families are well served by home health care for an extended period but then find at a certain stage that the specialized expertise of a hospice is what the child needs as death approaches. Interviews with home health care personnel indicate that they often would like to obtain consultations on symptom management from hospice personnel, but Medicaid and most private health plans will not pay for such consultations (Huskamp et al., 2001). Chapter 7 recommends changes in such policies to make palliative care expertise more widely accessible.

Many hospices provide home care under both their hospice license and separate home health care licenses. Under their home care license, these organizations may serve some patients who have fatal illnesses but who do not fit the traditional hospice model and coverage rules. They may not fit because their course to death is unpredictable and could be lengthy or because they want to continue curative or life-prolonging treatments. Service under the home care umbrella may also be less painful emotionally for families. If formal referral to the affiliated hospice eventually occurs, care can usually be continued with minimal disruption of continuity in trusted relationships.

Availability of Pediatric Home Hospice Care

In 1983, only 4 of the 1,400 hospice programs in the United States reported that they offered any pediatric services (Armstrong-Daley and Zarbock, 2001). The number has undoubtedly grown, but the committee found no firm count or estimate of the number of hospices that routinely provide care to a sufficient number of children to support specialized staffing, training, and outreach efforts.

Of the 3,000-plus existing hospice programs in the United States, 450 reported in a recent survey that they were prepared to offer hospice services to children (ChIPPS, 2001). The survey results do not, however, make clear whether these hospices actually have much or any experience providing such care. Based on discussions with staff of the National Hospice and Palliative Care Organization (NHPCO) and others and on its members' professional experience, the committee suspects that fewer than 100 hospices have active pediatric programs with trained personnel, protocols, policies, and outreach efforts. As discussed elsewhere in this report, the federal government's Center for Medicare and Medicaid Services is funding demonstration projects to test programs that provide more comprehensive services than those covered by current Medicaid hospice benefits.

Pediatric Home Hospice: Program Elements and Focus

In the United States, the first program of home-based care for dying children originated in the mid-1970s in Minneapolis under the joint sponsorship of a university hospital, a children's hospital, and a large multispecialty physician practice (Martinson, I., 1993). (The original program no longer exists.) The first U.S. hospice also dates to the mid-1970s. In 1979, Edmarc was established as a community-based home hospice serving children (Armstrong-Dailey and Zarbock, 2001). In 1983, the nonprofit Children's Hospice International began to provide resources to support the development of hospice services specifically for children. In recent years, the national association of hospices (NHPCO) has also supported efforts to develop pediatric hospice programs through the Children's International Project on Palliative/Hospice Services (ChIPPS, 2001).

Hospice care for children differs from that for adults in a number of areas: patient characteristics, family concerns and decisionmaking, funding, and organizational resources. As discussed earlier, children's needs are particularly variable, reflecting both developmental differences and differences in underlying medical problems and their course. In most situations, parents are legally responsible for decisions about their child's care. Decisions to limit curative or life-prolonging efforts and focus exclusively on palliative care—as required for Medicaid and some private health coverage—are particularly difficult when the patient is a child.

Reflecting these differences, home hospice care for children builds on traditional hospice principles and practices but adapts them to accommodate the developmental characteristics and needs of children and the values and goals of their families (see, e.g., Goldman, 1996, 1999; ChIPPS, 2001; Armstrong-Daley and Zarbok, 2001; Sumner, 2001). Some hospices may develop special pediatric programs, but smaller hospices may make adjustments to incorporate children in programs that are adult-oriented or refer children to hospices with pediatric programs (Orloff, 2001). Hospice nurses and other personnel need special training to prepare them for the special requirements of working with young patients and supporting the families who are facing the exceptional stress of a child's death. As noted earlier, even experienced pediatric and hospice nurses may have qualms about taking on this role. They may need moral support beyond that ordinarily recognized as necessary for the emotionally demanding work of hospice care.

Models and principles for pediatric hospice care are still being developed and tested. At a minimum, regardless of the patient population, turning palliative care principles into consistent, effective care at home involves certain core organizational capacities. These include

1. offering support for patients and families 24 hours a day, 7 days a week;

2. developing, evaluating, and improving organizational procedures and protocols for reliably and effectively meeting the physical, emotional, spiritual, and practical needs of terminally ill children and their families;

3. constructing interdisciplinary care teams that, taken together, have the necessary knowledge and skills needed to provide comprehensive and continuous care for a child at home under most circumstances;

4. providing reliable and immediate access to inpatient pediatric palliative care and other services for patients and families who require them;

5. training and assisting family caregivers; and

6 working, as appropriate, with the child's specialist care team and general pediatrician.

When a child's family and physicians have recognized that curative and life-prolonging care will fail or is failing, unfamiliarity with hospice and misunderstandings about hospice services may discourage families from fully evaluating the option of hospice care. Sumner (2001) has identified several such misunderstandings and argued that hospice personnel may have to make clear to families and clinicians—and ensure in practice—that hospice personnel do not take over the home or usurp normal parental care and authority but, rather, advise on ways to increase the child's comfort and ease stresses on all members of the family. Further, hospice enrollment should not require or encourage the severing of all relationships with the primary care and specialist personnel who have been caring for the child and family, although health plan rules may limit relationships to unpaid consultations and emotional support. Perhaps most important, families should be assured that parents continue to make the decisions about the child's care with information, consultation, and support from the child's care team, including hospice personnel.

Box 6.4 presents a number of questions, similar to those for inpatient palliative care, that may serve as a guide for those concerned about the adequacy of palliative care and end-of-life care at home. Again, the questions were adapted from a set that focused on adult care, but the committee believes that the basic concerns apply to adults and children alike. The questions were framed somewhat generally so as not to exclude services provided by home health agencies. Given the mission of hospices and regulatory requirements, families whose child needs palliative or end-of-life care will probably find that hospices (and home health agencies closely affiliated with hospices) have more resources, clinical protocols, and experience in palliative, end-of-life, and bereavement care in general. Nonetheless, families cannot assume that all hospices are adequately prepared to care for children.

For children perhaps more than adults, broader access to home hospice care will depend on trusting relationships between hospice personnel and inpatient care personnel in neonatal and pediatric intensive care units, specialized cancer and other centers, and even obstetrical units. The latter relationship has become important as prenatal diagnosis has expanded the number of children diagnosed before birth with fatal medical conditions, and some hospices have begun to offer support to families that want to continue the pregnancy and achieve whatever time they can with their infant in the hospital or at home. Families cannot reliably be offered the option of such care without substantial cooperation from obstetricians and hospital obstetrical facilities and personnel.

Given the relatively small potential base of child hospice patients, a hospice that wants to create a pediatric program will often have to establish relationships with a number of hospitals, each of which will have its own procedures and conventions. If these hospitals have or are developing

---

BOX 6.4
Questions About Palliative Home Health and Hospice Care for Children and Their Families

Training and Preparation

• Are staff trained and prepared to care for children with life-threatening medical conditions? What continuing education and training related to pediatric palliative and end-of-life care are available to staff?

• What clinical practice guidelines, symptom assessment protocols, referral and consulting arrangements, and other supports are in place to guide staff in assessing and meeting children's needs for care?

• Have practices for limiting life-support interventions been reviewed to determine whether they should be modified to reduce distress for child patients, families, and staff?

• Are resources and procedures available to help staff cope with the stresses of caring for gravely ill and dying children?

Staffing, Facilities, and Other Resources

• What internal and external resources and expertise are available to provide 24-hour coverage, physical and emotional care, spiritual support and counseling, practical assistance, and other aid for children and families? Is residential care available?

• What practice guidelines, symptom assessment protocols, and other tools are used to guide patient assessment and care?

• What are the criteria for accepting children as patients? Are families with a prenatal diagnosis of a fatal congenital problem accepted? Has the organization a made an effort to identify resources that will allow more flexible and comprehensive care than allowed under the coverage policies of Medicare, Medicaid, and some private health plans?

• How is physician support for patient care organized? Are children's primary care or specialist physicians encouraged to continue involvement with the child and family after enrollment in hospice?

• If home care proves insufficient for a patient's needs, what are the arrangements for inpatient care?

---

inpatient palliative care programs, that good news may be offset by concerns about competition for patients. In building relationships with hospitals and hospital-based specialists, hospice personnel will have be careful not to provoke a defensive reaction among hospital-based physicians, nurses, and others who may feel that their skills in symptom management or family support are being questioned.

Some hospices have actively pursued community and philanthropic contributions that allow them important flexibility in meeting the needs of children and their families. Although the committee recommends changes

Responsiveness

• How well are children and families informed about who is responsible for care, what they can expect, and to whom they can look for information and assistance? Is continuity in relationships supported?

• How specifically are the preferences and circumstances of children and their families determined, assessed, recorded, and accommodated? Are care processes focused narrowly on written orders or more broadly on a comprehensive care plan?

• What support, including bereavement care, is available for parents and siblings?

• What structures and processes are in place to prevent, moderate, or mediate conflicts involving families, children, or home health or hospice staff?

• What provisions are made for non-English speakers, cultural minorities, and others who may not fit routine administrative and clinical procedures?

Continuity, Coordination, and Community Resources

• What protocols and procedures are in place to promote continuity of care, for example, if hospitalization is required?

• What relationships and referral arrangements exist with other health care organizations, for example, hospitals?

Information Systems and Evaluation

• Are clinical information systems in place that reliably document and update treatment decisions (including orders about resuscitation and other life support interventions), symptom assessments, care processes, patient responses and outcomes, and similar matters?

• What structures and processes are in place to evaluate and improve the quality of care?

SOURCE: Adapted from IOM, 1997; see also Armstrong-Dailey and Zarbock, 2001; Sumner, 2001.

in restrictive Medicaid and private health plan policies (see Chapter 7) and recognizes real fiscal constraints on hospice services, it also urges hospices not to define themselves and their mission in terms of Medicare and Medicaid coverage policies.[10] A hospice's refusal to accept a child can be a

---

[10]Some palliative care and hospice programs have been very sensitive to the risk that coverage will distort their mission. For example, in discussing one of the older inpatient hospice programs at Northwestern Memorial Hospital, Charles Von Gunten recalls that "the

bitter blow, especially when hospice managers are perceived as showing not the "the least sensitivity" to the gulf between their policies and the needs of parents to do the best for their child (Avila, S., 2001). Every hospice may not be able to mobilize resources to care for children not covered by public or private insurance or who do not fit payer's requirements, but Medicaid policies do not preclude them from making the effort.

Hospices with smaller service areas may, in particular, find it financially and otherwise impractical to routinely extend their capabilities to children. Even for larger hospices, maintaining a high level of pediatric expertise 24 hours a day, 7 days a week can be a challenge. As recommended at the end of this chapter, the development of regional or national telephone or on-line consultation services can provide additional expert resources to hospices as well as generalist pediatricians or family practitioners and community hospitals.

Other Sites of Care

Residential Hospice Services

A few residential care programs are intended specifically to serve dying children and their families. Helen House, the world's first residential children's hospice, was founded in England in 1982, and some 20 additional freestanding hospices have since been established in Great Britain (Goldman, 2000a). These hospices may receive revenue from government sources, but they are private organizations that depend significantly and deliberately on private contributions and philanthropy.

Some hospices in the United States that serve children offer residential services. Examples include the Hospice of the Florida Suncoast, the San Diego Hospice, and Edmarc. A freestanding, residential hospice for children is scheduled to open in the San Francisco Bay Area in 2003 (George Marks Children's House).

One goal of residential hospice care is to offer a short-term alternative to hospitalization for dying children and their families when a child requires more intensive assessment, symptom management, and care planning than can be successfully provided at home. Another goal of residential hospice care, particularly in the United Kingdom, is to provide respite care when families need relief from the demands of caring for their child. Respite services can also be provided at the family home while the parents, siblings, and other family members vacation or visit distant loved ones. Residential

---

program resisted becoming certified for the Medicare Hospice Benefit until 1991 because of the risk that palliative care would be defined by a reimbursement mechanism rather than by the principles of good practice" (Von Gunten, 2000, p.166).

respite care offers families the opportunity to rest, attend to neglected family relationships and chores, and do things together without leaving home. As discussed in Chapter 7, funding for this kind of respite care is very limited in the United States.

Long-Term Residential Care Facilities

No matter how much they are loved and cherished, children with severe physical and mental disabilities can create tremendous emotional and financial burdens on their families, whose lives may be completely overwhelmed by a child's care needs or by psychological stress resulting from a child's violent or otherwise disruptive behavior. In 1997 an estimated 24,000 children aged 0 to 21 with mental retardation and developmental disabilities were being cared for outside the family home in residential facilities (Lakin et al., 1998). Another 83,000 were awaiting placement. Facilities range from small home-like settings to larger intermediate care facilities, although the latter have declined substantially in numbers and census in recent decades.

Children in these residential care settings have serious to severe mental retardation and developmental disabilities and suffer from multiple severe chronic conditions such as cerebral palsy, epilepsy, and impairment of hearing, vision, speech, or language. Many are expected to and do live into adulthood, but others are at high risk of death in childhood. The acceptable setting of care for children with severe disabilities is an important and often controversial issue (see, e.g., Rosenau, 2000) that is beyond the scope of this report.

The role and provision of palliative and end-of-life care for adults or children in residential care settings has received little attention. A recently published review of records of deaths at a center for people with severe development disabilities reported during a 30-month period, 38 of 850 residents died and that of this group, 10 deaths involved end-of-life decisions (defined as decisions about end-of-life care that followed formal discussions of what care is in a resident's best interests) (Lohiya et al., 2002). Among all residents, decisions about end-of-life care had been made for 16 individuals, 12 of which involved do-not-resuscitate orders and 4 of which involved continued full medical treatment. Decisions, which could be requested by employees or family members, were made by committee consisting of the resident, attending physician, resident-rights advocate, an uninvolved physician, social worker, clergy, psychologist, caretakers, and family or surrogate, legal conservator, or guardian. Decisions to forgo intrusive care had to be unanimous.

Quality of life is a concern for all residents of long-term care facilities, but comfort care is a particular concern for children who are bed bound or technology dependent. Children who are unable to turn over in bed and those being tube fed appear to be at highest risk of death (Eyman et al., 1993, but see Strauss et al., 1997). Researchers involved in longitudinal studies of one large group of California children have called for controlled trials of tube feeding in these children to help clarify the benefits and burdens of that practice for this group of children (Strauss and Kastner, 1996; Strauss et al., 1996). Although focused on a special group of children in a special setting, such research is potentially relevant to decisions about appropriate palliative and end-of-life care for children being cared for at home and in hospitals.

Schools

The main objective of schools is education not health care. Nonetheless, various federal and state laws, reinforced by judicial decisions, require public schools to educate and assist increasing numbers of children with special health care needs (NICCY, 1996).[11] Some of these children have conditions that are likely to end in death in childhood, but most do not. As discussed in Chapters 4 and 5, a central goal of care for ill children is the maintenance, insofar as possible, of normal life, and school is a major part of normal life for school-age children.

As specified by law, schools must provide or arrange for the provision of appropriate health care services and make appropriate alterations to their physical plant, furnishings and equipment, and procedures to accommodate children with special health care needs. In some cases, this may mean providing individual aides to assist them with movement or other needs; in other cases, school nurses may provide medications and assist in emergencies. Both the American Academy of Pediatrics and the National Association of School Nurses assert that procedures such as the administration of intravenous medicines, catheterization, tracheostomy care, or gastrostomy tube feeding can all be undertaken in the school setting by a school nurse or an appropriately trained and supervised aide (AAP, 1987; NASN, 1996). Chapter 8 discusses legal issues involving family requests that schools respect care plans for their child, including do-not-resuscitate orders.

Perhaps more important than the provision of medical services in school are the efforts of teachers and other school personnel to offer a child with a

---

[11]The Individuals with Disabilities Education Act (20 USC §1400) includes several pieces of legislation that, in combination with judicial decisions, establish requirements for public schools to serve children with disabilities. Separate sections of the law cover children age 3 and younger and children age 4 and older.

serious medical condition as normal and supportive an environment as possible given the child's condition and need for assistance. This will normally mean preparing classmates and other children for condition- or treatment-related changes or differences in a child's appearance or functioning. Some children's hospitals, pediatric oncology teams, and other groups have established formal programs to assist families and schools with a child's reentry. School systems and related programs can also offer support to an ill child's sisters and brothers by educating teachers and classmates about children's experiences living with a sibling who has life-threatening medical condition.

These kinds of support and preparation are important because children can be cruel to those who are different. One parent told the committee that he learned after his 11-year-old daughter's death that kids had made fun of her because of her hair loss and were afraid of her because she had cancer— "and the teachers did not how to handle it" (Weil, 2001). His response was to develop a comprehensive educational program—"using cancer as a metaphor for all difference"—to help teach understanding, respect, compassion, and acceptance (Washburne, 2000, p. 2; Weil, 2001). The program gets its name and theme from a short story that the daughter, Kelly Weil, wrote three months before her death about Zink the Zebra, who had spots instead of stripes and was treated differently by other zebras. The program is now available to and being used by preschool programs, schools (kindergarten through eight grade), and scout troops (Weil, 1996).

When a child dies or leaves school for what is expected to be the terminal phase of his or her illness, schools may facilitate support groups for classmates of the child and help the children express their sadness, for example, by making cards for the dying child or for the family after the child's death. Following a child's sudden and unexpected death, for example, from violence or a car crash, schools may organize counseling and bereavement services for classmates. Especially upon the death of older children, classmates and friends may attend the funeral.

Camps

A number of camps have been organized to serve children living with serious medical problems that preclude participation in traditional camp programs. Camps vary in emphasis, but some focus on children with life-threatening conditions such as cancer, end-stage renal disease, cystic fibrosis, or AIDS. Some camps invite siblings to participate or provide special sessions especially for brothers and sisters of children with a life-threatening condition. Unlike their ill brother or sister, siblings may have no contact with other children facing similar circumstances, and thus a special summer camp can be an important resource for them.

Special camps usually rely on trained volunteers, led by just a few paid specialists. Nurses and doctors may volunteer their time, valuing the opportunity to see children other than "on the wrong side of a sharp object." Nurses provide most of the medical care, including distribution of medications, but a physician is available in case of emergencies and serious changes in a camper's health status. Camps may be staffed and equipped to provide chemotherapy, blood and platelet transfusions, intravenous fluid therapy, hemophilia factor replacement, pain therapy, and other curative or palliative therapies. In addition, they may aim to improve the child's medical status, for example, by helping children with cystic fibrosis gain weight (Rubin and Geiger, 1991).

Staff of these special camps must be actively aware of the particular circumstances of each camper. Sometimes they must restrict certain activities for the safety of other campers, for example, excluding HIV-positive children with open sores from the swimming pool (Pearson et al., 1997).

Such camps can be very significant to seriously ill children, important enough to make one of their goals be to live long enough to attend camp again before they die. Occasionally, children do die while at camp. Most camps memorialize campers who have died as a way to recognize their lives, however brief. For instance, a tree may be planted to honor the children who died during the year and then it can be decorated with friendship bracelets or painted rocks made by campers and staff. Such memorials also provide a means of helping other campers and counselors discuss their own feelings and fears about progressive illness and death.

COMMUNITY AND REGIONAL SYSTEMS OF CARE

General

Beyond individual professionals and institutions, special care teams, and medical homes, children who die and their families need community systems of care that respond to the differences in child and family circumstances and values and that provide a range of services and settings of care to accommodate these differences. For some children and families, care provided by home health organizations will be welcome; for others, hospice will better meet their needs. Some children may move from one to the other as their needs change. Flexibility, however, can come at the cost of complexity and fragmentation. This puts a premium on coordinating strategies, including the medical home and improved versions of older mechanisms such as hospital discharge planning and insurer case management.

Box 6.5 presents the basic objectives of a community-focused approach to care at the end of life. A community approach to care that supports these objectives would include a mix of inpatient and home care resources—

BOX 6.5
Objectives of Community Systems of Palliative, End-of-Life, and Bereavement Care

• Making palliative care available wherever and whenever needed by child and family from the time of diagnosis through death and, for the family, after death
• Providing sufficient flexibility in attitudes and procedures that special needs of child and family can be recognized and accommodated insofar as possible at home or in the hospital
• Encouraging timely referral to home hospice for children whose medical problems and personal circumstances make such care feasible and desirable
• Allowing flexible arrangements for home health care for patients whose prognosis is uncertain but for whom palliative services at home would be valuable in preventing and relieving symptoms and discouraging unwanted or inappropriate life-prolonging interventions
• Encouraging, when possible, the continued involvement of the child's primary care physician through the course of the child's life and the continued involvement of specialist physicians and health care teams as valued by children and families after the goals of care have shifted away from cure toward comfort
• Developing protocols and procedures for transition planning that prepare clinicians and others to manage common child and family situations (related to, e.g., medical condition, place of residence, comfort with managing care at home, financial resources)
• Making necessary and helpful information readily available to families and clinicians (e.g., truly portable and accessible records of care plans and preferences, training programs or materials for family caregivers)
• Supporting activities and programs that respond to nonmedical needs of children and families (e.g., camps, schools, religious programs)

SOURCE: Adapted from IOM, 1997.

organizations, personnel, programs, policies, and procedures. In the foreseeable future, it would have to be constructed within and around this country's existing arrangements for organizing and delivering care, which are—on the whole—decidedly nonintegrated, uncoordinated, and yet often inflexible. Rural and smaller communities present particular challenges that call for regional consulting and other supportive services, which are recommended at the end of this chapter.

In some communities, children's hospitals can play a central role in developing programs to coordinate palliative and other care across inpatient, outpatient, and home settings. For example, the Pediatric Advanced Care Team at Dana-Farber Cancer Institute and Children's Hospital Boston involves a multidisciplinary team to advise and assist in the development and implementation of plans of care for seriously ill children and their families before, during, and after the child's hospitalization (Dana-Farber, 2001). It is primarily a consultative service for children admitted to the hospital but includes educational and outreach activities to increase awareness among physicians, families, and the community. An important element of the program is bereavement support for both families and clinician caregivers. For the latter, the program conducts weekly "caregiver bereavement rounds" that encourage reflection on the death of a patient and review of the care plan's adequacy. Like a number of other pediatric programs, it has been funded in part by private foundation grants.

Where community size and resources limit what can be done locally, regional responses may be needed. For example, when a child has returned home after specialized treatment, children's hospitals can provide consulting assistance on pain management and other topics to primary care physicians and community hospitals. Some of this assistance could be provided through on-line clinical practice guidelines and other written resources, but telephone consultations would also be required similar to those provided by hospices. Start-up resources for such programs might be found through government and private grants, but maintenance of a program could be difficult without some kind of health plan reimbursement for consultative services, including those provided by telephone.

Telemedicine as an Option

One option to extend services into rural areas and smaller communities is telemedicine. Defined broadly, telemedicine is the use of electronic information and communications technologies to provide and support health care when distance separates the participants (IOM, 1996b; Field and Grigsby, 2002). Given insurance traditions and limited evidence of cost-effectiveness (see, e.g., AHRQ, 2001c), health insurance coverage is limited for most telemedicine applications beyond radiology, where direct patient contact has not been part of usual consultative practice.

Several projects have tested or are testing telemedicine to support intensive management of serious chronic conditions. Although not designed for patients who are dying, they could provide some useful lessons about benefits, limitations, and costs of such care. Some projects focus on rural areas, and Congress has authorized Medicare payment for certain telemedicine services in rural areas (HCFA, 2001g). An increasing number of Medicaid programs and some private health plans also cover telemedicine services under certain circumstances, and a few states prohibit insurers from reimbursing differently for telemedicine and regular medical services (OAT, 2001).

Some of the telemedicine applications being tested provide both medical monitoring and hardware and software (e.g., sensitive videocameras, instruments to measure heart rate and other physiological parameters that are connected to telephone modems that can transmit the information; software that alerts clinicians to atypical findings). Some also include individual patient Web sites that link patients with physicians, nurse practitioners, and other health care personnel, and some include links to other patients and families. To support patient self-care activities, the Web sites may also provide easy Internet access to targeted clinical and educational information and links.

A two-year study involving hospices in Kansas and Michigan and researchers at Michigan State University and the University of Kansas has been investigating telemedicine to support hospice care. (Whitten et al., 2001). In a preliminary report, the researchers concluded that hospice personnel were cautious but supportive whereas patients and families were uniformly positive, although some families declined the service. The state of Florida is funding Hope Hospice to test a videoconferencing application that will allow a nurse to visually check the patient, medical equipment, and caregiving procedures (Hospice, 2001).

At Beth-Israel Deaconess Hospital in Boston, a federally funded, randomized controlled trial of an intervention for families with very low birth weight infants reported improved family satisfaction and lower costs for the intervention group (Gray et al., 2000). A central feature of this application was an electronic communications link for parents that provided information about their hospitalized infants, including daily photographs, daily progress reports, scheduled live video visits with babies and their nurses, and e-mail access to clinicians. With the end of federal support, the hospital is marketing the program to large employers and Medicaid, and several other hospitals are reported to be trying the program. This program was not designed for children who are not expected to survive, but it could nonetheless provide useful lessons (Halamka, 2001).

Interactive and noninteractive telemedicine has grown slowly in the face of insurer wariness, unfriendly technologies, and physician disinterest. As technological development continues and research clarifies its benefits, limitations, and costs, remote patient monitoring applications of telemedicine are likely to grow.

DIRECTIONS FOR PROFESSIONALS AND INSTITUTIONS

The discussion in this and preceding chapters has identified concerns about the quality and consistency of palliative, end-of-life, and bereavement care in several areas. These include the provision of timely and accurate information, the formulation of goals and plans of care, the effective management of pain and other symptoms, the management of the end-stage of a fatal condition, and the offering of bereavement care.

The experience of advocates of better pain management can help guide the development of strategies to improve other aspects of adult and pediatric palliative and end-of-life care. As described by one leader in national and international initiatives to improve pain management for adults and children, cancer pain was identified in the 1980s as a "wedge issue" because of a strong professional and public perspective that pain relief in cancer patients should be a priority (Kathleen Foley, M.D., Memorial Sloan-Kettering Cancer Center, personal communication, June 19, 2002). As cancer pain relief strategies evolved, it became clear that clinicians could not provide comprehensive, consistent, and effective care for patients with pain without attending to their multiple symptoms and other needs and without considering the needs of their families. That is, the focus needed to expand to patient- and family-centered palliative care conceived broadly. For example, what began in 1986 as a World Health Organization monograph on cancer pain was later broadened to include comprehensive care including palliative services (WHO, 1998).

As part of a comprehensive strategy for care improvement, advocates identified multiple targets for action: government policies including payment for palliative care and access to effective medications; public education to create awareness that effective strategies were available to prevent and relieve pain; professional education about effective use of existing knowledge to prevent suffering; and scientific research to build new knowledge. The strategies were pragmatic and operated on the principle that "nothing would have a greater impact on improving the care of patients with pain than institutionalizing the knowledge we have now." Institutionalizing knowledge meant, for example, developing and implementing evidence- and consensus-based practice guidelines, creating and refining tools for assessing pain and measuring desired outcomes of care, forging collaborations among groups and institutions to develop and test pain management protocols, and formulating supportive public and private policies, including accreditation standards.

Although recognizing that deficits in pain care persist and that more progress is needed on all fronts, advocates of improved palliative, end-of-life, and bereavement care—including many who led efforts to improve pain management—have learned from the pain management experience. The web sites of the Open Society Institute's Project on Death in America (http://www.soros.org/death), the Last Acts program initiated by the Robert Wood Johnson Foundation (http://www.lastacts.org), and other linked sites document their multifaceted approach to care improvement.

The discussion below focuses on steps clinicians, administrators, and others can take—usually in collaboration with others in the community and nationally—to define responsibilities and implement and test strategies for improving care. All those involved in care for children with fatal or potentially fatal conditions should act to remedy deficits in care. However, because care for such children is often concentrated in neonatal and pediatric intensive care units, these units and their governing institutions must play a central role.

Communication, Goal Setting, and Care Processes

Practice guidelines and administrative protocols are, as discussed earlier, one means of providing direction and defining expectations and responsibilities for the health care professionals and organizations that care for children with fatal or potentially fatal medical conditions. If implemented, they should increase the consistency of services and provide a base for evaluation of the effectiveness of the recommended practices and procedures.

Existing literature and committee experience suggest that even hospitals that regularly care for children who die often lack protocols and procedures to guide such basic aspects of palliative and end-of-life care as the assessment and management of pain and other symptoms, the communication of diagnosis, prognosis, and treatment options, and the ethical and competent management of end-of-life decisions and interventions. The committee recognizes that the evidence base is limited but believes that "institutionalizing" existing knowledge and experience is an important step in improving care and building better knowledge to guide future care.

Recommendation: Pediatric professionals, children's hospitals, hospices, home health agencies, professional societies, family advocacy groups, government agencies, and others should work together to develop and implement clinical practice guidelines and institutional protocols and procedures for palliative, end-of-life, and bereavement care that meet the needs of children and families for

• **complete, timely, understandable information about diagnosis, prognosis, treatments (including their potential benefits and burdens), and palliative care options;**
• **early and continuing discussion of goals and preferences for care that will be honored wherever care is provided;**
• **effective and timely prevention, assessment, and treatment of physical and psychological symptoms and other distress whatever the goals of care and wherever care is provided; and**
• **competent, fair, and compassionate clinical management of end-of-life decisions about such interventions as resuscitation and mechanical ventilation.**

As discussed earlier in this chapter, guidelines and protocols should be based on systematically developed expert consensus and on scientific evidence to the extent it is available. Guidelines and similar statements developed by reputable national organizations should be a starting point when possible, but local review and adaptation will often be necessary and helpful to meet local needs and win support from those who must implement guidelines and protocols. Given this country's cultural, religious, and ethnic diversity, guidelines and protocols should also be sensitive to this diversity and flexible enough to accommodate departures from usually advised procedures.

Depending on the aspect of care in question, clinical practice guidelines and institutional protocols may include or be supplemented by ethical guidance, model conversations, checklists, and documentation standards. Once adopted, guidelines and protocols are one obvious candidate for quality improvement projects as discussed earlier.

Bereavement Care

Although many families will rely primarily on support from other family members, friends, neighbors, and spiritual advisors after a child's death, they may also seek care from their primary care physician, hospice personnel, psychotherapists, grief counselors, or family support groups. Still, the child's specialist care team—physicians, nurses, social workers, and others—can meaningfully "be with" the family in a variety of ways in the days and months following a child's death in the hospital or at home. As observed in Chapter 5, an abrupt end to contact soon after the child's death can feel like—and be—a kind of abandonment.

Despite the shortfalls in the research base and the need for more research on bereavement interventions (see Chapter 10), the committee concludes that enough experience and judgment is available to guide the development, implementation, and assessment of systematic processes for offering and providing bereavement support. Such support should become a more consistent and reliable service of hospitals that routinely care for children who die and their families.

Recommendation: Children's hospitals and other hospitals that care for children who die should work with hospices and other relevant community organizations to develop and implement protocols and procedures for

- identifying and coordinating culturally sensitive bereavement services for parents, siblings, and other survivors, whether the child dies after a prolonged illness or after a sudden event;

- defining bereavement support roles for hospital-based and out-of-hospital personnel, including emergency medical services providers, law enforcement officers, hospital pathologists, and staff in medical examiners' offices; and
- responding to the bereavement needs and stresses of professionals, including emergency services and law enforcement personnel, who assist dying children and their families.

Coordination and Continuity of Care

Parents repeatedly cite the frustrations they experienced in coordinating the care needed by a very ill child. Reducing the burdens of care coordination is a formidable challenge. This is especially true for children with complex, chronic problems that require inpatient, home, and community-based services from many different professionals and organizations that may be separated geographically, institutionally, and even culturally from each other. As described earlier in this chapter, interdisciplinary care teams, case managers, disease management programs, and medical homes are important but still incomplete foundations or strategies for care coordination and continuity. These strategies themselves have to be coordinated or linked within and across organizations and sites of care.

The committee recognizes that the development and institutional adoption of guidelines or protocols as recommended above is but one step toward changing practice and improving outcomes. Other steps include the assignment of institutional accountability for the implementation of protocols (including the identification of barriers to implementation), the development of programs to train personnel in the basis and use of the guidelines, and the creation of information systems to make adherence to the guidelines easier and assessment of their consequences—both expected and unexpected—routine.

Recommendation: Children's hospitals, hospices, home health agencies, and other organizations that care for seriously ill or injured children should collaborate to assign specific responsibilities for implementing clinical and administrative protocols and procedures for palliative, end-of-life, and bereavement care. In addition to supporting competent clinical services, protocols should promote the coordination and continuity of care and the timely flow of information among caregivers and within and among care sites including hospitals, family homes, residential care facilities, and injury scenes.

An essential foundation for improved coordination of care—and improvements in the quality and efficiency of health care generally—is better medical information systems that make patient information available when-ever and wherever it is needed (see, e.g., the reports and citations in IOM, 1991, 2000c, 2001b and resources listed at http://www.amia.org/resource/pubs/f3.html). Such systems are not yet in place within most individual health care systems much less in forms that allow quick, reliable, and secure access to information across sites of care. Interim information strategies—including paper-based techniques—are also needed.

In addition to investing in better medical information systems, it is also important to continue public and private investments in other system changes that will make it easier for local institutions and communities to improve palliative, end-of-life, and bereavement care for children and fami-lies. Chapter 7 outlines directions for change in the financing of care, and Chapters 9 and 10 discuss educational changes and research directions.

Regional Support for Rural and Small Communities

Children with life-threatening medical conditions are often referred to specialized centers for treatment. Some will need little follow-up care, but others will require considerable amounts of care after they return home. Families in rural areas and small towns and the local health care profession-als, community hospitals, and other organizations that serve them may need special support in caring for such children. Such support may involve a mix of written protocols, family guides, telephone consultations, Internet-based information, interactive videoconferencing, and other tools. Children's hospitals have an important role to play in developing such consultation and information resources. They may require collaboration with or assistance from state officials, national and state associations and professional groups, community business and philanthropic entities, and other groups.

Recommendation: Children's hospitals, hospices with established pedi-atric programs, and other institutions that care for children with fatal or potentially fatal medical conditions should work with professional societies, state agencies, and other organizations to develop regional information programs and other resources to assist clinicians and fami-lies in local and outlying communities and rural areas. These resources should include the following:

• consultative services to advise a child's primary physician or local hospice staff on all aspects of care for the child and the family from diagnosis through death and bereavement;

- clinical, organizational, and other guides and information resources to help families to advocate for appropriate care for their children and themselves; and
- professional education and other programs to support palliative, end-of-life, and bereavement care that is competent, continuous, and coordinated across settings, among providers, and over time (regardless of duration of illness).

Neither regional support services nor actions to improve the coordination and continuity of care are free. In some cases, these activities and others recommended here may promise and produce savings (e.g., from avoided hospitalizations or transfers) that cover or exceed their costs. The costs and savings may, however, sometimes accrue to different parties (e.g., program costs for hospitals and savings for insurers or families). State and local governments and philanthropic and other organizations may provide funds or services in kind to help establish telemedicine and other supportive programs. If, however, the system for financing the provision of services to individual patients and families fails to cover the kinds of palliative, end-of-life, and bereavement services advised in this report, professionals and organizations may struggle merely to provide basic services much less coordinate them and support them regionally. Chapter 7 examines this country's system for financing health care as it relates to pediatric care and palliative care generally and to pediatric palliative, end-of-life, and bereavement care specifically.

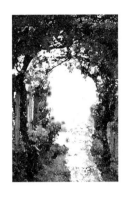

CHAPTER 7

Financing of Palliative and End-of-Life Care for Children and Their Families

[Let me mention] the frustrations that we did have with insurance. You need to have a business degree, I think, to deal with these things.

Winona Kittiko, parent, 2001

Wearing my administrator's hat, I myself see [hospital palliative care] programs as a major risk. They . . . require short-term renovation costs and continuing personnel costs, and invite concern about lost long-term opportunities: What if we had put a profitable cardiac [catheterization] unit into the same space or a chemo infusion center?"

Thomas J. Smith (Lyckholm et al., 2001)

Health insurance—whether public or private—has traditionally focused on acute care services intended to cure disease, prolong life, or restore functioning lost due to illness or injury. It has excluded most preventive services as well as extended care for long-term, chronic illness. Medicaid has been the major exception. From the outset, this federal-state program has covered many long-term care services for beneficiaries with serious chronic health problems and disabilities. Early on, it added a range of preventive services, particularly for children. Medicare and private insurers have gradually added coverage for various preventive services (e.g., screening mammography), influenced in part by contentions that such services could reduce subsequent spending on disease treatment. Medicare and most Medicaid programs and private insurers also now cover at least one form of supportive care—hospice—for patients who are dying.

234

Nevertheless, gaps and other problems in the financing of palliative and end-of-life services contribute to access and quality concerns for adults and children living with life-threatening conditions. Complete lack of insurance is an obvious problem. Yet, even when a person is insured, coverage limitations, financing methods and rules, and administrative practices can create incentives for undertreatment, overtreatment, inappropriate transitions between settings of care, inadequate coordination of care, and poor overall quality of care. Low levels of payment to providers can discourage them from providing certain treatments and from treating some patients at all.

Obtaining a good picture of financing for palliative and end-of-life care services for children is difficult. Unlike virtually all elderly Americans, children are covered not by a single insurance program (Medicare) but, instead, by thousands of private insurers and a multitude of state Medicaid and other public programs that have differing eligibility and coverage policies. These policies are poorly or not conveniently documented and constantly changing, so such information as is available on private health plans and Medicaid programs may be incomplete or out of date.[1] Further, because death in childhood is relatively uncommon, data from surveys (e.g., of hospice and home care services) may not provide reliable estimates. Insofar as available data permit, this chapter

- describes payment sources for palliative, end-of-life, and bereavement care for children and their families;
- reviews relevant coverage and reimbursement policies for private health plans and Medicaid; and
- recommends directions for changes in coverage and reimbursement policies.

---

[1]For those covered by Medicare (particularly the almost 90 percent who are enrolled in the traditional fee-for-service Medicare program), fairly good claims information is available about payment for most kinds of hospital, physician, and other covered services. In addition, the Current Beneficiary Survey tracks service use, out-of-pocket payment, supplemental coverage, health status, and other information that provides a broader picture of health care use and spending for Medicare beneficiaries. These data have been analyzed to determine the share of Medicare spending accounted for by care during the last six months of life, assess the proportion of expenses for different kinds of health services not paid by Medicare, and evaluate beneficiary use of hospice and other services. No such data are available for children.

WHO PAYS FOR PALLIATIVE AND
END OF LIFE CARE FOR CHILDREN?

General

Sources of Payment

Policymakers have long made children, especially poor and sick children, a special focus of programs that promote healthy growth and provide access to needed health services. At the national level, the creation of the Maternal and Child Health Bureau in 1935 (Title V of the Social Security Act) was an important affirmation of the federal government's interest and involvement in services for pregnant women, infants, and "crippled" children (Gittler, 1998).[2] Since then, the program has expanded its focus to include other children with serious chronic health problems. The creation of Medicaid in 1965 significantly expanded access to health insurance and health services for children in low-income families, whether or not they had medical problems. Recently, the State Children's Health Insurance Program (SCHIP) has sought to extend coverage for poor children through Medicaid expansions or other strategies.

Most children (and adults) are, however, covered by private health plans sponsored by employers. As summarized in Figure 7.1, in 2000, almost two-thirds of this country's 72 million children (under age 19) were covered by employment-based or other private health insurance (AHRQ, 2001b). An estimated 20 percent of children had public insurance (primarily Medicaid and then SCHIP).[3] A significant proportion of children—some 15 percent of those under age 19—were not insured. (For those aged 19 to 24, the figure is 33 percent.)

National figures on coverage do not reflect the substantial variation across states. For example, in Maryland in 1997, approximately 78 percent

---

[2]An earlier Maternity and Infancy Act, which was passed in 1921, expired in 1929. The Children's Bureau dates back to 1912. In 1985, Congress changed the terminology for the relevant Title V components from "crippled children" to "children with special health care needs" to reflect expansions in the program's focus and changing attitudes. (see www.ssa.gov/history/childb2.html and www.mchdata.net/LEARN_More/Title_V_History/title_v_history.html).

[3]Under special provisions, Medicare covers those diagnosed with end-stage renal disease who are insured under Social Security or who are spouses or dependent children of such insured persons. In 1997, approximately 2,200 individuals under age 15 were receiving Medicare-covered dialysis (see http://www.hcfa.gov/medicare/esrdtab1.htm). According to the United Network for Organ Sharing, about 600 children under age 18 received kidney transplants in 2000 (http://www.unos.org/Newsroom/critdata_transplants_age.htm#kidney).

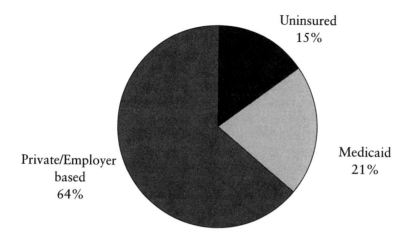

FIGURE 7.1   Source of health insurance coverage for children ages 0 to 18.
NOTE: Figure combines data reported separately for the 0–17 and the 18-year-old age groups.
SOURCE: Compiled from data from Center for Cost and Financing Studies, Agency for Healthcare Research and Quality: Medical Expenditure Panel Survey Household Component, 2000.

of children were covered by private insurance, 6 percent by Medicaid, and 16 percent had no insurance (Tang et al., 2000). In neighboring West Virginia, the comparable figures are 54 percent, 35 percent, and 11 percent, respectively. Arizona, Alaska, and Texas had more than 25 percent of children uninsured compared to less than 8 percent in Hawaii, Minnesota, Vermont, and Washington state. These variations reflect a mix of factors including state economic conditions, immigration, demographics, and political choices about such matters as taxation and spending priorities.

In 1999, of children in poor families (at or below 100 percent of the poverty level or $13,290 for a family of three in that year), an estimated 26 percent were uninsured. Of children in near-poor families (up to 200 percent of the poverty level), an estimated 21 percent were uninsured (Broaddus and Ku, 2000).[4] In 1999, an estimated 85 to 94 percent of low-income,

---

[4]One study of high-cost children in California (including those with conditions not likely to cause death in childhood) suggested that children with high health costs were more likely than other children to be covered by private insurance (about one-half) than by Medicaid (about one-third) or other sources (Ku, 1990). In this study, which included individuals up to age 25, younger children were more likely to have costs covered by private insurance and older children (over age 17) were more likely to be uninsured.

uninsured children were eligible for Medicaid or SCHIP, but their parents or guardians had not enrolled them (Broaddus and Ku, 2000; Dubay et al., 2002a). Approximately two-thirds of the eligible but uninsured children were eligible for Medicaid and the other third for SCHIP. Among children identified as eligible for Medicaid, participation in the program ranges from a high of 93 percent in Massachusetts to a low of 59 percent in Texas (Dubay et al., 2002b; see also HCFA/CMS, 2000g). For children with serious medical problems, hospital social workers or other health care personnel often assist low-income families in enrolling the child in Medicaid, SCHIP, or any other special programs. A recent survey indicated that from 1997 to 2001 the number of uninsured children (under age 18) dropped from 12.1 percent to 9.2 percent while the percentage of children reported to have difficulty getting care dropped from 6.3 to 5.1 percent during this period (Strunk and Cunningham, 2002).

Access to Care: More Than Just Insurance Coverage

Lack of insurance does not necessarily mean the lack of access to all health care, especially for children with life-threatening medical conditions. Uninsured children may have some care paid for or provided by their families, "safety-net providers," philanthropy, and other sources, but they may also go without needed services. Improved financing of care is one cornerstone of improved access to care for children, including children and families living with life-threatening medical conditions (IOM, 1998; Lambrew, 2001).

When children are insured and parents are not, children may still suffer. For example, some research suggests that insured children are less likely to have preventive care if their parents are uninsured (Gifford et al., 2001). As a result, some federal and state insurance initiatives are also reaching out to parents. For example, states can apply for waivers of SCHIP or Medicaid requirements to cover parents directly or through subsidies for enrollment in employer-based plans (AHSRHP, 2001).

Variability in Coverage of Palliative, End-of-Life, and Bereavement Care

Coverage of end-of-life and palliative care services for children who die and their families varies tremendously, both across payer types (e.g., private insurance, Medicaid) and among payers of the same type. Regional variation in coverage policies and their day-to-day interpretation is substantial, as is variation by size and other characteristics of employers. Moving across a state border or changing jobs can result in substantial changes in services covered for seriously ill children and their families.

The next sections of this report review what is known about how three major sources of insurance (private, Medicaid, and SCHIP) cover important palliative, end-of-life, and bereavement services. Other sources of funding for children's care—including federal Title V programs, safety-net providers, philanthropy, family out-of-pocket payments, and clinical trials—are discussed briefly. The focus is on coverage of hospice, home health care, inpatient care, pharmaceuticals, psychosocial services, and respite care. Provider payment methods and levels and other important financing issues are discussed in subsequent sections.

Employment-Based and Other Private Insurance

General

As noted above, almost two-thirds of children in the United States are covered by private health insurance, mostly through plans sponsored by employers that also offer—usually for an additional charge—coverage for an employee's family. Many employers, especially small, low-wage employers, do not offer health insurance, in part because their profit margins are slender and in part because premiums are typically much higher for small firms. Even when employers offer insurance, some employees do not "take up" coverage because the required employee contribution is too high or because better or less expensive coverage is available through a spouse.

Some self-employed and other parents are able to buy family coverage individually. These individuals tend to face high premiums, and those with past medical problems may have difficulty obtaining any coverage. Older children may be able to obtain coverage in their own right as an employee or college student. Some states have programs to help provide private insurance to uninsured individuals.

Summary data on coverage rates do not depict the extent of instability in employer-sponsored coverage. Insurance coverage for children and families may be interrupted or altered for a variety of reasons. Parents may lose their jobs or take new jobs that either offer coverage from different health plans or do not include health benefits at all.[5] In addition, employers may change the scope of benefits they offer or switch health plans, which may mean changes in provider networks or administrative procedures. This can affect continuity of care, a particular concern for families with a seriously ill child. As discussed in Chapter 5, other employer-provided benefits, includ-

---

[5]Federal law generally requires that firms with 20 or more employees allow eligible former employees and covered spouses and children to pay for continued coverage at group rates (actually, at 102 percent of the group premium) for up to 18 or 36 months, depending on the circumstances (http://www.dol.gov/dol/pwba/public/pubs/COBRA/cobra99.pdf). Not all individuals or families can, however, afford such continuation coverage.

ing paid or unpaid leave, may help children with serious medical conditions and their families. Flexible spending accounts, funded with pre-tax dollars, can pay for health care services not covered by an employee's health plan and for deductibles, copayments, and coinsurance that are required for covered services.

Many states have laws requiring that private health plans cover or offer coverage for a wide range of services (e.g., infertility treatments, breast implant removal), some of which (e.g., hospice, mental health care) are relevant to palliative and end-of-life care. Self-insured employers generally claim freedom from such requirements under the Employee Retirement Income Security Act of 1974, commonly referred to as ERISA. Most large and many middle-sized employers are self-insured.

Private Insurance Coverage of Home Hospice Care

As an insurance benefit, hospice coverage normally includes home-based nursing care, physician services, physical or occupational therapy, respiratory therapy, medical social services, medical supplies and certain equipment, and prescription drugs. The benefit usually includes a limited amount of inpatient care if needed for respite or symptom management.

A study by Gabel and colleagues (1998) analyzed information about private hospice coverage from a national random sample of more than 1,500 employers with 200 or more employees each. It also drew on information from focus groups that included employee benefits managers and their insurance advisers. The researchers found that a substantial majority of employers surveyed (83 percent) offered formal hospice benefits. Most of the rest covered a similar range of services through high-cost case management programs that allow case managers discretion to pay for and assist in arranging services not otherwise covered by a health plan. Large employers were more likely to offer hospice benefits than were mid-size employers.

Many private insurance plans have adopted the hospice eligibility and coverage rules used by the Medicare program. Almost half of respondents to the survey by Gabel and colleagues reported that their health plan hospice benefit restricted eligibility to individuals with a life expectancy of six months or less. Another 30 percent did not know whether such a requirement existed in their plan. Unlike Medicare, 28 percent of the plans were reported to include an individual dollar cap on hospice benefits (e.g., $5,000), and 31 percent limited the length of stay.

A second study by Jackson and colleagues (2000) reported an analysis of booklets that summarized benefit plans for 70 large employers. According to these summaries, most employers (88 percent) offered hospice benefits. Most required a physician's certification of a terminal illness, but only half specified a prognosis of six months or less of remaining life. Most plans did not require cost sharing (e.g., paying a fixed amount per visit or a percentage of the charge) for the services, and the majority did not set lifetime day or dollar maximums. Further, in interviews with nine employer representatives, the researchers found more flexibility in the administration of benefits than was suggested by the written plan summaries. The typical comment was that waiving certain benefit restrictions on hospice care was "the right thing to do" (Jackson et al., 2000, p. 4).

Based on their interviews, Jackson and colleagues categorized the nine employer plans as following a Medicare-like model, a comprehensive model, or an unbundled approach. Only two plans followed the Medicare approach of requiring the suspension of curative treatment. Two of the three managed care plans used an unbundled approach, placing the plan's case manager in a central position to enroll individuals in hospice and approve individual care plans and services.

In contrast to the studies described above, Bureau of Labor Statistics (BLS) data, which are based on a large sample of large- and medium-sized private employers (those with 100 or more workers), showed lower rates of hospice coverage in 1997—just 60 percent across all categories (BLS, 1999). The BLS data indicated that health maintenance organization (HMO) plans were more likely to cover hospice than other plans (69 percent versus 43 percent, respectively). A separate BLS survey of state and local government employers reported that 64 percent offered hospice coverage in 1998 (BLS, 2000).

No individual employer example can represent the variability described above, but as an illustration, Table 7.1 presents the hospice coverage listed in the 2002 benefits description for the large Blue Cross Blue Shield options for federal employees. Among other restrictions, the plan requires prior approval. Coverage excludes bereavement services but includes inpatient care to provide brief respite for family members. As with all the other health plans offered to federal employees, the benefit structure is approved and sometimes directed by the federal Office of Personnel Management rather than unilaterally determined by the insurer or health plan.

Private Insurance Coverage of Home Health Care

Health plan rules, licensure regulations, and physician and family reluctance to accept hospice can make home hospice coverage less helpful than it might otherwise be for children who die and their families. For these children and families, home health care providers, including those affiliated with hospices, may offer an array of supportive medical and other services including home nursing care. Also, home health agencies may start providing care before a child is recognized as dying. Continuity with the same organization and personnel may be reassuring to a child and family, even

TABLE 7.1   2002 Hospice Coverage Benefits for Blue Cross Blue Shield
Federal Employees Health Insurance Plan

Hospice Care	You Pay– Standard Option	You Pay– Basic Option
Hospice care is an integrated set of services and supplies designed to provide palliative and supportive care to terminally ill patients in their homes. We provide the following **home hospice care** benefits for members with a life expectancy of six months or less **when prior approval is obtained from the Local Plan** and the home hospice agency is approved by the Local Plan: • Physician visits • Nursing care • Medical social services • Physical therapy • Services of home health aides • Durable medical equipment rental • Prescription drugs • Medical supplies	Nothing	Nothing
Inpatient hospice for members receiving home hospice care benefits: Benefits are provided	Preferred: $100 per admission copayment	Preferred: $100 per day copayment up to $500 per admission

when home hospice care is covered by the family's health plan and would otherwise be acceptable to parents.

The Bureau of Labor Statistics reported that 85 percent of large and medium-sized private employers provided some home health care coverage (BLS, 1999). HMO plans were more likely to cover these services than other plans (93 percent versus 81 percent).

Health plans that pay for home health care may, however, exclude certain services that are often or sometimes included in hospice benefits (e.g., physical therapy, bereavement care). Moreover, state licensure requirements may restrict licensed home health care providers from providing certain end-of-life services such as bereavement care. In addition, employer-sponsored plans often limit coverage for home health care to a certain

TABLE 7.1 Continued

Hospice Care	You Pay– Standard Option	You Pay– Basic Option
for up to five (5) consecutive days in a hospice inpatient facility. Each inpatient stay must be separated by at least 21 days. These covered inpatient hospice benefits are available only when inpatient services are necessary to: • Control pain and manage the patient's symptoms; or • provide an interval of relief (respite) to the family Note: **You are responsible for making sure that the home hospice care provider has received prior approval from the Local Plan.** Please check with your Local Plan and/or your PPO directory for listings of approved agencies.	Member: $300 per admission copayment Non-member: $300 per admission copayment plus 30% of the Plan allowance, and any remaining balance after our payment	Member/Non-member: You pay all charges
Not covered: Homemaker or bereavement services	All charges	All charges

NOTE: PPO = preferred provider organization.
SOURCE: Blue Cross and Blue Shield, 2002 Service Benefit Plan, p. 63, http://www.fepblue.org/pdf/2002sbp.pdf (emphasis in the original).

number of nursing or therapy visits (e.g., 60 visits per year) or require that care be expected to lead to improvement in the health condition. Thus, services needed by chronically or terminally ill patients on an ongoing basis such as nursing visits, respiratory therapy, and physical therapy may be limited or excluded altogether under an employer's plan.

In one study of Medicare financing of end-of-life services, end-of-life care providers (including home health agencies as well as hospices) reported the need for end-of-life consults from a hospice team for dying patients not enrolled in hospice in order to assist in symptom management and end-of-life care planning (Huskamp et al., 2001). Such consultative services for a patient receiving home health care would not ordinarily be covered by private health insurance (unless the health plan waived coverage restrictions as described earlier). In these situations, lack of coverage for consultations by hospice or other palliative care experts may lead to avoidable pain and other suffering for dying children and their families.

As discussed in Chapter 6, telemedicine could help extend information and advice to support home health providers for children and families in smaller communities and rural areas. Private insurer coverage for telemedicine services is limited (OAT, 2001).

Private Insurance Coverage of Inpatient Hospital Care

The centerpiece of most private health insurance has traditionally been coverage for inpatient hospital services, which continue to be generously covered compared to other services. Thus, much of the emergency, intensive, and palliative care—including nursing care, diagnostic tests, medications, and many other services—that is provided to children with life-threatening conditions is routinely covered.

If, however, patients, families, and physicians choose to forgo curative or life-prolonging care in favor of inpatient care that is exclusively but intensively palliative, some health plans may refuse to pay if the plan limits inpatient coverage to treatment intended to cure or restore function. (As discussed later, even if coverage is not an issue, the case-based and other payment systems for hospitals are based on data and assumptions that exclude modern palliative services, which is a disincentive for hospitals to provide these services.) The committee found no systematic information on the extent to which coverage is approved or denied when inpatient pediatric care is exclusively palliative.

Private Insurance Coverage of Outpatient Prescription Drugs

Unlike Medicare, most employers that offer insurance to employees cover outpatient prescription drugs, subject to various limitations such as cost sharing requirements. Information from a large survey of employers indicates that nearly all employees (96 percent) covered by employer health plans had prescription drug coverage in 1997 (Marquis and Long, 2000). Even for small employers and low-wage employers, more than 85 percent provided outpatient drug coverage.

BLS data for medium- and large-sized private employers also show very high levels of employer coverage of outpatient prescription drugs (BLS, 1999). For nearly 80 percent of covered workers, the level of cost sharing for prescription drugs was no higher than for physician services; about 18 percent faced higher cost sharing for drugs.

Spending for prescription drugs has increased dramatically during the last decade. Health plans have responded by increasing the level of cost sharing and using pharmacy benefit managers (PBMs) to manage drug benefits separate from their general health plan or plans (Cook et al., 2000; Mays et al., 2001). Elements of these programs typically include negotiated price discounts with manufacturers, a mail order service, drug utilization review to detect inappropriate prescribing patterns, processing of drug claims, and formulary management. In an insurance context, a formulary is a list of covered drugs.

Most HMOs, preferred provider organizations (PPOs), and PBMs report using some kind of formulary that sets forth what prescription drugs are routinely covered and what exceptions are permitted under specified circumstances (Wyeth-Ayerst, 1999). Some plans have closed formularies, meaning that they refuse to pay for drugs not on the list. These plans often offer an exemption process that allows coverage of an unlisted drug if a patient's physician provides documentation that the particular drug is medically necessary for the patient. The flexibility of this "exemption" process varies across plans.

A three-tier approach to pharmacy benefits has become increasingly common. Although the specifics vary, the first tier, with the lowest copayments, typically consists of generic drugs (e.g., generic amoxicillin). The second tier consists of brand-name drugs that the organization considers to be safe, effective, and reasonably priced. The third tier consists of nonpreferred brand drugs, for example, those that the plan judges not to provide better outcomes for their extra cost. Drugs considered to be primarily "lifestyle-enhancing" in nature (e.g., Propecia for baldness, Viagra for sexual dysfunction) may also be included in the third tier, or they may be excluded from coverage altogether.

Depending on the values, knowledge, and choices of the health plan and the PBM about, for example, pain medications, these programs could make effective drugs more or less costly for children with serious medical problems (Motheral and Henderson, 2000; Motheral and Fairman, 2001). Formulary provisions could also lead parents and physicians to select less costly drugs that are also less effective for a particular child given, for example, his or her ability to metabolize certain opioids or other drugs.[6]

A separate and often controversial issue with employment-based health plans is the introduction of therapeutic substitution policies. Such policies

---

[6]Not all persons are created equal in the enzymes needed to metabolize medications. The absence of certain enzymes can render some drugs pharmacologically inert. One example is codeine, a pain medication suited to mild-to-moderate pain that is commonly prescribed for children (although other medications may have fewer side effects). Recently, researchers reported that that 10 percent of Caucasians, 3 percent of Asians, and 1 percent of African-Americans in the United States lack the liver enzyme CYP2D6 need to convert codeine to its active form, morphine. Neonates and infants also have lower levels of this enzyme (see the review in Williams et al., 2001a).

allow pharmacists to substitute an alternative drug (a different chemical entity) considered therapeutically equivalent[7] in place of the drug prescribed by the physician. Such policies are controversial because designations of therapeutic equivalence may not adequately reflect the physiological variability that a clinician may recognize in an individual patient's response to a drug but that has not yet been demonstrated scientifically.

Private Insurance Coverage of Psychosocial, Respite, and Other Services

Most employer health plans provide coverage for mental health services that may help children with life-threatening medical problems and assist families before and after a child's death. Some health plans cover (i.e., allow direct billing by and payment to) for services provided by a clinical psychologist or clinical social worker. Child-life specialists, art therapists, music therapists, chaplains, or other personnel are rarely if ever reimbursed directly for their professional services.

Except through hospice, health insurance plans generally do not cover bereavement care as such, although insured parents or siblings may be covered for services to treat depression, anxiety, and certain other emotional problems experienced during bereavement. One disadvantage of coverage contingent on these diagnoses is that bereaved family members may receive a diagnostic label that could jeopardize their future ability to qualify for health insurance, especially individually purchased insurance. Even as part of their hospice benefits, private health plans do not universally cover

---

[7]The Food and Drug Administration (FDA) "classifies as therapeutically equivalent those products that meet the following general criteria: (1) they are approved as safe and effective; (2) they are pharmaceutical equivalents in that they (a) contain identical amounts of the same active drug ingredient in the same dosage form and route of administration, and (b) meet compendial or other applicable standards of strength, quality, purity, and identity; (3) they are bioequivalent in that (a) they do not present a known or potential bioequivalence problem, and they meet an acceptable in vitro standard, or (b) if they do present such a known or potential problem, they are shown to meet an appropriate bioequivalence standard; (4) they are adequately labeled; and (5) they are manufactured in compliance with Current Good Manufacturing Practice regulations. The concept of therapeutic equivalence, as used to develop the List, applies only to drug products containing the same active ingredient(s) and does not encompass a comparison of different therapeutic agents used for the same condition (e.g., propoxyphene hydrochloride vs. pentazocine hydrochloride for the treatment of pain). Any drug product in the List repackaged and/or distributed by other than the application holder is considered to be therapeutically equivalent to the application holder's drug product even if the application holder's drug product is single source or coded as non-equivalent (e.g., BN). Also, distributors or repackagers of an application holder's drug product are considered to have the same code as the application holder. Therapeutic equivalence determinations are not made for unapproved, off-label indications." (FDA Orange Book; http://www.fda.gov/cder/ob/docs/preface/ecpreface.htm#Therapeutic Equivalence-Related Terms).

bereavement counseling for family members. (See, e.g., Table 7.1 and other illustrative examples at Presbyterian Health, 2001; and Aetna Insurance, 2001).

Traditionally, most private insurance plans have imposed special benefit limits (e.g., higher copayments or coinsurance, caps on the number of visits or total payments during a year or lifetime) for mental health services that they did not apply to other types of covered health care services. In the Mental Health Parity Act of 1996 (P.L. 104-204, reauthorized for one year in 2001), Congress required that if an employee health benefit plan covers mental illness, the plan cannot set lower annual or lifetime spending limits for mental health services than those set for services for physical or surgical illnesses (Otten, 1998).[8]

Employer plans may cover limited amounts of respite care as part of hospice benefits. Otherwise, benefits for respite care appear to be rare.[9] Most discussions of expansion in respite services focus on public programs (see, e.g., Silberberg, 2001). When a child has a severe chronic condition, families may bear extraordinary physical, emotional, and financial burdens because neither regular paid assistance nor occasional respite care is covered.

Innovations in Coverage

Some private health plans have developed or are testing innovative programs of coverage for palliative and end-of-life care focused on adults. For example, a recent publication sponsored by the Robert Wood Johnson Foundation (RWJF) described nine programs involving Blue Cross and Blue Shield plans in various parts of the country (Butler and Twohig, 2001).

Two plans (Regence Blue Shield and Premera Blue Cross) participated with the state of Washington in an RWJF-sponsored research project led by the Children's Hospital and Medical Center of Seattle. Regence's program covered any child under age 21 in a health plan that included a benefits management clause that allows waivers of certain plan restrictions under certain circumstances. After the project began, the plan added payment for

---

[8]Plans can, however, set lower limits on the number of covered outpatient visits or hospital stays and can require higher cost sharing (deductibles, coinsurance, or copayments) by patients (Aston, 2001). They can also choose not to offer coverage at all. More than 30 states have some kind of mental health parity legislation, some going beyond current federal law. Some restrict parity to a subset of mental health diagnoses only, whereas others encompass substance abuse as well as mental health services. As noted earlier, ERISA frees self-insured employers from these mandates.

[9]Limited respite care benefits may be provided as part of long-term care insurance plans, which usually must be purchased directly by individuals. These policies are intended for adults who are basically healthy at the time of purchase.

a child's participation in well-designed clinical research as a case management option, and it is developing a palliative care "add-on" feature to offer as part of future benefits packages. The Premera program was designed to assist early access to hospice care, promote active case management, and encourage creative use of home care benefits. Both plans used a "decision-making tool" (developed by medical ethicists at the University of Washington) that provided a comprehensive framework for discussing all aspects of a child's care and taking into account medical circumstances, family preferences and situations, quality of life, and financial issues. Challenges identified by the two health plans included early identification of children and families who might benefit from hospice care and changing the relationship with hospices from adversarial to cooperative. Cost and satisfaction data are still being collected and analyzed.

Blue Cross Blue Shield of Montana is participating in a multisite project, this one testing the Advanced Illness Coordinated Care model that was developed by the Life Institute and is described in its pediatric format in Chapter 6. This program is unusual because the plan will fund participation in the program of 120 people under age 65, whether or not they have coverage from the plan. The program is organized around six to nine home visits made by case managers to individuals who have a fatal diagnosis but do not meet hospice criteria. The case management services are paid for by the plan under a contract with the Life Institute. The plan anticipates that the discussions will lead to some cost savings based on advance care planning and avoidable hospitalization.

In addition, as one outgrowth of its involvement in community initiatives to improve end-of-life care, the Blue Cross Blue Shield plan (Excellus) in Rochester, New York, recently established payment for palliative care consultations by physicians certified in hospice and palliative medicine (BCBSRA, 2002). The plan also has established a program called CompassionNet aimed at children who meet one of the following criteria:

- a diagnosis of a potentially life threatening illness,
- two unplanned hospitalizations in the preceding six months (other than for asthma),
- an acute exacerbation of a chronic illness that creates an extreme risk, or
- a prognosis of three years of life or less.

Medicaid

General

The state–federal Medicaid program is a critical source of funding for services to low-income children. It covers large numbers of children with chronic illnesses and serious disabilities. [10] Consistent with Title XIX of the Social Security Act, federal law establishes requirements for states that participate in Medicaid, which all states now do. Among other services, states must cover

- children ages 6 to 18 with family incomes at or below 100 percent of the federal poverty level (in 2001, $14,630 for a family of three) (to be fully phased in as of 2002) and
- children under age 6 and pregnant women with family incomes at or below 133 percent of the federal poverty level.

About 80 percent of Medicaid-enrolled children are covered under the mandatory categories. The remainder, whose families have higher incomes, are covered at the discretion of states. The optional coverage categories for children include

- infants up to age 1 and pregnant women, who are not covered under the mandatory rules and whose family income is no more than 185 percent of the federal poverty level (with the specific percentage set by each state),
- children under age 21 who meet the income and resources requirements for Aid to Families with Dependent Children (AFDC) that were in effect in their state on July 16, 1996, and
- children under age 18 who qualify under complicated federal and state rules as "medically needy."

In general, the option for "medically needy" children allows a state to extend Medicaid coverage when the family's income is too high to qualify otherwise but the child has very high medical expenses. The family "spends down" to eligibility because the child's medical expenses reduce the family's income below the state Medicaid maximum. If a state has a medically needy program, it must include certain children under age 18 and pregnant women who would otherwise be eligible as "categorically needy" under the optional coverage requirements.[11]

Overall, children comprise just over half of Medicaid enrollees, roughly 21 million out of 40 million total in 1998. Reflecting their generally good

---

[10]Unless otherwise indicated, data in this section come from HCFA/CMS (2000b; 2001d).

[11]States may also allow families to establish eligibility as medically needy by paying monthly premiums to the state in an amount equal to the difference between family income (reduced by unpaid expenses, if any, incurred for medical care in previous months) and the income eligibility standard (HCFA/CMS, 1997; http://www.hcfa.gov/medicaid/meligib.htm).

health, however, children accounted for only about 14 percent of Medicaid expenditures of nearly $170 billion dollars that year (Kaiser Commission on Medicaid and the Uninsured, 2001).

Within federal requirements (and monitoring capabilities), states have considerable discretion to establish eligibility for Medicaid, determine the scope of services covered (e.g., number of physician office visits during a year), set levels of enrollee cost sharing for adults except pregnant women (e.g., $5 per office visit), establish methods and rates of payment for services, and administer the program. Federal law requires, however, that state Medicaid programs cover a generally broader array of services for children than for adults. The major vehicle for achieving this objective was 1969 legislation (P.L. 90-248) and subsequent amendments requiring coverage for early periodic screening, detection, and treatment (EPSDT) services for those under age 21. In 1989, Congress specifically defined the required EPSDT benefits (P.L. 101-239). It also required states to provide necessary health care, diagnostic services, treatment, and other measures to "correct or ameliorate defects and physical and mental illnesses and conditions discovered by the screening services, whether or not such services are covered under the State plan" (42 USC §1396d(r)(5)). (See also HCFA/CMS, 2001c). Some states responded by expanding their list of covered services; other states provided that decisions about services not usually covered be made on a case-by-case basis (NASMD, 1999). Box 7.1 lists the services specified in the 1989 legislation.

The EPSDT provisions would seem to require states to provide children (including those with life-threatening medical conditions) access to almost any medical and supportive service identified as needed through screening.[12] In practice, reflecting the potentially large additional costs they would face, states have often been slow to implement EPSDT provisions or have been very restrictive in their interpretations of the provisions (Perkins, 1999; O'Connell and Watson, 2001). These responses have prompted a number of lawsuits, several of which have focused on services for children with mental or developmental disabilities, including those on waiting lists for

---

[12]Screening has been unconventionally defined in this context to include certain visits prompted by symptoms. "Interperiodic EPSDT Screening Services are physical, mental, dental, vision or hearing screens described in subsection (b) that, in furtherance of the preventive purpose of the EPSDT benefit: (i) occur at a time other than the applicable periodic EPSDT screening services referenced in subparagraph (A); and (ii) is requested by an enrolled child's family or caregiver or by an individual who comes into regular contact with the child and who suspects the existence of a physical, mental or developmental health problem (or possible worsening of a preexisting physical, mental or developmental health condition)"(CHSRP, 1999, http://www.gwumc.edu/chpr/sps/part1.htm). See also the State Medicaid Manual discussion of medically necessary interperiodic screening (HCFA/CMS Publication 45; http://www.hcfa.gov/pubforms/progman.htm).

home and community-based services. In any case, it is not clear what EPSDT services are effectively available to Medicaid-covered children in each state.

Adding to the complexity of summarizing state Medicaid coverage, most states have been rapidly enrolling beneficiaries in managed care programs, whose specific coverage and other policies also vary. Under Section 1915(b) waivers of "freedom-of-choice" provisions of Title XIX, states can require Medicaid enrollees to enroll in comprehensive or specialized (e.g., behavioral health) managed care plans (HCFA/CMS, 2001a). The Balanced Budget Act of 1997 allows states to institute mandatory enrollment through an amendment to their state plan and thereby bypass this waiver process. One exception is that states must still get a waiver to require managed care enrollment for children with special health care needs, a group that will include some children with fatal or potentially fatal medical conditions (Gruttadaro et al., 2001). This restriction recognizes the particular care requirements and vulnerabilities of special needs children.

In 2000, 56 percent of Medicaid beneficiaries were enrolled in some form of managed care, up from 40 percent in 1996 (HCFA/CMS, 2000b).[13] These percentages include some who were enrolled in more than one kind of plan. In 1998, the percentage of Medicaid beneficiaries enrolled in managed care plans ranged from zero in Alaska and Wyoming to more than 75 percent in a dozen states (HCFA/CMS, 2000b). More than 55 percent of all Medicaid managed care enrollees were children.

In addition to the freedom-of-choice waivers, states can also obtain waivers that allow them to include additional populations or services not otherwise covered under Medicaid. As discussed further below, under Section 1915(c) waivers, states can provide additional home and community-

---

[13]As defined by the Health Care Financing Administration (HCFA), now CMS, several Medicaid managed care options exist. *PCCM* (primary care case management) provider is usually a physician, physician group practice, or an entity employing or having other arrangements with such physicians who contracts to locate, coordinate, and monitor covered primary care (and sometimes additional services). This category includes PCCMs and those prepaid health plans that act as PCCMs. *PHP* (prepaid health plan) provides less than comprehensive services on an at-risk basis or provides any benefit package on a nonrisk basis. For example, medical-only PHP, dental PHP, transportation PHP, mental health PHP, substance abuse PHP, etc. *Commercial MCO* (managed care organization) is an HMO, an eligible organization with a contract under Section 1876 or a Medicare+Choice organization, a provider-sponsored organization, or any other private or public organization that meets the requirements of Section 1902(w). These MCOs provide comprehensive services to commercial and/or Medicare enrollees, as well as Medicaid enrollees. *Medicaid MCO* provides comprehensive services to Medicaid beneficiaries, but not to commercial or Medicare enrollees. *HIO* (health insuring organization) provides or arranges for the provision of care and contracts on a prepaid capitated risk basis to provide a comprehensive set of services. *"Other" managed care entity* is used if the plan is not considered a PCCM, PHP, MCO or HIO.

Box 7.1
Scope of Medicaid EPSDT Services for Enrolled Children
Required by Federal Statute (42 U.S.C. § 1396d(a)(22))

- Inpatient hospital services (other than services in an institution for mental disease)
- Outpatient hospital services
- Rural health clinic services (including home visits for homebound individuals)
- Federally qualified health center services
- Other laboratory and x-ray services (in an office or similar facility)
- EPSDT services
- Family planning services and supplies
- Physician services (in office, patient's home, hospital, nursing facility, or elsewhere)
- Medical and surgical services furnished by a dentist
- Medical care or any other type of remedial care
- Home health care services (in place of residence)
- Private duty nursing services (in the home, hospital, and/or skilled nursing facility)
- Clinic services (including services outside of clinic for eligible homeless individuals)
- Dental services
- Physical therapy and related services (including occupational therapy and services for individuals with speech, hearing, and language disorders)
- Prescribed drugs
- Dentures
- Prosthetic devices
- Eyeglasses

based services as an alternative to institutional care (Smith et al., 2000).[14] Waiver services do not have to be provided on a statewide basis or to all those with similar levels of need.

Under yet another waiver authority (Section 1115), states can undertake demonstration projects to test innovative program ideas or service concepts. As noted in Chapter 1 and discussed further below, Congress has authorized several state demonstration projects to test innovative approaches to providing comprehensive palliative and end-of-life care for

---

[14]When developed for children with disabilities, Section 1915(c) waiver programs are often referred to as Katie Beckett programs for the child dependent on a ventilator whose situation prompted national attention and initial legislative action (Federal Tax Equity and Fiscal Responsibility Act of 1982, P.L. 97-248).

- Other diagnostic, screening, preventive, and rehabilitative services, including medical or remedial services recommended for the maximum reduction of physical or mental disability and restoration of an individual to the best possible functional level (in a facility, home, or other setting)
  - Services in an intermediate care facility for the mentally retarded
  - Inpatient psychiatric hospital services for individuals under age 21
- Services furnished by a midwife, which the nurse-midwife is legally authorized to perform under state law, without regard to whether or not the services are performed in the area of management of the care of mothers and babies throughout the maternity cycle
  - Hospice care
  - Case management services
  - Tuberculosis-related services
  - Respiratory care services
- Services furnished by a certified pediatric nurse practitioner or certified family nurse practitioner that the practitioner is legally authorized to perform under state law
- Community-supported living arrangement services (e.g., personal assistance, habilitation services, assistive technology), to the extent allowed and defined in 42 U.S.C. §1396u
- Personal care services (in a home or other location) furnished to an individual who is not an inpatient or resident of a hospital, nursing facility, intermediate care facility for the mentally retarded, or institution for mental disease
  - Primary care case management services
- Any other medical care, and any other type of remedial care recognized under state law, specified by the secretary (includes transportation and personal care services in a recipient's home)

SOURCE: Perkins, 1999.

children and families. Eligibility for services provided under this demonstration waiver authority is not restricted to low-income families. A condition for both Section 1915(c) and Section 1115 waivers is that they be budget neutral (i.e., not generate costs to the federal government more than occur without the waiver).

As discussed in a later section on professional and provider payment, Medicaid coverage for specific services is less an issue for many physicians, hospitals, and Medicaid enrollees than is the level and predictability of payments. A significant fraction of physicians do not accept Medicaid patients because payment levels are low and claims administration can be frustratingly inconsistent (Yudowsky et al., 2000; see also AAP, 1999d). This can result in access problems for children covered by Medicaid.

Medicaid Coverage of Home Hospice

Under federal Medicaid requirements, hospice is an optional benefit for adults. Most state Medicaid programs include hospice, but programs in Connecticut, Nebraska, New Hampshire, Oklahoma, and South Dakota do not (Tilly and Weiner, 2001). For children, however, the 1989 EPSDT amendments cited earlier include hospice as a covered service. Therefore, children should have coverage for hospice even in states that do not provide hospice coverage to adult Medicaid enrollees.

The Medicaid hospice benefit follows the Medicare benefit in defining covered services, payment categories, and payment rates. Like Medicare enrollees, Medicaid enrollees must be certified as having a life expectancy of six months or less and must agree to forgo curative treatment (interpreted to include life-prolonging therapies) of their terminal illness in order to be eligible for the hospice benefit (MedPAC, 2002). Even when children are enrolled in Medicaid, hospice services may not be covered because the physician is unable or reluctant to certify a six-month prognosis. As discussed in Chapter 4, determining prognosis is even more difficult and uncertain for children than for adults. Also, families seeking assistance from hospice may still want the option of potentially life-prolonging interventions for their child. Medicaid home health benefits (discussed below) may cover some but not all of the services provided by hospices.

Although Medicaid beneficiaries have to forgo curative care to receive hospice benefits, federal law no longer requires that Medicaid beneficiaries receiving hospice care give up other supportive Medicaid services. Specifically, the Omnibus Budget Reconciliation Act of 1990 (P.L.101-508) allows "payment for Medicaid services related to the treatment of the terminal condition and other medical services that would be equivalent to or duplicative of hospice care, so long as the services would not be covered under the Medicare hospice program. This means that Medicaid can cover certain services which Medicare does not cover" (HCFA/CMS, 2001b).

Nonetheless, it appears that some state Medicaid programs (e.g., New York) may force families to choose between hospice and more benefits for home and community-based services (Tilly and Weiner, 2001). Hospice personnel have repeatedly mentioned this as a concern in discussions with committee members and staff. The apparent divergence between federal policy and some state practice requires further attention as an inappropriate barrier to needed services for dying children.

In addition, Huskamp and colleagues (2001) have noted access problems for some high-cost hospice patients (e.g., those requiring expensive pain medications, blood transfusions[15]) enrolled in Medicare. Providers

---

[15]The committee understands that some hospices lack staff expertise to manage blood or platelet transfusions and that some view transfusions as too aggressive for a palliative inter-

reported that hospices would not enroll some patients because the hospice felt it could not afford to provide the high-cost services needed by a patient, given the Medicare (and Medicaid) per diem rates for hospice care. Alternatively, patients might be enrolled under the condition that certain high-cost items would not be provided by the hospice. The extent to which Medicaid patients—adults or children—experience this kind of access problem warrants investigation.

Medicaid Coverage of Home Health Care

A child's eligibility for home care services under Medicaid can be difficult to determine given the complexity of federal Medicaid provisions and the variability in state Medicaid policies (see, e.g., Smith et al., 2000). Under federal law, required home health services for eligible beneficiaries include nursing care, home health aides, and medical supplies and equipment.[16] Optional home health services include physical and occupational therapy. States have the option to cover personal care services, including assistance with bathing, dressing, and other routine daily activities.

Nearly all state Medicaid programs also provide some home care coverage under Section 1915(c) waivers that—as noted earlier—encourage a wide range of home and community-based services as an alternative to institutional care. The federal waiver provisions specifically mention home health, personal care, case management, respite care, adult day health services, habilitation services, and homemaker services. Eligibility for services provided to children under this waiver authority is not necessarily restricted to low-income families, but coverage need not be state wide, and the groups targeted for assistance may be quite narrow (e.g., persons with brain injuries).

Again, notwithstanding general Medicaid policies, EPSDT provisions would appear to require that a range of home care and home health services

---

vention. Other hospice and palliative care experts believe that such transfusions are appropriate (but costly) ways to prevent or manage serious visible bleeding associated with the late stages of certain cancers and other diseases (see, e.g., Goldman, 1999).

[16]A recent report has noted confusion about Medicaid home health benefits. "Since 1970, home health services have been mandatory for persons entitled to nursing facility care. Confusion about eligibility for home health services has arisen because the term entitled to nursing facility care has sometimes been erroneously interpreted to mean that people must be eligible for nursing facility care—i.e., that they must meet a state's nursing facility level-of-care criteria—in order to receive home health benefits. This erroneous interpretation has persisted notwithstanding its conflict with home health regulations prohibiting a state from conditioning eligibility for home health services on the need for or discharge from institutional care" (Smith et al., 2000, no page number).

be covered for children for whom such services are necessary. Also, as discussed below, other federal and state programs—primarily those funded by Title V—may assist with home and other services for children with special health care needs and their families. Medicaid coverage for telemedicine services in the home is limited. Compared to private insurers, however, states appear to have been somewhat more receptive to arguments for such coverage (OAT, 2001; see also http://www.hcfa.gov/medicaid/telemed.htm).

Medicaid Coverage of Inpatient Hospital Care

As is the case for private insurance, much of the emergency, intensive, and palliative care provided to children who die is covered as an inpatient service. The EPSDT services listed earlier in Box 7.1 do not include inpatient palliative care specifically, but EPSDT coverage requirements would seem to extend to almost any medical and supportive service identified as needed by a child. The committee found no information on coverage in practice for hospitalized children receiving only palliative services. The same kinds of reimbursement issues mentioned in the review of private coverage of inpatient palliative services apply in a general sense to Medicaid and are discussed further below.

Medicaid Coverage of Outpatient Prescription Drugs

Prescription drug coverage is optional for adults covered by Medicaid, but federal EPSDT policy requires coverage for children and also prohibits cost-sharing requirements (Bruen, 2000, 2002). Some states set no restrictions on the number of covered prescriptions for children, whereas others require prior authorization once a numerical limit is reached. For example, a South Carolina survey reported that five of eight southeastern states had no restrictions on the number of prescriptions for children, but three required preauthorization for prescriptions above a specified number (e.g., six per month in Georgia and North Carolina) (Legislative Audit Council, 2000). Limits on the number of prescriptions covered could create a barrier to effective symptom management for children with life-threatening medical problems and multiple or difficult symptoms.[17]

Federal legislation passed in 1993 (P.L. 103-66) allowed states to institute a number of restrictions on coverage of prescription drugs, including

---

[17]As discussed in Chapter 10, many drugs approved for use with adults do not have dosing information for children, and recent legislation includes incentives and requirements to stimulate the research needed to provide such information.

prior authorization requirements and closed formularies (Kaiser Commission, 2001).[18] If a drug is excluded from a formulary, patients must still be able to seek coverage through a prior approval process. Several state Medicaid programs (e.g., Michigan, Florida) recently announced an intention to implement a closed formulary (Bruen, 2002). As is true for private health plans, one goal of formulary implementation is to negotiate lower drug prices or additional services (e.g., chronic disease management programs in Florida) with manufacturers.

How restrictive closed Medicaid formularies are or will be is still unclear, as is how they may affect children with life-threatening medical conditions and their families. Their restrictiveness will depend on the burden imposed by the prior approval process and on the extent to which the formulary includes an adequate number and choice of drugs effective for the palliation of pain and other symptoms.

Managed care introduces another complication for assessments of outpatient prescription drug coverage. A 1999 report on Medicaid formularies concluded that "some states do not monitor to see whether managed care organizations are assuring that Medicaid recipients receive the Medicaid pharmacy benefit. Since often only a closed formulary is available to their commercial members, providers [managed care plans] may not treat Medicaid recipients differently" (Bazelon, 1999, online, no page number).

Legislation in 1990 (P.L.101-508) required states to develop retrospective and prospective Medicaid drug utilization review programs. A retrospective program could, for example, involve profiling of providers in an attempt to reduce inappropriate prescribing patterns. A prospective program could involve the use of automated systems that produce an alert when prescriptions might result in drug–drug interactions for a patient. The goals of these programs can include monitoring safety and quality of care as well as cost containment (Kaiser Commission, 2001). The effects on children living with life-threatening conditions could be positive or negative depending on which drugs were monitored and what safety or quality criteria were used.

Medicaid Coverage of Psychosocial, Respite, and Other Services

State Medicaid programs are required to cover a broader range of mental health services for children than for adults. Most attention has

---

[18]Federal law allows Medicaid programs to exclude drugs from their formulary under two conditions: (1) when the exclusion is based on labeling or information in official medical compendia and (2) when the drug offers no clinically significant advantage related to safety, effectiveness, or health outcome over other drugs (Omnibus Budget Reconciliation Act of 1993, P.L. 103-66).

focused on EPSDT-required services for the early identification and treatment of children's mental health problems and on long-term services for children with developmental disabilities or mental illness.

A number of different categories of professionals provide mental health services, but state policies vary on whether they directly reimburse psychologists, social workers, clinical nurse specialists (psychiatric), and other nonphysicians for services provided to Medicaid beneficiaries. According to a 1995 analysis by the American Psychological Association, 42 states allowed direct payment to psychologists for EPSDT services (APA, 1995).

With increasing numbers of children enrolled in managed care plans, scrutiny of these plans includes contract provisions and plan practices (e.g., prior authorization based on "medical necessity" determinations) that may affect the availability and quality of mental health services for children, especially those with special needs (see, e.g., NIMH, 1998; Stroul et al., 1998). Scrutiny is also being directed at the practices of specialized managed behavioral health organizations into which states have directed Medicaid beneficiaries with behavioral health problems. Some studies suggest that families tend to have difficulties getting timely referrals from Medicaid managed care plans for mental health services—even short-term services—for children with special needs (see, e.g., Fox et al., 2000).

Although problems with Medicaid coverage of mental health services will affect some children who die and their families, they do not appear to be high-priority concerns for this population. Clinicians and families are generally focused on other issues.

Bereavement services for family members of a child who dies are not explicitly covered by Medicaid outside the hospice benefit. (As discussed later, payment for such services is included in the per diem payments to hospices, which end with the patient's death.) A parent or sibling covered by Medicaid in his or her own right might, however, be able to receive supportive mental health services upon referral for a diagnosis of depression or certain other emotional problems.

As Box 7.1 indicates, state Medicaid programs are not required under federal law to provide respite care, which offers family members rest and relief from the demands of caring at home for a child with major health care needs. Some states have applied for waivers to cover such services, but these are usually limited to a subset of diagnoses or conditions (e.g., severe mental retardation) (see, e.g., http://ddd.state.wy.us/Documents/kathy1.htm and http://www.dhs.state.tx.us/programs/communitycare/mdcp/services.html). In reality, Medicaid in-home services for a child may provide respite to the child's family caregivers, but this is not their explicit purpose.

Innovations in Medicaid Coverage

In 1999, Congress appropriated funds for a series of demonstration projects to support the development of children's hospice programs that provide integrated medical, social, and other services to children with life-threatening medical conditions (CHI, 2002). A major task for these projects, called Programs for All-Inclusive Care for Children and their Families (PACC), is to identify obstacles to such integrated care that are related to Medicaid and other regulations. In its solicitation of proposals from these states (HCFA/CMS, 2000c), the government described the most burdensome obstacles to pediatric palliative care:

- requirements that limit hospice eligibility to children certified by a physician as being within six months of death;
- regulatory limits on the array of services that a child may need, including skilled, intermittent, and 24-hour nursing care, respite care, music and other therapies designed to meet children's developmental needs, and bereavement care;
- payment limits that discourage hospices from accepting children who require expensive care;
- waiver program provisions (e.g., requirements that a child needs an institutional level of care) that are not fitted to the needs of children who could benefit from hospice care; and
- EPSDT programs that are inconsistent or too narrow.

The goals of the demonstration projects include (1) identifying children and families who could benefit from better integration and coordination of palliative, end-of-life, and bereavement services; (2) devising integrated care strategies and identifying necessary waivers of restrictive regulations; (3) reducing hospital use by increasing services in the community; and (4) increasing awareness of state officials, providers, and health care professionals of unmet needs and stimulating interest in further initiatives to meet those needs. Projects must show that the programs are not expected to increase a state's Medicaid costs.

As specified in the appropriations conference agreement for FY 2000, the five initial projects are located in Florida, Kentucky, New York, Utah, and Virginia. A project in Colorado has since been approved. The projects differ in scope and strategies (CHI, 2002). Appendix H describes the approach in New York state to developing the demonstration project.

State Children's Health Insurance Program

Congress created the State Children's Health Insurance Program in 1997 as Title XXI of the Social Security Act.[19] The objective was to increase health insurance coverage for lower-income children through Medicaid expansions or creation of separate state programs or both. (If a child is legally eligible under a state's Medicaid program requirements, he or she is supposed to be enrolled in Medicaid as such.)

With federal matching funds, states can extend coverage to children in families with incomes that are 200 percent of the federal poverty level. For states that had already expanded Medicaid eligibility to optional groups, the law raised the income threshold to 50 percent above the state's existing limit. Certain technical actions (i.e., use of "income disregards" allowed for in Medicaid under Section 1931 of Title XIX) can allow other states to exceed the 200 percent figures (AHSRHP, 2001). State SCHIP programs are, like state Medicaid programs, highly variable.

Separate SCHIP programs may or may not provide the same covered benefits as the state Medicaid program and may or may not use state-approved Medicaid managed care plans to provide services. A recent analysis indicated that "among the 34 states with separately administered SCHIP programs in effect in 2000, 32 states use coverage exclusions that would not be permissible in Medicaid" (Rosenbaum et al., 2001, p. 2). Services that tended to be excluded from separate SCHIP programs were hospice, case management services, and home and community-based services. Depending on the availability of other support, the result could be inadequate palliative and end-of-life care for children and their families. Also, if the state creates a separate SCHIP program, it is not precluded—as it would be for its Medicaid program—from requiring copayments.

For states with separate SCHIP programs, coverage may be part of the basic program or part of a program designed specifically for children with special needs. Some state programs, for example, Wisconsin's BadgerCare program, also offer coverage to low-income uninsured parents who have a child under age 19 living with them (see http://www.dhfs.state.wi.us/badgercare).

---

[19]For general information about SCHIP, several Web sites provide useful descriptions or analyses including CMS/HCFA (http://www.hcfa.gov/init/children.htm); George Washington University's Center for Health Services Research and Policy (http://gwhealthpolicy.org); American Academy of Pediatrics (http://www.aap.org/advocacy/schip.htm); and American Public Health Association (http://www.apha.org/ppp/schip/); and Health Services Research (http://www.hsrnet.com/pubs/pub04.htm).

Other Sources of Financing

Title V Maternal and Child Health Block Grants

In addition to public insurance programs such as Medicaid and SCHIP, Title V block grant programs in each state provide services directly to a broad range of chronically ill children (Gittler, 1998; MCHB, 1998).[20] In 1989, Congress required state Title V programs for children with special needs "to provide and promote family-centered, community-based, coordinated care . . . and to facilitate the development of community-based systems of services for such children and their families" (MCHB, 2000b, online, no page number; P.L. 101-239).

As discussed in Chapter 2, children with special needs are those who have or are at increased risk of a chronic physical, developmental, behavioral, or emotional condition and who also require health and related services of a type or amount beyond that required by children generally. Children covered by Title V programs have conditions that tend to fall into three broad, overlapping groups: (1) developmental disabilities or delays (e.g., mental retardation); (2) chronic illnesses or ongoing medical disorders (e.g., diabetes, severe asthma); and (3) emotional or behavioral problems (e.g., attention deficit disorder). Depending on state eligibility criteria, children who have diagnoses such as fatal neurodegenerative diseases and certain cancers could be eligible for Title V services. Overall, however, most children covered by Title V programs have chronic conditions and disabilities that are not usually expected to lead to death in childhood, and the programs are not explicitly intended to provide or assist end-of-life care.

The Maternal and Child Health Bureau administers the federal Title V program. It conceptualizes Title V-supported activities as a "pyramid" consisting of (1) direct personal services, (2) enabling services that assist children and families in obtaining coverage or services, (3) population-based preventive services, and (4) infrastructure-building activities (e.g., support for information systems, standards development, program evaluation). One long-standing positive feature of state programs for children with special health care needs is their concern with the organization, coordination, and availability of services (Ireys, 1996).

Children with special health care needs may be identified for assistance in many ways, including family inquiries about the availability of assistance, referral by physicians and other care providers, and state outreach

---

[20]In addition to information from the Maternal and Child Health Bureau, this discussion draws on reports and analyses prepared by Ireys, 1996; Fox et al., 1998; Fox et al., 2000; Kaye et al., 2000; and AHRQ, 2001a.

programs. In addition, when the Social Security Administration determines that a child under age 18 is eligible for Supplemental Security Income (SSI),[21] the child and family are referred to state programs for children with special health care needs for assistance in securing needed services and enrolling children in Medicaid. In some states, Medicaid enrollment for children with SSI is automatic.

Within the requirements of federal law, states have considerable discretion to establish the scope and organization of programs for children with special health care needs. They have different criteria for financial eligibility, provide different services in different ways, and vary in the definition of qualifying diagnoses or conditions. Congress has, however, required state programs to provide and promote family-centered, community-based, coordinated care. A major recent emphasis of Title V programs has been on promoting enrollment of children with special health care needs in managed care plans, monitoring results, and encouraging program and plan adjustments to better serve these children and their families.

Family Payments and Caregiving

Figure 7.1, presented earlier, includes information on the source of insurance coverage for children rather than the source of payment for services. Thus, it does not refer to out-of-pocket payments by families. Little specific information is available on the share of palliative and end-of-life care for children that is paid for by families out-of-pocket, although some hospices can identify the share of their income derived from family or individual payments.

Young families with children often have limited resources—both income and savings—to cover the considerable health care costs generated by a child's serious illness or injury. Some qualify for Medicaid coverage or other public programs only after they have "spent down" their own financial resources, lost or given up their jobs to care for a child, or otherwise impoverished themselves.

As described in Chapters 4, 5, and 6, families also support their ill or injured children by personally providing much health and supportive care. Although the care provided by a mother, father, or other relative cannot be valued merely in economic terms, a comprehensive analysis of the economic

---

[21]Under the Social Security Act, a child is eligible for SSI payments if he or she has a physical or mental condition or conditions that can be medically proven and that can result in marked and severe functional limitations and that must last, or be expected to last, at least 12 months or be expected to result in death.

aspects of child illnesses would include not only out-of-pocket payments but also unpaid care and time lost from caregiver's paid work.

In addition to initiatives to extend insurance coverage for children, efforts to assist family caregivers through training, respite services, and other support have been growing. Public and private financing of assistance for caregivers is, however, still limited and often offered only to narrowly defined groups, such as families of children with severe developmental disabilities or adults with dementia. A recent review for the American Associated of Retired People of 25 state programs for caregivers concluded that many have such limited budgets that they can serve only a small number of caregivers. The review also concluded that increased funding would help more people seeking to keep a family member at home, but increased flexibility is also needed to fit the diverse circumstances and needs of family caregivers (Coleman, 2000).

Health Care Safety Net

This country's so-called health care safety net for the uninsured and underinsured has been characterized as "a patchwork of providers, funding, and programs tenuously held together by the power of demonstrated need, community support, and political acumen" (IOM, 2000a, p.17).[22] In addition to direct Medicaid and Medicare payments for patient services, the resources for safety-net providers are a variable and often unreliable mixture that includes other local and state government support, patient payments, philanthropy, volunteer services, and federal payments for hospitals caring for a "disproportionate" share of low-income patients.

As defined in a recent Institute of Medicine (IOM) report, the health care safety net consists of "those providers that organize and deliver a significant level of health care and other related services to uninsured, Medicaid, and other vulnerable patients" (IOM, 2000a, p. 3). Core safety-net providers are those that "either by legal mandate or explicitly adopted mission . . . maintain an 'open door,' offering access to services for patients regardless of their ability to pay" (p. 3–4).

For many seriously ill children, children's hospitals, academic medical centers, community hospital emergency departments, and other providers act as an important but precarious safety net. Nonetheless, given its un-

---

[22]In decades past, public and private insurance payments subsidized care to the uninsured. Today, the opportunities for such cross-subsidies are limited or nonexistent in a world of competitive markets, health plan contracts, discounts from charges, global per-case payments related to diagnosis, and other cost-control strategies (see, e.g., IOM, 2000a; MedPAC, 2000a).

stable financial base, this system cannot promise reliable, continuing, coordinated care to uninsured and underinsured children with life-threatening conditions.

Philanthropy and Volunteer Funding and Services

Philanthropy clearly plays a role in funding some palliative and end-of-life services for children and their families, but no data on the level or trends in such funding are available. Examples of philanthropic support for pediatric palliative care include

- targeted community events to raise funds for palliative and hospice services for children and families,
- inclusion of pediatric hospices in United Way campaigns,
- foundation grants to support pediatric palliative care programs in children's hospitals,
- sponsorship of "make-a-wish" and similar programs,
- grants and fundraising for camp programs that serve sick children or siblings, and
- organization of community-based and on-line support groups.

Faith communities also support grieving families spiritually and emotionally. In addition, many enlist clergy and volunteers to provide counseling, visiting, transportation, meal delivery, and other services to families with sick children. Some also fund parish nurse and other programs that provide health and supportive services.

Some philanthropic contributions support direct services for individuals. Other funds go to projects intended to improve the quality of such services, for example, through the assessment of community needs or the development of tools for assessing symptoms and the adequacy of symptom management.

Even in countries in which most health services are financed publicly, hospices may out of choice or necessity rely substantially on private philanthropic contributions and volunteer services. For example, in England, most children's hospice programs were established outside the structure of the National Health Service, although they may receive government payments as well as philanthropic grants and volunteer services.

Clinical Trials

Most clinical trials are designed to test therapies that researchers hope will prevent, cure, or slow the progression of disease or save injured persons from death or disability. Some trials are intended to test therapies that will prevent or relieve pain, nausea, and other symptoms that arise from illnesses and injuries or their treatment. Trials may involve problems that are not life threatening, but many enroll patients with very serious conditions. Thus, although usually not intentionally, some end-of-life care is financed by research grants and other funds for clinical trials.

Insurance payments for those participating in clinical trials have long been controversial. Some private insurers have agreed to pay for certain trials or for routine care associated with trials, although many today and in the past have undoubtedly paid for such care without knowing it (IOM, 2000d; NCI, 2001b).[23] In June of 2000, the President directed that Medicare explicitly authorize payment for routine patient care costs and costs to treat complications associated with participation in clinical trials.[24] A recent study found that nearly 90 percent of Blue Cross Blue Shield plans already pay for routine care in clinical trials, and some encourage the creation of clinical trials to test certain therapies (IOM, 2000d). Coverage of investigational drugs is permitted by a few Medicaid plans, but the committee found no comprehensive information on such policies.

HOW PHYSICIANS, HOSPITALS, AND OTHER PROVIDERS ARE PAID

Overview

How insurers pay providers and how much they pay them can significantly affect child and family access to palliative and end-of-life care and

---

[23]Routine costs have been defined to be those items or services that are "(1) typically provided absent a clinical trial (e.g., conventional care); (2) required solely for provision of the investigational item or service (e.g., administration of a noncovered chemotherapeutic agent), the clinically appropriate monitoring of the effects of the item or service, or the prevention of complications; and (3) needed for reasonable and necessary care arising from the provision of an investigational item or service—in particular, for the diagnosis or treatment of complications" (HCFA/CMS, 2000d).

[24]The Health Care Financing Administration (HCFA), now the Centers for Medicare and Medicaid Services announced in September 2000 that clinical trials with a therapeutic purpose that will qualify automatically include "1. Trials funded by NIH [National Institutes of Health], CDC [Centers for Disease Control and Prevention], AHRQ [Agency for Healthcare Research and Quality], HCFA, DOD [Department of Defense], and VA [Department of Veterans Affairs]; 2. Trials supported by centers or cooperative groups that are funded by the NIH, CDC, AHRQ, HCFA, DOD and VA; 3. Trials conducted under an investigational new drug application (IND) reviewed by the Food and Drug Administration [FDA]; and 4. Drug trials that are exempt from having an IND under 21 CFR 312.2(b)(1) will be deemed automatically qualified until the qualifying criteria are developed and the certification process is in place" (announcement at www.hcfa.gov/coverage/8d2.htm). Because Medicare covers few children, this program change will have little impact on children and their families unless Medicaid and private payers adopt similar policies.

also influence the quality of that care. Depending on the specifics, methods and levels of payment can encourage undertreatment, overtreatment, inappropriate transitions between settings of care, and inadequate coordination of care.

The past two decades have seen major changes in the way Medicare pays physicians, hospitals, and other care providers for their services. Many Medicaid and private insurers in the United States have followed Medicare's lead and changed their payment methods to mirror those of Medicare. Even when other payers have not adopted the same payment methods as Medicare, they may use elements of those methods for analytic and monitoring purposes. Thus, even though Medicare covers few children,[25] Medicare payment policies may have significant spillover effects on children and adults covered by Medicaid or private payers. Further, because Medicare is such an important payer, providers may develop perceptions and standard operating procedures based on Medicare policies that they then apply to patients covered by other payers and other payment methods. For these reasons, it is useful to understand Medicare payment policies and methods.

In 1983, Medicare adopted a prospective payment system (PPS) for inpatient hospital care. Under the PPS, Medicare reimburses hospitals a fixed payment per inpatient discharge regardless of length of stay. As explained below, the level of payment for each discharge varies based on the diagnosis-related group (DRG) into which the discharge is classified. The Balanced Budget Act of 1997 mandated the adoption of PPSs for other services, including home health care and skilled nursing facility care. Later legislation modified some provisions, but the basic direction of change—toward prospective payment—remains.

The primary goals of prospective payment methods have been to limit the rate of increase in health care costs, increase efficiency in health care, and make cost trends more predictable. In addition, they also may reduce certain kinds of administrative burdens and allow health plans more flexibility. Depending on how providers react, the quality of care could improve (e.g., if unnecessary services are cut) or decrease (e.g., if beneficial services are curbed or patients are discharged before they or their out-of-hospital care providers are ready).

Prospective reimbursement systems can, however, threaten access to care for patients with particularly high-cost needs (i.e., needs for which the cost considerably exceeds the fixed payment for care). As noted above, Huskamp and colleagues (2001) documented reports from multiple loca-

---

[25]As noted in an earlier footnote, the Medicare End-Stage Renal Disease Program covers a small number of children (HCFA/CMS. 2000e).

tions of patients with high-cost care needs being denied access to hospice because the cost of the services required would far exceed the hospice per diem payment. Efforts to "risk-adjust" Medicare payments to match patient characteristics continue, but no approach is yet considered satisfactory (MedPAC, 2000a).

The use of separate payment systems by Medicare and other payers for different types of services also creates incentives for shifts in the setting of care that may not be most appropriate for patients. Huskamp and colleagues (2001) documented providers' reports of transitions between care settings that were attributable to financial incentives in the Medicare fee-for-service program and that negatively affected the quality of care for the dying patient in the view of the provider.

The choice of payment method inevitably involves trade-offs between desired goals such as cost containment and other goals such as equity or quality of care. Methods that put hospitals and physicians at greater risk (e.g., DRGs, capitation) have the potential to stimulate reductions in both appropriate and inappropriate care. Quality monitoring systems can identify some unwanted responses, but these systems have their own costs and limits. Payment methods that put providers at higher risk also may jeopardize the survival of needed safety-net institutions, rural providers, or others whose services are not easily replaced.

The choice of payment level also involves trade-offs. On the one hand, stringent payment levels may promote efficiency and economy. On the other hand, if a health plan's payments are below costs for an efficient provider or are less than what other plans pay, providers may refuse to serve that plan's enrollees. Such payments may also threaten the survival of physician practices and hospitals, especially in low-income areas where few patients are covered by better-paying health plans.

Hospital Payment

Hospitals are paid by a variety of methods. The per-discharge DRG method used by Medicare is important because Medicare is the major source of inpatient revenue for most acute care hospitals serving adults. Some other payers have adopted DRG-based payment methods. Others use older cost-based reimbursement methods (usually in the form of a per diem payment), pay a specified percentage of hospital charges, or use hybrid methods. Many managed care plans have negotiated general or specialty capitation rates with hospitals. To the extent they can pay anything, individuals without health insurance (or with insurance that does not pay for certain care) may have to pay hospital charges, which do not necessarily bear much relationship to the cost of providing services and are typically significantly higher than DRG, cost-based, or negotiated payment rates.

Initially, children's hospitals, as well as psychiatric, rehabilitation, long-term care, and cancer hospitals, were excluded from Medicare's shift to prospective case-based payment. In the Balanced Budget Act of 1997 (P.L. 105-33) Congress specified that a PPS be implemented beginning in 2001 for rehabilitation hospitals and in 2002 for long-term care hospitals. In the Balanced Budget Refinement Act of 1999 (P.L. 106-113), Congress also required the Health Care Financing Administration (HCFA), now the Centers for Medicare and Medicaid Services (CMS), to report on a modified prospective payment system (per diem) for psychiatric hospitals and psychiatric units of other hospitals. Medicare payments to children's hospitals continue to be based on current costs or historical costs adjusted for inflation, whichever is less.

The move by Medicare—and other payers—from cost-based, retrospective reimbursement to prospective payment has had many effects on hospitals and other parts of the health care system (see, e.g., ProPAC, 1989, 1996; MedPAC, 2000b, 2001).[26] It has put pressure on hospital operating margins, encouraging efficiency but also affecting hospitals' willingness and ability to subsidize care for patients unable to pay for services. Hospitals have raised charges for privately insured patients, and private insurers have reacted by also adopting DRGs, negotiating discounts or capitation payments, and taking other protective steps. These steps have, in turn, made uncompensated care an even more critical problem and generally put services perceived as "nonessential" or "not contributing to the bottom line" in jeopardy. Safety-net providers, who serve many poor children, have been particularly affected.

Prospective per-case payment provides strong incentives for covered hospitals to shorten lengths of stay, and this effect or mind-set may extend to patients covered by other programs. In the 1980s, reductions in lengths of stay led to concerns that some patients were being discharged prematurely. Research has been mixed on this point (see, e.g., ProPAC, 1989; Kosecoff et al., 1990; Rubenstein et al., 1990). In any case, many patients who were discharged to nursing homes, personal homes, or elsewhere clearly had greater needs for out-of-hospital care than such patients previously did.

Because hospital care is generally better insured than other care, shifting care to nonhospital settings often increases the financial burden on patients and families. The pressure for quick discharges may make it difficult to mobilize appropriate hospice care or other alternatives promptly

---

[26]Medicare uses an outlier payment mechanism to reimburse hospitals for particularly high-cost inpatient hospital stays. Hospitals are reimbursed 80 percent of expenses above the hospital threshold for the DRG, a number based on estimates of marginal costs for a hospital. Medicare also adjusts payments to reflect differences in local wage rates as well as other factors.

enough. It also limits time for teaching the family about how to provide needed, sometimes complex, care at home. This has been a frequent concern of hospital palliative care teams and hospices (IOM, 1997).

Concerns about possible negative effects of DRG-based payment on quality of care reinforced Medicare's efforts to develop better methods for measuring, monitoring, and improving the quality of hospital and other services provided to Medicare beneficiaries (see, e.g., IOM, 1990b; MedPAC, 2000a). Like the introduction of the payment method itself, this focus on quality measurement and monitoring appears to have had spillover effects, influencing the care for other patients.

Payments for Hospital Care Provided to Children

General Children's hospitals and other acute care hospitals serving children are most directly affected by DRGs to the extent that they are used by Medicaid and private payers. Medicare accounts for less than 0.5 percent of discharges from children's hospitals (MedPAC, 2000b), mainly for children with end-stage renal disease (ESRD) and young adults with serious disabling conditions who are continuing with pediatric providers.[27] The committee did not locate information on the proportion of children's hospital discharges (or discharges of children from general hospitals) accounted for by Medicaid programs and other payers using DRG-based payments.

For children not covered by a payer using some form of DRG-based payment, hospitals face an array of other Medicaid, private insurer, and other payment methods and rates. Within a state, Medicaid and other state programs may use different payment strategies for urban and rural hospitals, make exceptions or adjustments for children's hospitals or safety-net hospitals, or treat certain classes of patients or services (e.g., children with special needs, labor and delivery, neonatal) differently. For Medicaid-covered children enrolled in a private managed care plan, the plan's payment strategy will apply, subject to any requirements specified in the contract with the state.

DRGs and Pediatric Care For professionals and institutional providers serving children, a central issue has been the appropriateness of using DRGs

---

[27]Because Medicare covers few children, teaching hospitals serving them do not benefit from the payments for graduate medical education (GME) incorporated in Medicare payments. In 1999, Congress provided for a two-year program of GME payments to 56 independent children's hospitals. The Health Resources and Services Administration, which administers the payments, provided almost $40 million in FY 2000 and $265 million in FY 2001, (http://bhpr.hrsa.gov/childrenshospitalgme/).

designed primarily for adults to pay for children's care or to analyze or monitor that care. Although the original analyses on which DRGs were based created groupings for neonatal care, they were based on data from a small sample of community hospitals and did not adjust for birth weight of infants (Schwartz et al., 1991).

Concerned by these methodological problems, researchers have worked to develop appropriate adjustments for infants' and children's care (see, e.g., Payne and Restuccia, 1987; Schwartz et al., 1991; Vertrees and Pollatsek, 1993; Hanson et al., 1998; Muldoon, 1999). In the 1980s, the National Association of Children's Hospitals and Related Institutions (NACHRI) sponsored analyses to develop "pediatric-modified" DRGs (PM-DRGs) and other adjustments (Averill et al., 1998). This project expanded the seven initial neonatal DRGs to 46 DRGs that took into account birth weight and use of surgery or mechanical ventilation. The Department of Defense adopted these modified neonatal DRGs for its civilian health insurance program, which uses its own DRG-based payment method (DOD, 1999). An Internet search suggested that at least three states (Michigan, Iowa, and North Carolina) had devised adjustments for neonatal DRGs. Several Nordic countries are also supporting a project to improve neonatal and pediatric DRGs (NCCD, 2001). An Australian analysis suggested the need to focus on higher costs associated with children less than three years of age and children with congenital anomalies and chronic illnesses (Hanson et al., 1998).

A more general effort to modify DRGs for care provided to patients under age 65 led to work on "all-patient" DRGs (AP-DRGs), since evolved to become all-patient-refined DRGs (APR-DRGs). This work, which takes comorbidities and complications more fully into account, has built on DRG adjustments that NACHRI developed for pediatric care (Averill et al., 1998). Although several states are using the APR-DRG system for various purposes, it is not clear whether any state (other than Maryland) is using it in setting Medicaid payments for hospitals.

An analysis of several DRG systems (sponsored, in part, by NACHRI) concluded that the use of Medicare DRGs for nonMedicare patients would result in underpayments, especially for hospital care provided to "nonnormal" newborns and chronically ill and other children (Averill et al., 1998). To the extent that care for chronically ill children is concentrated in a subset of children's and other hospitals, Medicaid and other payments based on Medicare DRGs will more seriously affect these institutions. (In principle, this could be mitigated with provision for outlier payments and possibly other adjustments.)

A subsequent analysis undertaken by NACHRI concluded that Medicare DRGs overpaid for normal newborns but substantially underpaid for newborns treated surgically, neonates transferred from other facilities or discharged to home health care, and neonates who died (Muldoon, 1999). The analysis also concluded that Medicare DRGs underpaid for care provided by freestanding acute care children's hospitals and major teaching general hospitals.[28]

Because the diagnosis component of DRGs is tied to the clinical modification (CM) of the International Classification of Diseases (ICD), weaknesses in this coding scheme can translate into weaknesses in DRGs. Experts on pediatric disease classification have criticized the current version of the classification system, ICD-9-CM, for the lack of specificity for many congenital anomalies and perinatal conditions. For example, a few codes contain as many as 100 different conditions. As one critic noted, "Although many of these diseases may be rare or low in prevalence they can account for extensive inpatient hospital stays, multiple surgical encounters and outpatient health care consumption" (Wing, 1997, p.1). ICD-9-CM codes undergo constant revision and adjustment, but pediatric groups have complained that the pace of revision is too slow. Implementation of a major revision of the codes, ICD-10-CM, is pending. NACHRI, in collaboration with Children's Hospital and Medical Center in Seattle, is developing a grouping system called Classification of Congenital and Chronic Health Conditions (CCCHC).

Even if an appropriate diagnosis-related classification and grouping scheme is used for inpatient care, the factors selected to convert relative values into actual payments may be set too low to cover the cost of efficient, appropriate services. Analyses show that Medicaid's payment-to-cost ratio improved during the 1990s, although the much higher ratios of private payers were beginning to drop (MedPAC, 2000b).

Payment for Inpatient Palliative Care

Although most inpatient palliative care programs will benefit adults (since adults account for most deaths), the development of more such pro-

---

[28]In June 2000, the commission that advises Congress on Medicare payment recommended that the Secretary of the Department of Health and Human Services direct the adoption of a system such as APR-DRGs so that payments would more accurately reflect differences in severity of illness for hospitalized patients (MedPAC, 2000b). The APR-DRG system has about 1,400 groups compared to about 500 for Medicare DRGs. The commission's analysis indicates that such a change, combined with other recommended changes related to calculation of DRG weights and outlier payments, would raise payments for hospitals that treat more seriously ill patients. In response, HCFA agreed that the change could reduce distortions in the current system. However, the agency stated that it would not propose such a change unless it had statutory authority to offset any increases in payments that resulted from changes in hospital DRG coding practices associated with a new classification system (HCFA, 2000f, p. 47103).

grams may stimulate greater attention to inpatient palliative care for children. As described in Chapter 6, approximately one-third of the children's hospitals responding to a recent survey reported that they provide palliative care services, but few have organized programs.

For those who have formally elected hospice care and need inpatient care related to their terminal condition, Medicare and Medicaid payments for inpatient care are made on a fixed per diem basis. The inpatient rate is higher for acute services (e.g., management of intractable pain) and lower for respite care.[29] One study found at least 20 percent of Medicare hospice beneficiaries who used the benefit in 1996 had at least one day of inpatient hospital care covered by the hospice benefit (Gage and Dao, 2000). The committee identified no equivalent information for Medicaid programs or private payers or for those children receiving inpatient hospice care. The commission that advises Medicare on provider payment has noted that hospice rates were developed in the 1980s and has recommended that they be reevaluated for adequacy (MedPAC, 2002).

DRG and other per case payments for other hospitalized patients are likewise based on analyses that largely predate modern palliative care services and technologies for gravely ill patients. Although Medicare adopted a secondary diagnosis code for palliative care in 1996, use of the code does not affect payment under a DRG. An analysis by HCFA concluded that a palliative care DRG was not needed, but the agency's analytic methods have been questioned (MedPAC, 1999). Because per case payment encourages early discharge, including patients who are near death and primarily in need of comfort measures, some hospitals have developed "compassionate nondischarge policies" to allow such patients to remain in the hospital when desired (Smits et al., 2002).

For adult or pediatric inpatient palliative care programs, the reality is that they will have to develop a case for hospital adoption that is based not only on clinical or ethical arguments but also on fiscal considerations.[30] In a world of DRGs, discounted payments, and other constraints, hospital executives for children's hospitals—like their adult hospital counterparts—

---

[29]For hospice patients receiving inpatient care, the Medicare per diem payment for acute care was $475.69 ($110.62 for inpatient respite care) in late FY 2001 (HCFA/CMS, 2001f). The aggregate number of inpatient days (general inpatient and inpatient respite) may not exceed 20 percent of the aggregate total number of days of care provided to all Medicare beneficiaries by a hospice during a year. How much the hospital receives would depend, for example, on whether the care was provided under a contract with a community-based hospice and what that contract specified.

[30]Helping palliative care experts develop the business analysis for inpatient programs is one objective of the Center to Advance Palliative Care at Mt. Sinai Medical School, funded in part by the Robert Wood Johnson Foundation (see, e.g., CAPC, 2001; Spragens and Wenneker, 2001).

may view organized palliative care programs as optional rather than as "a core service in the sense that it will help us survive" (Cassel et al., 2000, p. 169). In competing for scarce resources with existing services that already have been pared back to cut costs, advocates will have to develop information or credible arguments that a program

- will offset added costs by reducing other patient care costs (e.g., by allowing a patient to be discharged sooner or moved to a less resource-intensive inpatient area);
- has reliable sources of funding;
- can help the institution meet external accreditation or performance standards set by outside purchaser, patient advocacy, or regulatory groups;
- will increase patient or family satisfaction and attract desirable future admissions; or
- will have some combination of these characteristics.

Some hospitals report tapping foundation grants and philanthropy to fund adult inpatient palliative care programs. For example, Diane Meier, M.D., the director of Palliative Medicine at Mt. Sinai School of Medicine in New York City, described stresses in managing an inpatient palliative care program. "The fiscal environment in New York City teaching hospitals makes it nearly impossible to obtain hospital operations budget support for the program's clinical services. Billing income for physician services covers approximately 10 percent of clinical costs. The rest of the staff's salaries and benefits come from overlapping foundation and federal grants and from philanthropy. The head of nursing at our hospital recently agreed to cover 50 percent of the nurse coordinator's position and is considering covering 50 percent of a second nurse to be hired soon. We do not have enough money to hire a social worker, volunteer-program coordinator, or pastoral counselor" (Meier et al., 2000, p. 141). Meier noted that the lack of staffing raises the risk of burnout among existing personnel and compromises efforts to provide high-quality clinical and educational services. Philanthropy, which can be especially useful in supporting program development and initation, cannot substitute for adequate Medicare, Medicaid, and private insurer payments for inpatient palliative care.

Payment for Physicians and Certain Other Professionals

General

Physicians   Until fairly recently, insurers often linked payment for physicians' services directly or indirectly to charges physicians set for their services, although some of the links to an individual physician's fees became rather remote over time.[31] Surgeons and certain other physicians typically received "global payments" that bundled reimbursement for the procedure with some pre- and postprocedure services including time spent communicating with patients and their families. A few health plans (what later came to be called staff model HMOs) established physician groups whose physicians were salaried (as were many physicians working for government institutions).

In 1992, after years of planning and development work, Medicare began to implement a new physician payment system using a resource-based relative value scale (RBRVS) (PPRC, 1988, 1993). The relative values for a service are, in principle, based on (1) the amount of physician work (time, skill, mental effort, stress) that is involved in providing the service, (2) the practice expenses (e.g., office staff, equipment) associated with the service, and (3) the professional liability costs for the service. A conversion factor translates the relative value units associated with a specific service into an actual payment amount. Payments are also adjusted for geographic differences in expenses. The relative values are reexamined every five years and adjusted as appropriate.

A number of Medicaid and private payers have also moved to pay physicians based on elements of the RBRVS. A 1995 study reported that about 40 percent of Medicaid programs and 25 percent of managed care plans used some elements of the RBRVS to pay physicians and that one-quarter of managed care plans did (PPRC, 1995; see also Reisinger et al., 1994). According to the American Academy of Pediatrics (AAP), approximately 60 percent of Medicaid and private payers have adopted an RBRVS method of paying physicians (AAP, 2001e). Some payers have changed relative values to encourage provision of certain services (e.g., primary care). Payers may also use different conversion factors, with Medicaid, in particular, making adjustments to pay physicians less than Medicare.

In addition to or instead of adopting an RBRVS payment strategy, some health plans have negotiated contracts providing for payments to physicians based on substantial discounts from their charges. Other health plans have sought to capitate payment to physicians or physician groups for some (e.g., primary care) or all services using a prospectively set, per-person payment for a defined population, time period, and set of services.

A 1997 survey of 130 managed care plans serving Medicaid beneficiaries found that about 70 percent used capitation for primary care physi-

---

[31]For example, under private "usual, customary, and reasonable" methodologies, an individual physician would be paid the lesser of charges or an amount related to that physician's median past charge for the service, a percentile (e.g., the 75th or 90th) of other area physicians' charges for the service, or certain other factors. Medicare originally used a similar payment method.

cians with most of the remainder using discounted fees and a few paying physicians on a salaried basis (Landon and Epstein, 2001). About half of the plans also employed other financial incentives such as bonuses related to individual or group financial performance. A survey of its members by the AAP found that almost 32 percent of respondents reported that their state Medicaid program paid on a capitated basis, 42 percent reported payment on a discounted fee-for-service basis, and 22 percent reported payment on a traditional fee-for-service basis (Yudowsky et al., 2000). For SCHIP enrollees, respondents reported a generally similar distribution of payment methods: 32 percent capitated payment, 47 percent discounted fee-for-service payment, and 18 percent traditional fee-for-service payment. The survey did not cover payments from private health plans.

Other Professionals   Separate, direct reimbursement for inpatient services provided by pediatric nurse practitioners, clinical psychologists, clinical social workers, and other professionals is limited, although it has been expanding. Services by some professionals such as nurses, social workers, child life specialists and pastoral counselors are typically part of the overhead expenses for hospitals. They, thus, are vulnerable when hospitals are under financial pressure to look for ways to cut costs.

Pediatric physician groups also may employ various other health professionals who usually cannot bill directly for their services. This means that payments to physicians for their patient care services must also cover the services of these professionals or their employment will be discouraged (Hilden et al., 2001b). Approval to bill payers directly, which is a major objective of many nonphysician professionals, would almost certainly increase the provision of many psychosocial and other supportive services to children covered by Medicaid and private payers. Approval of payments to pediatricians for team conferences (without the patient present) to discuss a child's care could indirectly help support the patient care services provided by nonphysician professionals.

For other professionals who can bill directly, insurers may define the specified procedure or service codes for which they can bill. Payments for the same code may vary by type of professional. States also specify what level of physician supervision (e.g., general versus direct)[32] is required for services provided by nonphysicians.

---

[32] "*General supervision* means that the procedure is furnished under the physician's overall direction and control but the physician's presence is not required during performance of the procedure. The training of nonphysician personnel who actually perform the diagnostic procedure and the maintenance of the necessary equipment and supplies are the continuing

Payments to Pediatricians and Others Who Care for Children

RBRVS and Pediatric Care   As was the case for DRGs, the research and data analyses for the Medicare RBRVS emphasized services provided to adults by generalist and specialist physicians who care primarily or entirely for adults. Pediatrics was one of the 32 specialties studied, but relatively few services were examined in each specialty. The analyses, in general, did not consider differences in the work required to provide a service (e.g., a surgical procedure) to a child compared to an adult (AAP, 1998a).

Although systematic evidence is limited, providing services to a child may require more resources than providing similar care for an adult (Arnold and Alexander, 1997; AAP, 1998a). For example, it may take several tries to get a wiggling toddler to stay still for a physical examination, especially when some discomfort is involved. Similarly, it may require considerable probing and rephrasing of questions to elicit useful information about physical symptoms from an anxious or upset 6-year-old. Information from parents is often required, and treatment must be discussed with parents, who have legal authority to make treatment decisions and who often must implement them. The AAP (1998a) has also argued that practice expenses (one component of the RBRVS) may be higher for pediatricians than for comparable adult physicians because staff must spend extra time collecting laboratory samples, waiting for a child to dress or undress, and conducting telephone triage.[33]

Level of Payment   Internists, pediatricians, and other physicians who provide mostly nonprocedural services have long asserted that payers pay too little for these services compared to surgical, radiological, and other procedures (see, e.g., ASIM, 1981). One goal of physician payment reforms has been to realign payments to reflect resource use. Pediatricians caring for children with life-threatening medical problems continue to be concerned about recognition of the time needed for explanation and counseling of

---

responsibility of the physician. *Direct supervision* in the office setting means that the physician must be present in the office suite and immediately available to furnish assistance and direction throughout the performance of the procedure. It does not mean that the physician must be present in the room when the procedure is performed. *Personal supervision* means that a physician must be in attendance in the room during the performance of the procedure" (HCFA, 2001, http://www.noridian.com/medweb/notices/revised%20physician%20super.pdf).

[33]In 1999, HCFA expressed interest in whether there are pediatric services not described in the payment codes it uses or whether there are codes that describe both adult and pediatric services, but for which work varies between the two. Thus, the agency seems to have been receptive to the possibility of such differences (HCFA/CMS, 2001e).

children and parents, an especially critical element of palliative and end-of-life care. Reimbursement for this time-consuming and challenging care is typically very limited and may be entirely unavailable, for example, if the child is not present during discussions with parents (Hilden et al., 2001b).

Most complaints about level of payment focus on Medicaid. In 1994, a government commission concluded that Medicaid fees were still less than 75 percent of Medicare fees and less than half of what private insurers paid (PPRC, 1994). In 2001, the federal government's General Accounting Office reported to Congress that Medicaid fees in the states surveyed were only 29 to 61 percent of Medicare levels for the same services (U.S. GAO, 2001a). In 1997, Congress repealed Medicaid requirements that states reimburse pediatric services at rates sufficient to secure physician participation and access to care similar to that for the general population in the area (see the AAP analysis at http://www.aap.org/advocacy/schippro.htm#reim).

The variability and often low level of Medicaid payments is evident in AAP data on payments for services commonly provided by pediatricians (AAP, 1999d). For example, for a "high-complexity" evaluation and management visit for a new patient, Medicare paid $168 and Medicaid averaged $102 (AAP, 1999d). Among states, Medicaid payments for this visit category varied more than sixfold. New Jersey, Pennsylvania, and Missouri paid less than $25 for each visit, whereas Alaska, Arizona, and Connecticut paid more than $150. To cite another example, fees for newborn resuscitation (CPT 99440—see the explanation below of Current Procedural Terminology [CPT] codes) averaged $124 for all states but ranged from $29 in Maryland and $33 in Rhode Island to $243 in Idaho and $288 for Alaska (AAP, 1999d).

Some states provide higher payments for certain pediatric office and outpatient department visits than for corresponding adult visits (see, e.g., Prestowitz and Streett, 2000; Katz et al., 2001). This is consistent with Medicaid's usually more generous coverage of services for children compared to adults.

Some physicians respond to low levels of Medicaid reimbursement by choosing not to serve Medicaid patients or by limiting the number of such patients they will see. A recent survey of members of the AAP reported that 67 percent of pediatricians in direct patient care accepted all Medicaid patients, considerably higher than the 48 percent reported in the organization's 1993 survey (Yudowsky et al., 2000).[34] The figure varied among states from 48 percent in Oklahoma to 94 percent in Massachusetts.

---

[34]The response rate was 67 percent. Members of AAP account for about one-third of all pediatricians in the United States.

Of those responding, 69 percent reported accepting all SCHIP patients, and 76 percent reported accepting all private patients. Overall, nearly 90 percent of respondents reported participating in Medicaid and SCHIP and accepting some patients from these programs.

Of the AAP respondents who limited acceptance of Medicaid patients, 58 percent cited low reimbursement as a very important reason (Yudowsky et al., 2000). The next most common reasons cited were paperwork concerns and unpredictable payment, both cited by around 40 percent of respondents. Margolis and colleagues (1992) reported that participation decisions were also associated with location (higher participation rates in metropolitan areas), "busyness," and availability of other sites of care for Medicaid patients.

Payment, Procedure Codes, and Coverage Policies   Another continuing source of discontent among pediatricians as well as family practitioners, internists, and many other physicians is that most payers do not cover certain types of common physician services. Among pediatricians, two frequently mentioned omissions are telephone calls and team conferences. A few Medicaid programs cover telephone consultations, and some cover team conferences (CPT code 99361) as a separate service (AAP, 1999d). Team conferences are an important tool for managing the care of children with complex medical problems and complicated family situations.

Proponents of payment for these services may argue their case by noting that these services have Current Procedural Terminology (CPT) codes that are approved by the American Medical Association (AMA) and are required for billing purposes by Medicare, Medicaid, and other payers.[35] Payers, however, respond that just because the AMA provides a code does not automatically mean that a service is or ought to be covered by a health insurance plan. Although the primary use of the codes is in payment for clinical care, they are also used for internal practice management, research, and other billing purposes (e.g., billing for travel time or testimony in worker compensation or other legal proceedings). Thus, the coding system attempts to be very comprehensive. Establishing a CPT code for a service

---

[35]CMS/HCFA's Common Procedural Coding System (HCPCS) incorporates many but not all CPT codes. It also includes some additional codes (termed Level II codes) for nonphysician services that are covered under Medicare Part B (e.g., "J" codes for injectable drugs). Organizations that administer Medicare payment may establish local codes (Level III codes) under certain circumstances (e.g., for a new service not yet assigned a CPT or HCPCS code). In addition, various modifier codes can be added to the CPT codes to indicate special circumstances or provide additional information for payment or monitoring purposes. Use of HCPCS is required by Medicare and many Medicaid programs.

gives the service a certain legitimacy and may be one step in an effort to secure health insurance coverage. (CPT codes for telephone consultations were added in 1995.)

As noted earlier, one conventional principle of health insurance is that insurance is to cover services to cure or restore the functioning of the insured person. Thus, health insurance does not cover autopsies or purely custodial care. Insurance has, however, broadened in purpose to cover an increasing number of preventive services.

On the principle that insurance is for the insured person, Medicare and other payers generally refuse to pay for services when the patient is not physically present, for example, telephone conversations or discussions with family members only. Although limited, some exceptions to the "patient presence" rule exist, and they suggest rationales for some further exceptions that would recognize important realities of decision making and care for children with advanced illness. For example, in 2000, Medicare clarified that in determining payments to a physician for critical care services, it would include time spent with a family member to obtain a medical history, review the patient's condition, or discuss treatment (including limitations of treatment) when the patient was unable or incompetent to discuss his or her own care, provided such discussion was "absolutely necessary for treatment decisions under consideration that day" (HCFA/CMS, 1999). Except for the limitation to decisions on the day of the discussion, these circumstances characterize the situation for many pediatricians and parent decision makers who need to discuss and decide elements of a child's condition or treatment when the child is not present.

To cite another example of coverage for physician services when the patient is not physically present, Medicare began paying in 1995 for physicians (and recently nurse practitioners) to provide "care plan oversight" under certain circumstances for beneficiaries receiving home health or hospice services who require complex multidisciplinary care. The payment can cover a physician's time in discussions with other professionals (including telephone discussions), but it does *not* cover time in similar discussions with family caregivers. Given that family members are often central caregivers for patients at home, this restriction is a disincentive for physicians to oversee family members' understanding and performance of crucial, complicated tasks. Low payments rates are also a disincentive for physicians to provide such oversight (OIG, 2001). Some Medicaid and private plans pay for care plan oversight, but the committee found no comprehensive information about these policies or their implementation.

Claims Administration Claims administration is also a major source of confusion and problems for physicians and others who can bill insurers directly for their services. Procedures for documenting and filing claims for physician care are often complicated and burdensome. For example, for hospice patients, Medicare allows direct billing only by the physician of record. If another physician provides care related to the patient's terminal condition, the hospice must bill Medicare and pay the physician. Some physicians and hospices are unaware of this requirement and, thus, experience claims denials (Huskamp et al., 2001). Such denials may contribute to physician reluctance to care for hospice patients. (As noted earlier, Medicaid programs follow Medicare hospice policies and requirements.)

Another problem involves claims denials when a surgeon and a nonsurgical specialist appropriately provide care to a child on the same day. For example, even when a Medicaid program has explicitly stated a contrary policy, it appears that administrative entities sometimes deny payments to a pediatric oncologist or cardiologist for consultative services on the same day that a child undergoes a surgical or other procedure performed by another physician (Hilden et al., 2001b). In other situations, payment is denied for appropriate care because two physicians should use different procedure codes but their billing systems cannot coordinate this. Thus, when a surgeon concludes that surgery will not save a patient with cancer or a heart defect, the child's oncologist or cardiologist may find a claim denied for his or her difficult and time-consuming work of communicating the grim news and discussing care options with parents. Many groups provide seminars and other services to help physicians and physician office staff understand coding and billing procedures.

Other problems relate to the complex documentation required for claims, particularly physician evaluation and management services (MedPAC, 2000a).[36] These services constitute a large part of pediatric palliative care. (In general, the codes for evaluation and management services are used to categorize the intensity, comprehensiveness, and complexity of services that a physician provides during a patient visit. Different codes are used for new and established patients and for visits in different locations, such as hospitals or physicians' offices.)

Documentation issues are not well described for Medicaid programs and private payers, but these payers may follow claims administration procedures established for Medicare. The committee understood that claims for the EPSDT services that are covered for children but not adults sometimes cause confusion for Medicaid claims administrators. With payment levels for Medicaid often very low and not always consistent, physicians

---

[36]In a survey by the American Medical Association, three-fifths of the physicians responding reported that the Medicare guidelines for evaluation and management services were their biggest paperwork headache (Editorial, 2002).

may feel that it is not worth the staff administrative time to submit a claim for certain services (Hilden et al., 2001b).

Finally, one last concern for physicians, especially physicians in less well-paid fields of practice, is delayed payment of claims. A number of states have adopted "prompt payment laws" that establish varying definitions of and financial penalties for delays (see, e.g., NCSL, 2001a).

Payment for Palliative and End-of-Life Care by Physicians

For patients enrolled in hospice (which few children are), the physician of record can bill Medicare, Medicaid, or private insurance for services provided to that patient subject to certain conditions. Most hospice care is, however, provided and managed by nurses and other nonphysicians. Their services are covered under the hospice per diem payment. As suggested earlier, the adequacy of these payments needs examination in the context of modern palliative care practices, including the use of effective but very expensive medications.

For patients not enrolled in hospice, many palliative services (e.g., an inpatient or office visit to assess symptoms and adjust medications) fit within the evaluation and management services mentioned above. The same concerns about payment levels and claims administration practices, thus, apply. Although most home care is provided by nurses or other nonphysicians, very low payments for home visits may discourage physicians who judge that a home visit is the best way of managing child and family problems when a family wants a child at home but hospice care is not covered or available.

Physicians who provide palliative care will be especially affected by Medicaid or private health plan refusals to pay for team conferences, care plan oversight, telephone calls or consultation and information visits with parents when the child is not present. For children with life-threatening medical problems, consultations with parents are some of the most important, difficult, and time-consuming services provided by physicians.

As noted earlier, depending on the payer, the service, and the circumstances, pediatric nurse practitioners, child psychologists, and certain others who provide palliative services to children can bill directly. When such services are instead considered part of the overhead of a hospital or pediatric practice, these professionals must compete for resources with many other organizational priorities, and underprovision of their services is a frequent concern.

Because much physician care for children with life-threatening problems is provided in hospitals, payment for inpatient palliative care services provided by physicians is important. For example, medical centers and children's hospitals may track the collections of different clinical services in faculty practice plans as one indicator of a service's economic value to the institution. However valuable they may be to dying children and their families, services that are not reimbursed or are reimbursed at a low level put the services in jeopardy of understaffing or elimination.

Payment for Hospice Care

Under Medicare and Medicaid, hospices are paid on a per diem basis. These rates were based on data from a demonstration project that ended in the early 1980s and have not been adjusted to reflect the introduction of many effective but expensive palliative medications and other interventions (MedPAC, 2002).

Different per diem rates apply for four categories of hospice service: routine home care, continuous home care (for patients requiring eight or more hours of hospice care during a day), general inpatient care, and inpatient respite care.[37] In addition, hospices face caps on overall payments and on total payments for inpatient care (HCFA/CMS, 2001a). Use of these interventions could consume much of the current per diem for routine care (or exceed it). As noted above, this may create access problems for patients with particularly high-cost needs.

Private insurers may also use per diem payments, but some pay separately for certain expensive services such as palliative radiology, chemotherapy, durable medical equipment, and medications (Huskamp et al., 2001). To the extent that private payers cover such expensive services separately, hospices are under less pressure to restrict potentially effective palliative services or to refuse potentially expensive patients.

Concerns about prognostic and other requirements for Medicare and Medicaid coverage of hospice care were discussed above. The major issue related to hospice payments per se (not coverage and election requirements) has focused on the level of per diem payments and not the per diem method itself (Lynn and O'Mara, 2001). One advantage of per diem compared to per service payment is that it allows providers more flexibility to focus resources where patients need them most.

The level of per diem payments set by Medicare and Medicaid represent public policy decisions about the desired quality and type of hospice care. To increase legislators' understanding of the adequacy of per diems and to inform decisions about the need to re-base payments given signifi-

---

[37]For FY 2002, Medicaid rates are $110.56 for routine home care; $644.70 for continuous home care ($26.86 hourly rate); $120.23 for inpatient respite care; and $491.19 for general inpatient care (HCFA/CMS, 2001a).

cant changes in palliative care in the last two decades, Congress should direct CMS to undertake a comprehensive analysis of the costs of effective palliative care and then ensure that per diem rates reflect these costs.

MANAGED CARE AND END-OF-LIFE CARE

In many respects, health care in the United States has been transformed in the last decade by the growth of managed care. By 1999, 91 percent of individuals with employer-sponsored private insurance were enrolled in managed care, including HMOs, PPOs, and multiple variants on these structures. As indicated above, the use of managed care by state Medicaid programs has also become widespread, with more than half of the children covered by Medicaid now enrolled in managed care plans. Both across and within managed care plan types, benefit design and administrative practices vary greatly.

In general, the recent trend in employment-based plans has been somewhat away from the most restrictive or tightly managed plans toward plans that offer more flexibility in choice of provider and somewhat fewer administrative hurdles such as prior approval of services (Draper et al., 2002).[38] Such choice and flexibility often means higher costs.

Management Techniques with Implications for Palliative and End-of-Life Care

Managed care plans use a variety of techniques to control costs, including utilization review, restricted provider networks, and payment incentives for economical provider practice. Some techniques pose potential problems for patients and families, especially for children with fatal or potentially fatal medical problems (see, e.g., Sulmasy, 1995; Morrison and Meier, 1995; IOM, 1997; Fox, 1999; Huskamp et al., 2001).

Utilization Review

Managed care plans may employ several utilization review procedures to control costs. These procedures include requirements for authorization prior to the use of services and retrospective review of services. Plans will

---

[38]In 2001, 48 percent of insured individuals with private employer-sponsored coverage were enrolled in PPO plans (up from 41 percent in 2000), 23 percent were in HMO plans (down from 29 percent in 2000), 22 percent were in point-of service (POS) plans, and 7 percent were in indemnity plans (down from 27 percent in 1996 and 73 percent in 1988) (KFF, 2002).

usually require prior authorization for families with children needing home hospice care.

In managed care plans with tight utilization management processes and stringent criteria for authorizing services, the gap between nominal and meaningful coverage for certain services can be substantial. The committee found no systematic documentation of the extent to which children with life-threatening medical conditions and their families encounter serious problems with review requirements for hospice, home care, or other services to meet their needs for palliative or end-of-life care.

Provider Networks

Most managed care plans select a subset of providers in the area to be members of their provider network. These plans then provide patients financial incentives to use network providers as opposed to providers who are not members. More restrictive plans such as staff model HMOs cover services only if provided by network providers, with exceptions for emergency services under certain circumstances. Less restrictive plans typically require higher cost sharing when members use nonnetwork rather than network providers.

By creating networks, plans can negotiate discounted rates with many providers who are willing to accept lower fees in exchange for the higher level of patient volume likely to result from being listed as a network provider for a health plan. Plans may also choose to retain providers in the network based on analysis of the costs they generate or their practice patterns. A defined network of providers may make it more feasible for insurers to analyze and monitor provider practice patterns and outcomes and then design and institute remedies to identified problems.

The use of provider networks raises several concerns for dying children and their families. The breadth and depth of provider networks vary across plans. Some plans may not include specialists appropriate for treating a fatal or potentially fatal condition (e.g., the network may include a specialist in adult cases—but not child cases—of a particular condition) or may not include appropriate geographic representation of various specialists. Even if a plan's network includes appropriate specialties, it may not include a sufficient number of qualified physicians in each specialist category. This may create unacceptably long waiting times for children in need of specialized care. Arrangements may exist for referral to outside specialists, but families may find their options unsatisfactory. In general, free choice of physician and medical center is a particular issue when a child is seriously ill.

Other concerns include turnover of network providers, which can disrupt continuity of care and relationships of trust. An employer's switch to a new health plan can mean that new relationships must be established with a number of unfamiliar physicians and other providers. (In some regions and for less tightly controlled plans, overlap in provider networks may be substantial and thus minimize this problem.)

Shifting Financial Risk

A third type of cost-control tool involves passing financial risks for enrollee care to providers. As noted earlier, health plans are increasingly passing financial risks to groups of clinicians or, in some cases, to individual clinicians through the use of capitation, withholds, and bonuses.

Some health plans capitate primary care physicians for their own professional services, such that the physician absorbs all the extra costs if utilization is higher than expected. Under a withhold arrangement, a percentage of a clinician's payment is withheld at the time of service delivery. These funds are then distributed to clinicians if they meet certain performance targets, such as controlling pharmacy costs, controlling total health costs, or limiting the number of specialty referrals. Alternatively, plans may pay bonuses when such targets are met. These payment arrangements are intended to encourage cost-effective practice patterns. The concern is that these arrangements create incentives to reduce service provision or to reject sicker patients with higher-cost needs. Many children with fatal or potentially fatal problems fall in this category.

Medicaid Payment to Managed Care Plans

States initially found managed care plans receptive to enrolling Medicaid beneficiaries. More recently, like Medicare, state Medicaid programs have found less enthusiasm, particularly from plans with large private enrollments. Some plans are refusing to enter or continue in the Medicaid market, and others are limiting Medicaid enrollments. Particular complaints include low capitation rates and burdensome administrative requirements (Holahan et al., 1999). In a survey of state Medicaid agencies in late 2000, agency staff cited financing as the reason for about 70 percent of managed care plan departures from their state program (NASHP, 2001). Publicly held companies may be particularly sensitive to Wall Street assessments of their Medicaid participation (CSHSC, 1999).

States have argued, in part, that the plans were paid too much in the early days of voluntary enrollment, when they attracted healthier beneficiaries, and that rates are now more appropriate. In addition, federal requirements set upper limits on what states can pay relative to comparable populations with fee-for-service coverage. As a cost-containment feature, this provision makes sense, but it may not support some of the goals of Medicaid managed care, including greater coordination of care. According to Holahan and colleagues (1999), this provision is one reason why states with high Medicare capitation rates tend to have high Medicaid capitation rates. Other reasons for rate variations include a state's cost-containment objectives and the age of a program.

With new programs and voluntary programs, managed care plans may benefit from enrolling healthier beneficiaries, including those without established physician relationships (see, e.g., Freund et al., 1989; Leibowitz et al., 1992). With mandatory enrollment and more mature programs, the lack of satisfactory risk adjustment for the health status or riskiness of populations served becomes a serious concern for health plans (see, e.g., Buntin and Newhouse, 1998; MedPAC, 1998a). This is especially the case when Medicaid payment rates are well below Medicare and private rates.

Mandatory enrollment without a satisfactory risk adjustment strategy may create financial incentives for undertreatment, a particular threat to children with special health care needs. In establishing interim criteria for states enrolling these children in capitated managed care, HCFA (now CMS) required only that states use a payment mechanism that "accounts" for special needs populations (criterion quoted in Kaye et al., 2000, p. 149).

In 1999, just two state Medicaid programs—Colorado and Maryland—used health-related risk adjustments, although some states used elements of risk-adjustment for subsets of beneficiaries (e.g., Michigan for Title V children and Delaware for SSI enrollees [Kaye et al., 2000]). Some states use only demographic variables (e.g., age, sex) to adjust rates. In general, demographic variables alone do not perform well in predicting variation in beneficiary costs. Many state Medicaid programs use multiple rate categories as a blunt method of risk adjustment, although the rate categories are usually sufficiently broad that they achieve little risk adjustment. Even with adjustments based on health status, it may be difficult to set an adequate prospective capitation rate for high-risk children (Fowler and Anderson, 1996).

Some states deal with predictably high-expense groups, including children with special health care needs, by "carving out" special programs for them (Andrews et al., 1997; Inkelas, 2001). Payments for these programs may or may not be based on capitation and may or may not include adjustments for differences in population risks. One study in California of a carve-out for children with special health care needs suggested that the problem increased the identification of such children as eligible for services (Inkelas, 2001).

DIRECTIONS FOR POLICYMAKERS AND INSURERS

Positive Aspects of the Current Financing System

Notwithstanding its well-publicized inadequacies, this country's complex and unwieldy mix of public and private insurance, philanthropy, and other arrangements funds many needed medical and other supportive services for seriously ill or injured children and their families. In focusing on the system's weaknesses, it is important not to forget its strengths including access for many to helpful services and advanced technologies that save and extend lives, restore function, and otherwise prevent or reduce much illness and suffering.

Children whose parents are covered by health plans sponsored by large employers often have excellent access to care to cure or prolong life. Coverage for palliative and supportive care—often to supplement curative and life-prolonging care—may also be generous. Even when employer plans have restrictions on palliative and supportive care, plan administrators may waive or work around many of these restrictions to provide needed services to gravely ill children and their families.

For children in low-income families, Medicaid and other federal or state programs cover a wide range of services, including long-term home and community-based services, that are often excluded or very restricted in private insurance plans. This care is particularly important for children and families living with neurodegenerative disorders and other severe chronic conditions. State programs often include case management services that help families find and coordinate the complex array of services and providers needed by such children.

Required enrollment by Medicaid beneficiaries in managed care may have some negative features as discussed below, but it also may provide the foundation for more coordinated care and better monitoring of the quality of care for those with complex health problems. One reason that Title V programs are interested in managed care is that its structures should, in theory, make it easier to link children with special health care needs to a medical home that coordinates their complex care.

Finally, it is important to recognize that coverage limitations, payment limits, and other restrictions are not designed to cause suffering or to frustrate patients, families, and physicians—although they frequently do. Rather, the intent is to control the cost of health insurance and health services so that they are affordable for governments, employers, and individuals.

Problems with the Current Financing System

General

Perhaps the most obvious deficiency in this country's health care system is the lack of universal coverage—public or private—for all children and adults under age 65. Although public or private insurance does not guarantee access to reliable, effective, coordinated care and lack of coverage does not mean that care is unavailable, uninsurance does have negative consequences for children and families. For children with serious medical conditions and their families, lack of insurance and underinsurance can seriously disrupt the provision, coordination, and continuity of care—although most will receive at least crisis care. The struggle to find crisis care and other needed services may, however, drain family resources (and sometimes lead to bankruptcy), put parents' jobs in jeopardy if they must substitute for paid caregivers and case managers, trigger a frustrating search for so-called safety-net or free care providers, or all of these.

In addition, as employers or states restructure their programs, families are often subject to switches in health plans offered, revisions in a health plan's terms of coverage (e.g., reduction in home health care benefits), or changes in a plan's provider networks. These changes may be disruptive, resulting in the end of coverage for a valued service or the loss of continued access to trusted and familiar providers.

A less visible consequence of uninsurance or underinsurance is that physicians, hospital staff, and others may—instead of providing care—have to spend valuable (uncompensated) time trying to locate some source of payment or service for seriously ill children. Further, parents distracted by financial worries may find it difficult to provide all the emotional support their children need from them.

Finally, physicians, hospitals, and hospices may find levels of payment too low to allow them to provide the services they believe are needed by a child. In some cases, they may refuse to serve patients covered by a low-paying plan or program, notably state Medicaid programs, which typically pay providers considerably less than other public and private programs.

Although all of these problems affect seriously ill children and families, most can be addressed only by broad policy changes—for example, policies that extend public or private insurance to all—that are beyond the charge to this committee. The committee's recommendations deal with more specific deficits in the financing of palliative, end-of-life, and bereavement care for children and families. Based on its experience and judgment and review of relevant research and proposals of other groups, the committee recommends several changes in public and private coverage of hospice services for children, additional changes to encourage the integration of palliative services with curative or life-prolonging care, and analytic work to support the design and implementation of these changes. Chapter 10 includes directions for further research to refine and support these recommendations and assess their implementation and consequences.

Hospice

Several factors contribute to low use of hospice care by children who die, including physician and parent attitudes or lack of knowledge and the large proportion of child deaths that are sudden and unexpected. Coverage limitations also constitute a barrier in state Medicaid programs and some private insurance plans. In particular, although state Medicaid programs must (under EPSDT provisions) cover hospice care for children even if they do not cover it for adults, the six-month prognosis requirement and the requirement that curative care be forgone (both of which are federal rules) are a problem. If the federal government abandons or fails to enforce EPSDT requirements, then children in six states would, like adults in those states, not be covered for hospice care. Many private insurance plans also use the six-month prognosis requirement. Some hospices successfully rely on philanthropy to serve Medicaid-covered children who fall outside restrictive rules for hospice benefits; others cannot, or they may have other priorities.

Health plans may impose a variety of additional restrictions on hospice and other palliative services. These include caps on the number or amount of services covered, preauthorization requirements for each use of a service or use above a certain level, variable cost-sharing requirements, prescriptions restricted to a closed formulary, waiting lists, or limited "slots" for certain expensive services.

In general, hospices have been comfortable with the per diem payment method created when Medicare first added hospice coverage. Over the last two decades, however, the beneficial but often expensive advances in pain management and other palliative care strategies have strained hospice budgets and led some to limit acceptance of patients with high-cost needs or to forgo effective but costly palliative interventions. At a minimum, the adoption of an outlier payment provision should counter the incentive to refuse very high cost patients. Other options that should be considered include reevaluation of each category of per diem rates, higher per diems for the more expensive first two and last two days of care (a response to late referrals and short lengths of stay) and separate payment for pharmaceuticals, blood transfusions, and similar products. The federal advisory committee on Medicare payment policies recently recommended that the adequacy of Medicare's hospice payment rates be evaluated to determine whether they are adequate given the current costs of providing appropriate care (MedPAC, 2002).

Recommendation: Public and private insurers should restructure hospice benefits for children to

- add hospice care to the services required by Congress in Medicaid and other public insurance programs for children and to the services covered for children under private health plans;
- eliminate eligibility restrictions related to life expectancy, substitute criteria based on diagnosis and severity of illness, and drop rules requiring children to forgo curative or life-prolonging care (possibly in a case management framework); and
- include outlier payments for exceptionally costly hospice patients.

Extension and Integration of Palliative and Bereavement Care

Even with these recommended changes, additional reforms are needed to promote the integration of palliative care from the time of diagnosis through death and into bereavement and to make palliative care expertise more widely available. No child should die in pain or other distress because health plans fail to cover specialized expertise in symptom management. Families should also not have to face a choice between expert palliative care for their child and publicly funded home health assistance for children with special needs. When families choose home care for a seriously ill child, palliative care consultations should be available to children whose home care personnel lack the necessary expertise and experience to manage their physical or psychological symptoms.

Further, in recognition of the central role of parents and guardians in decisionmaking for children (as opposed to adults) with life-threatening conditions, physician reimbursement should cover extended and intensive communication and counseling of parents or guardians, whether or not the child is present. Informing and counseling parents of children with life-threatening conditions is a critical but time-consuming obligation for clinicians that is undervalued in current reimbursement policies.

Another pillar of competent and compassionate care for families who have suffered a child's death is bereavement care, which health plans should cover in its own right. Parents or siblings who seek counseling under their health plan's mental health benefits generally will be covered only under diagnoses such as depression and perhaps not even then, depending on health plan coverage criteria and practices. The recording of such diagnoses can result in later problems in securing health insurance, especially outside an employer-based plan.

The committee recognizes the cost pressures on employers, private health plans, and state Medicaid programs, particularly during periods of recession or slow economic growth. Because Medicaid covers many children with serious chronic health problems, the cost to states of even limited coverage expansions must be considered. Thus, the Centers for Medicare and Medicaid Services should develop estimates of the cost of adopting these recommendations in Medicaid, taking into account the possibility of avoided costs (e.g., hospitalization related to inadequately managed care at home). The analyses being undertaken for the demonstration projects described earlier in this report and in Appendix H should be helpful.

Recommendation: In addition to modifying hospice benefits, Medicaid and private insurers should modify policies restricting access to other palliative services related to a child's life-threatening medical condition or death. Such modifications should

- reimburse the time necessary for fully informing and counseling parents (whether or not the child is present) about their child's (1) diagnosis and prognosis, (2) options for care, including potential benefits and harms, and (3) plan of care, including end-of-life decisions and care for which the family is responsible;
- make the expertise of palliative care experts and hospice personnel more widely available by covering palliative care consultations;
- reimburse bereavement services for parents and surviving siblings of children who die;
- specify coverage and eligibility criteria for palliative inpatient, home health, and professional services based on diagnosis (and, for certain services, severity of illness) to guide specialized case managers and others involved in administering the benefits; and
- provide for the Centers for Medicare and Medicaid Services to develop estimates of the potential cost of implementing these modifications for Medicaid.

Implementation

To implement the recommendations related to improved benefits for palliative, end-of-life, and bereavement care, eligibility criteria must be defined. Federal officials should work with state Medicaid officials, pediatric organizations, and private insurers to define diagnosis and severity criteria to establish children's eligibility for pediatric palliative care and hospice services and family members' eligibility for bereavement services. In addition, federal officials should also take the lead in examining the appropriateness of diagnostic, procedure, and other payment-related classification schemes that were originally developed for adult services. These schemes include DRGs for hospital payment and an RBRVS for physician payment. Many private payers and Medicaid programs have adopted these classification schemes (although not necessarily the level of payment associated with them). Given the confusion about billing for palliative care services and the frequent denials of payment for improper coding or documentation, access to care may also be improved by providing clearer guidance about accurate coding and documentation of covered palliative services. Although providers faced with claims denials and hassles may sometimes render services without billing for them, they may also opt not to provide the services or to avoid patients that need such services.

> Recommendation: Federal and state Medicaid agencies, pediatric organizations, and private insurers should cooperate to (1) define diagnosis and, as appropriate, severity criteria for eligibility for expanded benefits for palliative, hospice, and bereavement services; (2) examine the appropriateness for reimbursing pediatric palliative and end-of-life care of diagnostic, procedure, and other classification systems that were developed for reimbursement of adult services; and (3) develop guidance for practitioners and administrative staff about accurate, consistent coding and documenting of palliative, end-of-life, and bereavement services.

Again, these recommendations target only a subset of financial barriers to competent and reliably available palliative, end-of-life, and bereavement care. Uninsurance, underinsurance, certain managed care requirements, and radically low levels of provider payment also constitute significant barriers. Reducing or removing these barriers will require far more comprehensive changes in policies.

CHAPTER 8

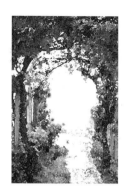

ETHICAL AND LEGAL ISSUES

> *I think in particular of two times when we made a particular request and were told that the ethics committee would be called. I'm now on the ethics committee at Children's Hospital here and . . . [I advocate there] that ethics committees not be viewed like the legal system. That's not helpful or open to families but one other thing to be really frightened about.*
>
> Deborah Dokken, parent, 2001

Questions and disagreements about what constitutes appropriate medical treatment or limitations of treatment for infants and children with severe and often fatal medical problems are a staple of the bioethics literature. They are rarely—but then very visibly—the subject of litigation and legislation. Even so, when parents question or disagree with the health care team or hospital management, they may perceive some responses as legalistic and intimidating rather than constructive and compassionate.

One goal of palliative and end-of-life care is to minimize avoidable conflicts related to poor communication, cultural misunderstandings, deficient clinical care, and approaches to decision making that fail to assure families that they and the health care team are doing their best for the child. Such failures can haunt family members and clinicians long after a child's death.

Not all conflict raises ethical or legal concerns, and ethical concerns about clinical decisionmaking certainly may arise in the absence of conflict. This chapter provides an overview of the ethical and legal context for decisions by clinicians, parents, and children about pediatric palliative and end-of-life care. It

• describes several categories of decisions that have prompted ethical or legal questions and disagreements;

• outlines the key ethical obligations of clinicians as commonly identified by clinicians and bioethicists;

• discusses the potential for conflicts among ethical obligations;

• identifies some strategies for preventing or resolving conflicts among those involved in decisions about a child's care; and

• reviews some ethical and legal questions about the care of children, including the status of children as decisionmakers and certain boundaries on parental authority.

This discussion focuses on clinicians' decisions rather than on parental obligations or societal issues of resource allocation and burden sharing. The discussion does not consider a number of ethical and legal controversies. These include the declaration of brain death in anencephalic newborns, continuation or discontinuation of pregnancy following prenatal diagnosis of a fatal medical problem, use of certain alternative or complementary therapies at the end of life, and euthanasia. The chapter also does not discuss licensure issues, some aspects of which are considered in Chapter 6. Chapter 10 examines ethical issues in research involving children. Although this chapter does not include formal recommendations, the committee believes that the strategies for preventing and resolving conflict discussed here should be considered and tested as institutions develop the procedures and protocols recommended in Chapters 4, 5, and 6.

Many legal and ethical questions considered here are relevant for palliative and end-of-life care for both adults and children. Some issues are, however, unique to children. One example is whether schools serving medically fragile children must honor parental requests that cardiopulmonary resuscitation not be attempted for their child. Another involves getting permission from an abusive parent to withdraw life support when the parent will be charged with murder after the child's death. Not unique but especially wrenching when a child is involved are questions about the ethics of using or forgoing certain medical interventions when disease is far advanced.

Although it is important to understand the limits that courts or legislatures have imposed on decisionmaking by clinicians or parents or both, these limits will not affect most decisions about palliative and end-of-life care for children. Similarly, the legal limits on children's decisions about medical treatment are not inconsequential, but they should not constrain efforts by clinicians and parents to inform children about their condition (consistent with their intellectual and emotional maturity) and to determine and consider children's treatment preferences. An assumption of this committee and most sources consulted by the committee is that litigation should be a last and rare resort when clinicians and family members disagree.

As with other aspects of palliative, end-of-life, and bereavement care, the legal system and ethical frameworks discussed here reflect this country's history and dominant culture. Although the legal system of the United States and arguments based in biomedical ethics may sometimes confuse or surprise those raised in this country, people raised in other cultures may find them incomprehensible or possibly shocking. Particularly in legal matters, flexibility to consider cultural differences may be limited. Nonetheless, it is still both humane and prudent for clinicians, social service personnel, and legal counsel to be sensitive to differences in cultural values and experiences and to try to minimize conflict and family distress related to such differences. (See Appendix D for additional discussion of cultural diversity.)

TYPES OF DECISIONS

In recent decades, many legal disputes and ethical debates about care for infants and children have involved decisions to start or stop medical interventions. Other disputes focus on the limits of parents' authority to decide about their child's care and on whether and to what extent quality-of-life and financial considerations should influence decisions about life-sustaining treatments. This section briefly describes these decisions and the questions they have raised. Much of the initial discussion of some of these issues, for example, withholding and withdrawing life-support technologies, occurred in the 1970s and 1980s and predated the increased attention to the techniques and benefits of palliative care. Again, the issues are not necessarily unique to children but tend to be more emotionally charged and difficult for all involved.

Decisions About Who Decides

In general, parents have the legal right to make decisions about medical care for their child. This parental authority is occasionally challenged, usually when parents refuse treatment recommended by their child's physician. In addition, adolescents have sometimes sought control over crucial decisions about their future, often in situations involving reproduction but sometimes involving care for far advanced illness. Sometimes they succeed. For example, in 1994, state officials unsuccessfully tried to force a 15-year-old boy, who had received two liver transplants, to take medications that he refused on grounds of unbearable pain (Penkower, 1996; see more generally McCabe, et al., 1996).[1]

---

[1] For the situation in which a child's participation in research is involved, federal regulations normally require both that parents give permission and that children also "assent" to participation. Chapter 10 discusses ethical issues related to the involvement of children in research.

That parents have the legal right to make decisions does not and should not, however, mean that parents and clinicians should simply exclude children from discussions and decisions about their care. Failing to provide children with information and the opportunity to discuss their fears, concerns, and preferences can isolate them and add to their anxiety and other distress. In Chapter 4, the committee recommended that children and adolescents be informed and involved in decisionmaking—consistent with their condition, maturity, and preferences and with sensitivity to the family's culture and values. Involving the child and trying to see care through the child's eyes is also an element of child- and family-centered care as discussed in Chapter 6. Particularly for adolescents, restricting participation in decisionmaking "may unnecessarily create tension where a therapeutic alliance is needed" (Burns and Truog, 1997, p. 73). Many medical care consent forms include a section documenting "assent" to care by adolescents.[2]

Care must, however, be taken not to give the false impression that parents will never override their child's expressed wishes. Decisions by child patients—and by parents and adult patients—may be constrained by organizational or governmental policies or by environmental factors. For example, state laws may require emergency medical services providers to attempt resuscitation even for adults or children with DNR orders (Sabatino, 1999). Likewise, deeply held cultural values may lead parents to reject proposals to involve the child or even provide the child with information about his or her condition. Clinicians may respect these values but still be dismayed. Years of experience may temper such reactions. As one clinician observed ". . . more and more I've realized that it's going to unfold the way that family needs it to unfold" (Mildred Solomon, Ed.D., Education Development Center, taken from interviews conducted for the Initiative for Pediatric Palliative Care, unpublished analysis by Hardart et al., 2002).

Although it is important to understand the ethical and legal context for decisionmaking, most disagreements about care are resolved informally through discussion and reflection. For example, the vignette about the Devane family in Chapter 3 described how an adolescent with recurrent cancer prevailed in refusing further burdensome experimental treatment (wanted by her physician and parents) and in living her remaining time doing what she wanted to do.

---

[2]The AAP defines the steps to securing assent to include helping the child understand his or her condition and what to expect, assessing the child's understanding of his or her situation and identifying any inappropriate pressure on the child, and seeking an expression of the child's willingness to accept treatment (Kohrman et al., 1995).

Decisions About Treatments

Stopping Versus Not Starting Treatment

Ethicists and judges generally agree that there is no meaningful ethical or legal difference between deciding not to initiate a treatment and deciding to discontinue a treatment (assuming that appropriate attention is paid to such matters as patient comfort) (see, e.g., President's Commission, 1983; see also AMA, 1994a).[3] Nonetheless, in the committee's experience, both clinicians and parents may find it more emotionally difficult and morally challenging to stop a treatment once begun than not to initiate it in the first place.

Implementing a decision to stop a life-sustaining medical intervention may also be technically challenging as demonstrated by ongoing discussions of which strategy for removing a ventilator or breathing tube best meets patient and family needs (see Chapter 5). These needs may vary, depending on the patient's condition and the family's values. Some clinicians may even be reluctant to start such interventions when they might be useful for fear of not being able to stop them if they prove nonbeneficial. Thus, it is important for those responsible for such interventions to be thoroughly knowledgeable about all clinical and ethical aspects of initiating and stopping them.

A recently reported survey of clinicians involved in pediatric intensive care found that although 78 percent of physicians agreed that the decision not to start an intervention (such as mechanical ventilation) and the decision to stop it were ethically the same, only 57 percent of nurses did (Burns et al., 2001). Another recent survey at seven children's hospitals or pediatric units of general hospitals found that majorities of nurses and residents and a near majority of attending physicians disagreed with this proposition of moral equivalence (Solomon et al., 2000c). Yet other research suggests that decisions about which interventions are forgone—and when—may not be supported by clear clinical or ethical rationales (see, e.g., Faber-Langendoen, 1996; Asch et al., 1999; Truog et al., 2000).

Clinicians' attitudes and practices related to the use of life-sustaining medical interventions may be influenced by a number of factors including their cultural or religious values and their emotional response to a child's grave illness or injury. Other factors include (1) ignorance or misunderstanding of the evidence about the benefits and burdens of specific interven-

---

[3]Some religious groups do make a major distinction between withholding and withdrawing (in non-brain dead patients) life-sustaining treatments at the end of life (see, e.g., Steinberg, 1998).

tions at the end of life, (2) insufficient education in clinical ethics and reinforcement of ethics in day-to-day practice, and (3) feelings of helplessness related, in part, to inadequate knowledge of palliative strategies to prevent or relieve distress when life-sustaining interventions are forgone. This lack of palliative knowledge may contribute both to the continuation of nonbeneficial interventions and to needless suffering when interventions are halted, for example, when the removal of a breathing tube is managed with paralytic agents that do not relieve distress but prevent the patient from communicating it (Rushton and Terry, 1995; Truog et al., 2000; Henig et al., 2001).

Life-Sustaining Treatments

With advances in medical technologies in the second half of the twentieth century has come increasing anxiety among clinicians, ethicists, and the informed public about the appropriate use of life-sustaining interventions, especially when a patient's chance of survival is very low. Cardiopulmonary resuscitation is perhaps the best known of an array of such interventions that may be attempted (or forgone) when death is imminent.[4] Other life-support measures include mechanical ventilation (for reasons in addition to respiratory arrest), mechanical provision of nutrients or fluids (artificial nutrition or hydration), blood transfusions, antibiotics, and dialysis.[5]

Decisions about life-sustaining interventions—especially resuscitation attempts—are often made in an atmosphere of crisis and even panic, but this is not always the case. For example, mechanical ventilation may be begun in a child with a progressive neuromuscular disease such as muscular dystrophy after extended discussion and profound reflection by the family, the child, and the care team on the benefits, risks, and burdens of this action.[6] Still, even when parents know that their child has an invariably

---

[4]Resuscitation involves aggressive measures to restore spontaneous breathing and blood circulation following cardiac or respiratory arrest. It may involve electric shocks to the heart, the insertion of breathing tubes to allow mechanical ventilation, and medications to stimulate the heart and restore breathing. Mouth-to-mouth respiration and chest compressions—which can be forceful enough to break a patient's ribs—may be used by either laypeople or medical personnel until more advanced technologies are available.

[5]Unlike resuscitation, these interventions are also used routinely in many noncritical situations. For example, during and following surgery with general anesthesia, life may be temporarily sustained by mechanical ventilation and intravenous administration of fluids (artificial hydration).

[6]Although some have questioned such care, most pediatricians believe it is appropriate when the child patient and the family have been fully informed about benefits, risks, and burdens (Orenstein, 2000; Gibson, 2001).

fatal condition, such as Tay-Sachs disease, and have been counseled that cardiac or respiratory arrest can be expected when functional and cognitive deterioration is advanced and even when they understand the ultimate futility of attempting resuscitation, they may still—in their distress at that stage—call "9-1-1," thereby triggering full-scale resuscitation efforts.

It is now generally accepted among clinicians, ethicists, policymakers, and the informed public that forgoing life-support measures is often appropriate as death approaches (see Chapter 5). Notwithstanding such consensus, the parents of a dying child may not accept a clinician's assessment that life-support no longer has the potential to benefit the child and may insist that it be continued. Much of the discussion later in this chapter focuses on strategies for understanding the reasons for family rejection of physician counsel and for resolving disagreements without harm to the patient, the family, or the health care team.

Some controversy about forgoing specific interventions persists. For example, discussion continues about whether artificial nutrition and hydration at the end of life are morally or clinically different from other interventions and whether they should be maintained when other life-support measures are forgone (see, e.g., Nelson et al., 1995; Burck, 1996; Post, 2001; Gillick, 2001). Surveys of pediatric specialists have found that specialists are much more willing to forgo resuscitation or mechanical ventilation than artificial hydration given the same clinical situations (Nelson et al., 1995; see also Smith and Wigton, 1987). Other studies suggest that clinicians may believe mistakenly that artificial nutrition and hydration are always legally required in situations or jurisdictions in which that is not the case (Meisel et al., 2000). Although research findings are limited and inconsistent, some suggest that artificial nutrition or hydration when death is near may be more burdensome than beneficial in some circumstances (Finucane et al., 1999; Brody, 2000; see also Chapter 5). Again, whatever clinicians may believe and whatever the evidence may be, family values and understandings may differ.

Another controversy, noted earlier, involves whether schools will honor do-not-resuscitate (DNR) orders for medically fragile children, an increasing number of whom attend school (see, e.g., NEA, 1994; Rushton et al., 1994; AAP, 2000d, Hoffpauir, 2001). Some districts have refused to honor parents' wishes, partly out of concern about the impact on staff and other students (see, e.g., Tucson Unified School District, 1996; Laramie County, 1996). Other districts have worked with parents on a case-by-case basis to develop a plan of care. State policies vary. In its discussion of this issue, the American Academy of Pediatrics (AAP, 2000d) does not make a blanket recommendation about what schools should do. Rather, it recommends that pediatricians and parents meet with relevant school personnel to explain the child's medical condition and the goals of care and to hear the concerns of other parents and school personnel, for example, about liability and effects on other children. It also urges that all parties be realistic, flexible, and ready to negotiate.

Other Treatments

Interventions such as resuscitation and mechanical ventilation are usually intended to sustain life temporarily, for example, when a patient is incapacitated as a result of surgery or injury and when recovery or prolonged meaningful life is a realistic goal. They are not intended to cure or to alter the underlying disease. Other interventions such as surgery, chemotherapy, or radiotherapy are usually intended to cure the child's medical problem or provide extended remission of disease.[7] Decisions about these interventions sometimes arise in emergency situations, but they ordinarily follow a less urgent assessment of the child's condition. Although the underlying ethical, legal, or clinical issues may be similar for decisions in both situations, the bias "to do something" (meaning something beyond providing comfort) seems most evident in an emergency.

Decisions About the Criteria for Decisions

Many ethical and legal criteria for decisions about end-of-life care are well accepted, although disagreement may exist about how to apply and weigh them in specific situations. Two criteria have, however, aroused particular controversy. One criterion involves the consideration of quality of life, particularly in decisions made on behalf of a patient who is not able to describe his or her own experience or preferences. The other criterion involves the consideration of organizational or societal costs in treatment decisions.

Quality of Life as a Criterion in Decisions

At both the societal level (when the well being of populations is the focus) and the clinical level (when the well being of individual patients and their families is the focus), there is more to health care decisionmaking than preserving life. As expressed by the American Academy of Pediatrics, "the goal [of palliative care] is to add life to the child's years, not simply years to

---

[7]They may also be used to relieve pain or other symptoms, but such palliative uses, in and of themselves, rarely generate ethical or legal conflicts. Palliative uses may, however, trigger disputes with insurers that argue that such care is not covered.

the child's life" (AAP, 2000g, p. 353). When physicians and others are identifying, explaining, and weighing the potential benefits and burdens of different courses of care, the implications for quality of life—not just the quantity of life—need attention. Chapters 4 and 9 and Appendix C discuss concepts and measures of quality of life (and their limitations) in more detail.

Judgments about quality of life involve both factual issues (e.g., what do data and experience suggest about a child's prognosis with or without the treatment in question) and subjective elements (e.g., when has a child's suffering become so great that it outweighs any benefits of the treatment). For infants and very young children as well as older children who are cognitively limited or comatose, judgments will rely on parents' or others' values and assessments.

Although ethicists, theologians, and clinicians may disagree among themselves about issues such as assisted suicide or euthanasia, most have come to agree that palliative actions intended to relieve suffering (i.e., protect the quality of life) are justified even when one unintended consequence or effect may be to hasten death (i.e., limit the quantity of life) (see, e.g., Cherny and Portenoy, 1994; Fleischman, 1998; Jonsen et al., 1998; Sulmasy, 2000; but see also Beauchamp and Childress, 1994, for a review of critiques of such arguments). Many professional organizations have also endorsed this perspective (see, e.g., AMA, 1994a; AAP, 2000g). As discussed in Chapter 5, the practice of terminal or palliative sedation involves this kind of "double-effect" reasoning.

Still, the role of quality-of-life considerations continues to prompt discussion (see, e.g., Kuhse, 1987; Beauchamp and Childress, 1994; Pellegrino, 2000). For example, are life-sustaining measures ethically or legally required for a permanently comatose infant? What about infants with profound impairment short of this state? Some take the position that, absent a double-effect situation, it is never acceptable to forgo life-sustaining treatments based on quality-of of-life considerations, regardless of family wishes. What are the obligations of clinicians to patients and families when unwanted interventions leave a patient profoundly impaired cognitively and physically? As described below, controversy over these questions has in a few instances prompted litigation and even legislation that has sought to preclude or restrict clinicians and families from considering quality of life in decisions about infants with severe birth defects.

Resources as a Criterion in Decisions

As health care costs have escalated since the 1960s, clinicians and others have become increasingly concerned about real or potential conflicts between clinicians' responsibilities to individual patients and their obligations to support the prudent use of limited societal or institutional re-sources. One view is that, by and large, so much nonbeneficial treatment exists that eliminating it will preclude the need to limit or ration beneficial care. An alternative perspective is that control of health care costs also requires decisions to limit or ration care that is thought to offer some benefit but not enough to warrant its provision, given higher priorities. Disagreements often arise, however, over the judgment that a service is not beneficial.[8] Many clinicians worry about the appropriateness of "bedside rationing."[9] The traditional consensus in the clinical community has been that resources should not enter into physicians' judgments about individual patients unless those judgments are governed by clear principles and proce-dures that follow public deliberation, reflect general community consensus, and are consistent with available scientific knowledge (see, e.g., Angell, 1985, Sulmasy 1992; AAP, 1996).

ETHICAL CONSIDERATIONS

Ethical analyses may focus on obligations at an individual or a collec-tive (organizational or societal) level. Regardless of the level of analysis, cultural diversity and sensitivity to individual and family differences must be factored into discussions, decisions, and practices.

Ethical Obligations at the Individual Level

At the individual level, ethical analyses generally focus on the obliga-tions of clinicians, first, to individual patients and, second and less often, to those close to or responsible for a patient. Most analyses of clinical decisionmaking devote little attention to parental responsibilities, focusing instead on the responsibility of clinicians and others to guide and redirect those parents who are viewed as acting against their child's best interests.

Notwithstanding children's stage of development or legal status, most

---

[8]Thus, the controversy over mammography screening, particularly for women under age 50, has pitted those who argue that no adequately controlled scientific research clearly docu-ments the benefits of such screening against those who agree that research is flawed but argue that the theoretical possibility of benefit is sufficient when such a dreaded disease is involved. Pediatrics has its share of disagreements over an array of interventions such as screening for scoliosis, metabolic screening for Gaucher's disease, and screening for conditions such as Huntington's chorea with no effective treatment (other than palliation).

[9]Ubel and Goold argue that "bedside rationing" occurs when these conditions are met. "The physician must 1) withhold, withdraw, or fail to recommend a service that, in the physician's best clinical judgment, is in the patient's best medical interests; 2) act primarily to promote the financial interests of someone other than the patient (including an organization, society at large, and the physician himself or herself); and 3) have control over the use of the beneficial service" (Ubel and Goold, 1997, p. 74).

issues related to their care can be considered within the same broad ethical frameworks that are widely applied to care for adults. During recent decades, general agreement has emerged on the core ethical obligations of clinicians to patients (see, e.g., Beauchamp and Childress, 1983; President's Commission for the Study of Ethical Problems in Medicine and Biomedical and Behavioral Research [hereafter, President's Commission], 1983; Jonsen and Toulmin, 1988; McCullough, 1988; Brennan, 1991). In common parlance,[10] these obligations are to

- do good (e.g., by relieving a child's pain or providing emotional support),
- avoid doing harm (e.g., by not providing life-sustaining treatments that impose burdens on a child without benefit),
- respect patient autonomy (e.g., by generally attempting to consider care "through the child's eyes" even though young children have no legal autonomy), and
- treat patients equitably (e.g., by seeking to provide or arrange needed care for children regardless of a family's ability to pay).

These ethical obligations may sometimes be in conflict and may not be equally weighed in practice. For example, a single action may involve both benefits and harms that have to be balanced in view of the patient's overall circumstances and understood preferences. The obligations to avoid harm and to respect autonomy have been exhaustively considered in debates about forgoing life-sustaining treatment. In contrast, one recent study of such situations concluded that the value of providing effective palliative care when life-sustaining treatment is forgone "remains underanalzyed and needs more rigorous examination" (Burns et al., 2000, p. 3060).

Other obligations or other formulations of clinical and, more generally, medical ethics exist.[11] Ethicists may, for example, cite the obligations of

---

[10]In the language of bioethics, these obligations are often described as *beneficence*, the obligation to provide care that improves health or well-being (or, as it is sometimes expressed, to do to others their good); *nonmaleficence*, the obligation to prevent or avoid harm; *autonomy*, the general duty to respect people's right of self-determination regarding choices about their life and body; and *justice*, the duty to avoid discrimination on the basis of irrelevant characteristics (sometimes expressed as treating individuals [or equals] equally in morally relevant situations) or, under the label *distributive justice*, the duty to distribute health care resources in ways that can be defended as fair and equitable and not arbitrary or capricious.

[11]Medical ethics extends beyond clinical practice to cover legal obligations, relationships with other professionals, and community responsibilities. For example, the American Medical Association's principles of medical ethics, among other provisions, state that physicians should report other physicians who have deficits in character or competence and that they should, except in emergencies, be free to choose the patients they serve (AMA, 2001).

"fidelity" and "professional integrity." Fidelity is the responsibility of health care professionals to place the interests of their patients first. Professional integrity can be viewed as a broad obligation of physicians to act ethically in all their relationships and to be faithful to their moral values when they are challenged (see, e.g., Beauchamp and Childress, 1994; Alpers and Lo, 1999).

The clinician's primary obligation is to his or her patient, and ethical discourse has focused on this obligation. In pediatrics, the principle that the "child and family are the unit of care" raises the issue of the clinician's obligations to parents and other family members. These obligations do not appear to have been systematically interpreted using the ethical framework outlined above, although the potential for conflict between a child's interests or preferences and a family member's interests or preferences has been discussed (see, e.g., Randall and Downie, 1999).

A few observations about clinical ethics in this context can be offered. First, the communication strategies discussed in Chapter 4 and the consensus building strategies described below should usually help clinicians to do good for parents (e.g., by helping parents to feel they have done their best for their child); avoid harming parents (e.g., by helping them avoid choices they will later regret); and treating parents fairly (e.g., by providing understandable information and generally respecting their values). Second, in most situations, when clinicians fulfill their obligations to a child of doing good, avoiding harm, and treating fairly, they are doing likewise for parents because parents usually want to advance their child's best interests. Third, in rare cases, as discussed further below, clinicians may conclude that doing good for the child requires opposing parental preferences and values.

Most discussions of clinical and medical ethics focus on the obligations of individual professionals rather than care teams. As discussed further below, different members of a child's care team may sometimes have different views of what constitutes ethical care. Although physicians usually have the legal and professional authority to prevail, the persistence of unresolved and unacknowledged conflict can compromise the implementation of decisions, damage team members, and subtly (sometimes explicitly) undermine patient and family trust in team members. Some conflicts may reflect individual values, characteristics, and personalities; others may be rooted in different professional socialization and norms.

Ethical Obligations at the Collective Level

Clinicians may sometimes perceive their obligations to their patients individually to be in conflict with their obligation to do good or avoid harm for patients collectively. To cite a dramatic but atypical example, in emergency departments and critical care units, an unusual surge in injured patients may outstrip available personnel, space, and equipment. In response, clinicians and others have established triage protocols to guide decisions about how to allocate—that is, ration—treatment resources in such situations. Appendix B describes how prognostic tools (e.g., assessments of a patient's likelihood of survival with or without treatment) have been developed to aid in formulating and applying such protocols (and for other purposes).

Debates about the appropriate use of limited resources arise across the spectrum of clinical decisions. Some involve routine elements of patient care, for example, how much physicians (and certain nonphysicians) should be paid for informing and educating patients compared to performing surgery or other procedures.

Once again, however, some of the most widely publicized disagreements about resource use focus on care for newborns who have conditions that—even with treatment—are incompatible with extended life or with neurological function beyond the most primitive level (Fost, 1999). One highly publicized case in the 1990s, that of "Baby K," raised questions about the limits of parental demands on community resources—and on providers who are convinced that such demands violate their professional ethics and integrity (16 F 3d 590, CCA 4, 1994; Glover and Rushton, 1995). In this case, which is discussed in more detail below, the mother of an anencephalic child (who lacked all parts of the brain except the brain stem) insisted on repeated resuscitation. Federal trial and appellate courts held that emergency care could not be denied under the federal Emergency Medicine and Active Labor Act. (See, e.g., Clayton, 1995; Brown, 1996; and Maragakis, 1996, for critiques of this interpretation of the legislation, which was passed to prevent emergency department "dumping" of uninsured patients.)

Often, physicians may join with parents in a desire to "do everything" to prolong the life of a gravely ill child, including providing some treatments of marginal or no benefit. They may argue that such care provides emotional comfort and hope to the parents and allows all involved freedom from any guilt they might experience had they not pursued every option. In other cases, physicians may resist such treatment because they believe it harms the child, violates their clinical values, and misuses limited community resources.[12]

Indeed, the effort to define a quantifiable concept of "futile" treatment

---

[12] These physicians may, however, accept that it is humane to provide a limited amount of care that cannot benefit a patient but that can reduce the suffering of family members. Thus, even when a child is, by clinical criteria, brain dead, a physician may delay removal of life support to give parents time to absorb the information, to come to terms with the decision to remove life-support equipment, and to say their good-byes in peace.

has been driven in considerable measure by physicians who want more protection against family demands for treatments with no or virtually no potential for benefit (see, e.g., the perspectives in Zucker and Zucker, 1997; see also Schneiderman et al., 1990; Rushton and Hogue, 1993; IOM 1997; Avery, 1998; Goldstein and Merkens, 2000). While accepting the concept that medical treatments are futile in certain situations, some ethicists, clinicians, and researchers have concluded that the term is so variably and imprecisely used that, in general, it ought to be avoided (Beauchamp and Childress, 1994).[13] Others have concluded, further, that it is impossible to craft a precise operational definition of futility that can reliably and validly govern subsequent real-world clinical decisions (see, e.g., Lantos et al., 1989; Truog et al., 1992; Waisel and Truog, 1995).[14] Rather, assessing futility is a judgmental process requiring "judicious balancing" of effectiveness, benefit, and burden specific to each patient and treatment (Pellegrino, 2000). In addition, some argue that proposals to limit futile treatment may mask "prejudices about those who are disabled, who come from disadvantaged social groups, or who are dying" (AAP, 1996, p.150; see also Krakauer and Truog, 1997).

Efforts to define futile care have also been motivated by the expectation or hope that the application of such a definition in practice could help control health care costs. Two studies of pediatric intensive care in single institutions concluded that only a small percentage of patients met any one of several definitions of futility and that their care generally involved relatively limited resources (Sachdeva et al., 1996; Goh and Mok, 2001).

The allocation of resources for medical care is just one element of a broader set of issues of about the allocation of community resources and responsibilities. Families of a seriously ill or injured child often must shoulder heavy financial burdens, sometimes extending to job loss, home loss, bankruptcy, and homelessness. Even if they have private health insurance, it will usually not cover all the home health care and nonmedical home care and other services needed by a child and family. Medicaid and other gov-

---

[13]Beauchamp and Childress (1994, pp. 212–213) list the many differing descriptions of what is futile: "whatever is highly unlikely to be efficacious (statistically the odds of success are exceedingly small), a low-grade outcome that is virtually certain (qualitatively the results are expected to be exceedingly poor), whatever is highly likely to be more burdensome than beneficial, and whatever is completely speculative because it is an untried 'treatment.'" They note that these interpretations go beyond situations in which benefit is physiologically impossible to situations that are characterized by competing value judgments and interpretations of probabilities.

[14]Although the American Medical Association has more recently offered guidance about the development of policies on medical futility (AMA, Policy E-2.037, 1997), it argued earlier that "denial of treatment should be justified by reliance on openly stated ethical principles and acceptable standards of care, . . . not on the concept of 'futility,' which cannot be meaningfully defined" (AMA, 1994a).

ernment programs may cover more services but, in most cases, only after a family's resources are virtually exhausted.

Ethics in Practice

Notwithstanding the moral passion and intellectual energy devoted to ethical analyses and positions, the greater challenge may be in matching practice to principles, even when the principles are, by and large, not in dispute. Financial constraints and time constraints may undermine ethical practice, for example, when clinicians face appointment schedules that leave them little time for the kind of consensus-building discussions described below.

Violations of ethical practice and avoidable patient and family suffering also may arise from missteps involving what should be routine organizational procedures and actions. For example, despite years of attention, patients and families cannot be guaranteed that decisions made in advance about the use of life-sustaining medical treatments will be honored because information about advance directives may not follow the patient, for example, during a transfer from home to hospital. Such failures prompted the Oregon effort, described in Chapter 6, to develop tools and implement procedures that have increased the likelihood that patients will have their wishes honored (Tolle et al., 2002).

In some cases, health care professionals and health care organizations may be constrained by licensure or other regulatory restrictions from providing care they believe appropriate. For example, hospices may be restricted not just by Medicare and Medicaid coverage limits but also by licensure from providing a broad range of palliative services to all adults and children in need. Eliminating or revising these restrictions would take state and national action.

Further, despite various educational efforts, it is clear that physicians and other care team members sometimes misunderstand both the evidence base and the ethical context for life-support interventions and are not properly prepared—intellectually or emotionally—to inform and advise patients and families. Even with a correct understanding of science and ethical principles, some clinicians may lack the skills and attitudes to provide compassionate and effective communication with seriously ill children and their families. Education is not sufficient to change practice but it is necessary to provide requisite skills and it can shape attitudes and values.

Consistent with studies of care for adults, studies of pediatric care have documented considerable variation in attitudes about and use of life-sustaining technologies in real or hypothetical situations (see, e.g., Levetown et al., 1994; Randolph et al., 1997, 1999; Keenan et al., 2000; see also Asch et al., 1995; Fins, 1999; Breen et al., 2001; Puntillo et al., 2001). Variations in attitudes can lead to variations in decisions and practices, although variations in knowledge, habits, and organizational protocols also may contribute. Patients and families may, as a result, be unable to expect consistency in care, fairness, and freedom from avoidable suffering.

Creating organizational and societal environments for ethical practice requires persistent, cooperative efforts to change virtually every dimension of medical care—including professional education, arrangements for institutional governance, mechanisms for professional collaboration, patient-clinician decisionmaking, information and performance evaluation systems, and financing principles and policies (see, e.g., Rushton and Brooks-Brunn, 1997; Brodeur, 1998; Jonsen et al., 1998). Although not identical in purpose or method, the principles and strategies for integrating ethical principles into organizational culture and routine professional practice have much in common with those guiding many of the continuous quality improvement initiatives discussed in Chapter 6.

The following section focuses on strategies for resolving conflicts. Some of these strategies, for example, the development and successful application of clinical practice guidelines, also can help in transforming statements of principles into effective practice.

STRATEGIES FOR PREVENTING OR RESOLVING PARENT–CLINICIAN AND OTHER CONFLICTS ABOUT CLINICAL CARE

As noted earlier, conflicts cannot always be avoided. Conflicts may even be productive or beneficial in some situations, for example, when parents pursue an issue in disagreement rather than capitulating to a course of action and later regretting their silence. The same point may hold when members of the health care team challenge and argue with each other. In the face of disagreement, overly confident or assertive clinicians may become more sensitive to parental concerns and values. Nonetheless, extended or severe conflict about care of a gravely ill or injured child may be very destructive to all involved and may subject children to needless suffering, for example, as clinicians and family argue about treatments.

Strategies to prevent or resolve conflicts about clinical care can operate at the individual level. That is, they come into play when a particular dispute arises or the potential for dispute exists, but they do not establish general rules or formal precedents to govern subsequent cases. Conflict resolution strategies can also operate at the organizational or system level, for example, in the form of ethics committees or ethics consultation protocols. In addition, research can be useful in preventing or resolving disputes, for example, by clarifying the benefits and burdens of specific medical interventions in different clinical situations. Although some efforts have been made to document the implementation and results of strategies to prevent or resolve conflict, more research is needed to assess their strengths and limitations and guide adjustments to produce better results.

Individual-Level Strategies

Continued Discussion and Involvement of New Parties

At the individual level, attempts to resolve conflicts involving specific clinicians, parents, and sometimes children typically involve continued discussion of the situation. Following the identification of a conflict, new participants may become involved in the discussion. Thus, a child's care team may meet as a group with the family and perhaps the child to discuss a disagreement that has arisen during discussions involving the family and the child's main physician. Sometimes, during such a team meeting, a nurse, social worker, or other physician may recognize that despite an individual physician's best efforts to communicate clearly, the family lacks or misunderstands crucial clinical or other information and terminology. The conflict, in essence, turns out to be not so much about differences in values as about differences in information or understanding of the "facts" of a situation or differences in the way language is understood. When organizations make family conferences or protocols for counseling routine elements of pediatric care, they become system-level strategies for preventing or managing conflict (see, e.g., Hansen et al., 1998; Curtis et al., 2001).

Team conferences without family members present may also be employed to deal with conflicts among care team members, for example, when physicians and nurses disagree about the use of a life-sustaining intervention. If such conflicts are routine, then system-level approaches may be appropriate and could include cooperative development of practice guidelines based on systematic assessments of evidence and consensus-building processes.

Counseling and Consultations

Some conflicts may be less about facts or values (e.g., whether it is ever morally acceptable to withhold medically provided hydration) than about emotional issues of power, loss, distrust, guilt, anger, or fear of abandonment. Psychological counseling (usually involving the patient or family but sometimes involving a physician or other clinician) may defuse these emotions and, thus, the conflict.

Sometimes, ethics consultants (see discussion below of ethics committees) are brought in to help resolve conflicts through continued discussion or, at minimum, to help provide a framework for the further discussion. Sometimes discussions may focus on information and exploration of values, but they may also uncover and address issues of trust, fear, anger, or other emotions, including personality conflicts.

Consensus Building Techniques

At the request of the American College of Physicians–American Society for Internal Medicine (ACP-ASIM), three experts in adult palliative care proposed a consensus-based approach to decisionmaking for those who are unable to make decisions about their own care (Karlawish et al., 1999; see also Hoffman, 2001). The authors also offer suggestions about how to handle situations when discussion has not resulted in a consensus about the care of a patient who cannot make decisions about his or her own care. These suggestions, which should be tested further, include the following:

- postponing decisions and recommending that those involved take more time to think about and discuss concerns and goals;
- seeking interim steps such as a time-limited trial of a medical intervention rather than insisting on an all-or-nothing decision;
- continuing to identify and understand each participant's views on the goals of medical care for the patient and the care options for achieving those goals;
- bringing in a trusted third party such as an ethics or palliative consultant or religious adviser; and
- avoiding language or actions that personalize conflicts, turn decisionmaking into a power struggle, or attack the religious, cultural, or other values of the participants.

Regardless of the specifics, discussion strategies place a premium on communication skills and advance care planning as discussed in Chapter 4. Poor communication skills as well as failures of empathy and compassion are undoubtedly behind some of the disputes with parents that require interventions of the kinds discussed here. Based on the guidance developed from the ACP-ASIM, Table 8.1 presents examples of discussion steps and illustrative language that can be employed to guide discussion toward consensus. Because the original guidance focused on adult care, the text has been slightly altered. Again, further assessment of these strategies is desirable.

Discussions of the kind outlined in Table 8.1 take time, which is often in short supply as clinicians respond to health systems, hospitals, hospices, private insurers, Medicaid programs, and other state programs that are trying to control costs. Nonetheless, investments in careful initial communications with families can help limit subsequent investments in discussions

TABLE 8.1 Structuring Discussions to Reach Consensus About Care for Patients Who Lack Decision-Making Capacity

Step	Discussion Lead
1. Identify the main participants	"We need to make some decisions about the care of [child's name]. Is everyone here who could help us think through what we should do?
2. Invite the participants to narrate how the patient has reached this stage	"Can you tell me how she's changed, how things have gone for all of you?" Or "I know I've been caring for [child's name] for some time, but it helps me if you can tell me how she's changed, how things have gone for each of you."
3. Teach the decisionmakers about the expected clinical course of the patient's disease	"[Child's name] has an incurable, progressive, and ultimately fatal disease. I can't say for sure when she'll die . . . but given [the situation], we shouldn't be surprised when she does."
4. Advocate the patient's quality of life and dignity	"We ought to care for her in a way that makes us confident that after she's gone, we can say we did the best for her."
5. Provide guidance on the basis of existing data and clinical experience	"For patients like [child's name], feeding with a tube does not significantly reduce the risk for pneumonia. On the basis of my experience, a speech therapist may give us some useful hints on ways to feed her that will allow her to continue to eat by mouth."

SOURCE: Adapted from Karlawish et al., 1999, for the American College of Physicians—American Society of Internal Medicine. Used with permission.

to provide fuller information, correct misunderstandings, and defuse conflicts over goals of care. In certain situations, they may also reduce the potential for expensive litigation. Nonetheless, when capitation payments for physician services or fee-for-service payments for physician office visits are unreasonably low, as is often the case with Medicaid, and when payment policies limit or preclude payment for counseling, team conferences, and other kinds of communication, financial incentives clearly do not support the communication strategies described here and in Chapter 4. Thus, just as research, professional education, and organization structures have to support good clinical practice, so must financing policies.

Organization- or System-Level Strategies

The discussion in the preceding section focuses on the resolution of disputes at the individual level but also points to the need for organizational- and system-level responses to prevent or resolve conflicts. If distrust related to ethnic or religious differences appears to be at the heart of some disputes, are there organizational or community sources of distrust or misunderstandings that should be investigated and responded to by health care organizations and their communities? If misunderstanding of facts or terminology is a consistent problem, can training programs and protocols be created to help clinicians communicate more successfully or might public education programs be helpful?

Ethics Committees

Ethics committees and similar groups constitute a system-level effort to assist in the resolution of disputes about clinical care (see, e.g, Fletcher, 1991; AAP, 1994b, 2001d; AMA, 1984, 1994b; Dugan, 2001). They developed as hospitals struggled with the increasingly difficult questions that advances in medical technology have created. In 1983, the President's Commission endorsed the creation of hospital ethics committees. Such committees are now part of the institutional fabric of most American hospitals. The Joint Commission on the Accreditation of Healthcare Organizations (JCAHO) accepts such committees as one approach to meeting certain of its requirements, for example, having a "functioning process to address ethical issues" (JCAHO, 1998, Standard RI.1). A number of organizations have set forth guidelines for the creation, composition, and operation of ethics committees. Box 8.1 presents the recommendations of the AAP.

To a considerable degree, ethics committees have focused on articulating processes and providing consultative resources for resolving disputes without necessarily establishing guidelines or rules to address the substance of such disputes. For example, committee consultants may be useful in identifying when a persistent conflict in values may be best handled by transferring responsibility for a child's care to another physician or trying to arrange for the child's transfer to another institution. More generally, they may set forth processes for attempting to determine when a dispute is grounded in misunderstanding of facts or terminology and when it is grounded in true differences in values about the goals of care or the benefits of treatments. Box 8.2 summarizes the elements of such a process.

Ethics committees may also propose and try to develop professional consensus on institutional policies for specific issues such as DNR orders. In addition, committees usually have an educational role in teaching other

BOX 8.1
Institutional Ethics Committees (IEC): Recommendations of the American Academy of Pediatrics

1. Membership on an IEC should be diverse and reflect different perspectives within the hospital and general community.
2. An IEC should have responsibility within an institution for clinical ethics consultation, review of policies, and education of professional, administrative, and support staff about ethical issues, regardless of whether these functions are delegated to other subcommittees or programs.
3. An IEC that is engaged in clinical ethics consultations should have policies and procedures that conform to ethical principles of fairness and confidentiality.
4. An IEC should establish continuing education and training programs that ensure that IEC members are qualified to perform their specific duties within the IEC.
5. Independent ethics committees, such as an infant care review committee, should be dissolved or restructured to report to the larger IEC.
6. IECs within a general hospital setting should ensure an adequate degree of multidisciplinary expertise for addressing ethical issues specific to pediatrics.

SOURCE: AAP, 2001d.

BOX 8.2
Due Process Approach to Disputes About End-of-Life Care

1. Earnest attempts should be made in advance to deliberate over and negotiate prior understandings between patient, proxy, and physician on what constitutes futile care for the patient and what falls within acceptable limits for the physician, family, and possibly also the institution.
2. Joint decisionmaking should occur between patient or proxy and physician to the maximum extent possible.
3. Attempts should be made to negotiate disagreements if they arise and to reach resolution within all parties' acceptable limits, with the assistance of consultants as appropriate.
4. Involvement of an institutional committee such as the ethics committee should be requested if disagreements are irresolvable.
5. If the institutional review supports the patient's position and the physician remains unpersuaded, transfer of care to another physician within the institution may be arranged.
6. If the process supports the physician's position and the patient or proxy remains unpersuaded, transfer to another institution may be sought and, if done, should be supported by both the transferring and the receiving institution.
7. If transfer is not possible, the intervention need not be offered.

SOURCE: AMA, 1997, Policy E2.037.

members of the hospital community about the application of ethical concepts in clinical situations.

A number of questions have been raised about the goals of ethics committees and their ability to meet the goals set for them (see, e.g., Povar, 1991; Nelson and Shapiro, 1995; Gillon, 1997; Casarett et al., 1998; Mitchell and Truog, 2000). Some questions involve who (e.g., nurses, social workers) can bring questions to these committees. Others concern whether committees have sufficient resources and expertise to provide ethics consultations.

Questions about the independence of ethics committees have also arisen. In an environment of fiscal stress and resource restrictions, ethics committees run the risk of becoming and being perceived as partisan institutional agents (see, e.g., Kelly et al., 1997; Howe, 1999).

Draft standards for ethics consultations have been developed by a task force that included the Society for Health and Human Values, the Society for Bioethics Consultation, and several other organizations (SHHV/SBC, 1998). Research on the consequences of ethics consultations or ethics committee involvement in decisions about patient care is limited, but some studies suggest a positive role (Dowdy et al., 1998; Schneiderman et al., 2000). Further research may guide these committees by identifying individual- and system-level factors that affect family perceptions about end-of-life decisions. For example, in retrospective interviews, Abbott and colleagues (2001) found that family members identified several sources of comfort and support, including pastoral care, prior discussion of treatment preferences, and lenient visiting rules.

Protocols for Communication and Decisionmaking

Organizational- or system-level strategies for preventing and resolving conflicts take varied forms. Box 8.3 summarizes one example of an organization-level strategy to reduce clinician–family conflict in the intensive care unit (ICU) by improving teamwork and communication with families of patients nearing death. Clinicians, administrators, and ethicists developed the approach in part to reduce the potential for certain troubling ethical dilemmas and in part to reduce institutional exposure to liability based on patient or family dissatisfaction with care. An evaluation of this process is under way.

The discussion below considers two other organizational or system approaches to preventing or resolving conflicts about clinical care: research- and evidence-based practice guidelines and public policy (litigation and legislation). In addition, although individual clinicians are obligated to consider how they may improve their skills and attitudes, corresponding action at the organizational and system levels also must be considered, for ex-

---

BOX 8.3
Conflict Prevention in the ICU: One Cooperative Strategy to Reduce Conflict by Improving Care for the Critically Ill

In combination with other strategies to either prevent or manage conflicts, several adult intensive care units associated with Harvard University have been cooperating to develop and implement a strategy to reduce conflicts between clinicians and families about aggressive use of life-sustaining technologies for patients nearing death. They began with a period of intensive data collection—both personal interviews and surveys—to better understand the experience of patients and families and to identify their characteristics, concerns, and areas of dissatisfaction. Based in part on this information and on information from physicians and nurses, they then developed a four-step process to prevent conflicts.

1. "The clinical team identifies families at high risk for conflict using four criteria: expressed anger or conflict, prolonged length of stay in the ICU, absence of an identified surrogate decisionmaker, or an ICU admission triggered by an iatrogenic event.

3. The unit social worker or another clinician skilled in interpersonal communication performs a structured interview with the patient or family, focusing upon four domains: information giving and understanding, communication, conflict, and psychosocial support.

3. The social worker or other clinician meets with the clinical team on rounds the following morning and provides feedback to the team about the findings from the structured interview.

4. The clinical team develops a list of recommendations that it will pursue, based on the information received. These recommendations may range from scheduling a team meeting, to obtaining a second opinion for the patient, to obtaining formal input from the hospital ethics committee."

Other elements of the strategy include developing palliative care guidelines and developing a procedural approach to assessing when care is "futile."

SOURCE: Summarized from Truog, 2000. Quoted material used with permission.

---

ample, in the form of continuing education programs, changes in undergraduate and graduate medical education, competency testing, and funding to support these initiatives.

As discussed throughout this report, the procedures and policies of managed care organizations, insurers, and cost-conscious hospitals or other providers can contribute to conflicts and misunderstandings. System-level finance reform is essential, although it will never provide all the resources that health care professionals and families want. Some conflict over resources is inevitable.

Strengthening the Knowledge Base for Decisionmaking

Better scientific knowledge will neither prevent nor resolve all debates and disputes. For example, in the Baby K case mentioned earlier, clinical facts were not central to the mother's insistence on repeated resuscitation of her infant with anencephaly. Likewise, as discussed in Chapter 6, efforts to synthesize scientific knowledge in the form of guidelines for clinical practice are important but implementation of guidelines cannot be assumed in the face of contrary institutional, financial, and cultural influences (Rushton and Brooks-Brunn, 1997).

Nonetheless, doing good is easier when practice is guided by research demonstrating what works and what does not work to produce desired outcomes—whether those outcomes are cure for a disease or relief from suffering. Scientific research can also help defuse some controversies by challenging contradictory factual premises (explicit or implicit) on different sides of a dispute.

For example, in the United States, the 1980s saw considerable discussion of the appropriateness of correcting physical defects in newborns with significant mental retardation and other severe physical deficits. In one notable case, after parents would not approve surgical repair of a correctable defect in a child with Down syndrome and after a judicial challenge to their decision failed, politicians responded with the so-called Baby Doe regulations, toll-free telephone hotlines for people to report similar cases, and subsequent legislation to require treatment of handicapped newborns except in specified situations (see, e.g., Pless, 1983; Lantos, 1987; AMA, 1992; Weir, 1992; Caplan et al., 1992). Since this episode, research has indicated that many affected infants have a better prognosis than clinicians and parents previously assumed (Teddell et al., 1996; State et al., 1997; Amark and Sunnegardh, 1999). That is, the infants often have reasonably good prospects for many years of dependent but apparently enjoyable life.

Clinical practice guidelines or protocols represent one focused system-level strategy to create a credible, authoritative, evidence-based framework to guide individual patient care decisions (IOM, 1990a, 1992). Procedures vary in rigor and credibility, and methods for developing guidelines continue to be debated and refined. Generally, the more rigorous processes for guideline development bring together clinicians, methodologists, and sometimes consumers, ethicists, and others to define the issues at stake, identify and evaluate relevant scientific evidence or facts, and set forth statements about appropriate care that are based on an explicitly described combination of evidence, clinical judgment, and values.

Recent international guidelines on cardiopulmonary resuscitation, for example, assessed a considerable body of research that attempts to link resuscitation outcomes (e.g., survival to hospital discharge, neurological function) to patient characteristics (e.g., diagnosis, age). These guidelines note that cardiac arrest in children, unlike adults, is uncommon and is rarely a sudden event. It typically results from other than a primary cardiac cause and often is the final event associated with progressive shock or respiratory failure related to trauma, respiratory or neurological disorders, sepsis, or unexplained causes (sudden infant death syndrome [SIDS]) (AHA, 2000a). Survival is uncommon, and children who survive are often neurologically devastated. The guidelines note these dismal outcomes and urge the development of a consensus definition of when resuscitation would be futile. The guidelines mention only two specific circumstances in which not initiating resuscitation is indicated: (1) when patients have a clear advance directive asking health care workers not to begin resuscitation in the event of a cardiac arrest and (2) when patients show signs of irreversible death such as rigor mortis, decapitation, and dependent lividity or postmortem hypostasis (purple coloration from pooling of blood in dependent body areas) as agreed upon by a consensus of the medical community. The guidelines emphasize the lack of rigorous research to support many common elements of resuscitation and identify many areas for further research.

To the extent that research helps to reduce disagreement among clinicians, this will be a benefit in itself. Further, reducing disagreements among clinicians should also reduce clinician–patient or clinician–family conflicts that are stimulated or reinforced by evident variations in clinician views and practices.

Throughout this report, the limited knowledge base for much pediatric palliative and end-of-life care is documented. Chapter 10 includes recommendations and directions for research to strengthen the knowledge base for effective palliative and end-of-life care for infants, children, and adolescents. The recommendations focus on knowledge to improve clinical care, but better knowledge is also important to inform ethical and legal decisionmaking.

Litigation and Legislation

Disputes about which values should prevail in a patient's care may end up in court when other conflict resolution approaches fail and death or another outcome has not intervened to make the conflict moot. The judicial system provides a socially sanctioned process for resolving individual disputes within a framework of statutes, regulations, and case law (i.e., precedents established by prior decisions). As courts have increasingly faced disputes that involve highly technical issues, judges and policymakers have struggled with questions about the ability of judges and juries to understand and weigh scientific and technical information, often presented by experts who differ in their presentation and assessment of this information.

In general, litigation tends to be a costly, disruptive, and unpredictable vehicle for resolving conflicts that is stressful for all parties.

Statutes or administrative regulations constitute a different kind of system-level response to controversies about clinical decisionmaking. The development of statutes or regulations may or may not take scientific evidence into account and may or may not attempt to reflect or create clinical or community consensus about an area of disagreement. For example, state laws about adolescent decisionmaking "form a patchwork quilt of rights and limitations" that neither reflects nor contributes to a coherent view of adolescent capacity to make medical decisions (Oberman, 1996, p. 127).

Oregon offers an example of the rare jurisdiction that set out—not without problems and controversies—to employ careful and explicit strategy to (1) develop community consensus on priorities for medical care; (2) use clinical research and judgment to assess the relative benefits of treatments for common medical problems; (3) cover the most beneficial treatments within predetermined spending levels; and (4) expand health coverage to more people using the savings from reductions in services of marginal or no benefit (see, e.g., Bodenheimer, 1997; IOM, 1997). The priority-setting framework explicitly included comfort care (e.g., hospice, pain management) among the essential services (Cotton, 1992). Oregon's strategy has provoked continuing political, ethical, and analytic debates as well as legal challenges that have limited its application to and beyond the state's Medicaid program. State budget problems have limited the move toward universal coverage (see, e.g., Rojas-Burke, 1999). Despite, or perhaps as a result of, the attention paid to the Oregon approach, it has not been replicated by other states.

Debates about rationing care often focus on expensive versus inexpensive health care services. The real issue, however, is not the expense per unit of *service* but, rather, the expense per unit of *benefit* (for example, years of life or days free from pain). High-volume services with low unit costs are less dramatic but not necessarily less important than very expensive, low-volume services. Systems must inevitably make trade-offs among alternative ways of using available resources to benefit large groups (their members), and different systems have made different choices. Some of the implicit means of rationing potentially beneficial services rely on price or inconvenience. The next section discusses legal issues related to several kinds of disputes that can arise in the treatment of children.

LEGAL CONSIDERATIONS

Although the committee views litigation as a last resort in cases of conflict about care for children with life-threatening medical problems, situations will arise that make recourse to the courts appropriate or unavoidable. Litigation often takes a significant emotional and financial toll on all involved and can result in decisions and precedents that have unanticipated repercussions far beyond the original case. The following discussion reviews various legal issues related to decisions about medical care for children.

Parent–Physician Conflict

Parental Refusal of Treatment

As medical care becomes more complex, so do the types of legal problems arising out of parental refusals of treatment (Holder, 1983). Some refusals stem from religious convictions; for example, some Jehovah's Witness members object to blood transfusions for children as well as adults (Stanfield et al., 2000). Other refusals are based on a parental view that a child with a serious illness (such as cancer) should not be subjected to the side effects of treatment and that "alternative therapies" such as laetrile offer as much benefit as chemotherapy without the side effects (see, e.g., *Schiff* v. *Prados*, 112 Cal Rptr 2d 171, 2001; *Marshall* v. *Sackett*, 907 SW 2d 925, Tex 1995; *Green* v. *Truman*, 459 F Supp 342, DC Mass 1978; see also Faw et al., 1977; Horwitz, 1979). Some parents, who accept the fact that their child is probably dying, want to stop painful or other unpleasant treatments to prolong the child's life in an effort to provide as much peace as possible (*Gerben* v. *Holsclaw*, 692 F Supp 557, DC ED Pa 1988; see also Nealy, 1995).

Court intervention, based on the legal principle that failure to obtain adequate medical care for a child is a violation of state child neglect laws, is always an option if physicians consider it appropriate. Until recently, when a physician testified that a child would die or be permanently disabled if treatment were not provided at once, the court order would be automatic. This is not so uniformly true today, but it is still clearly the case in situations where parents refuse treatments that would likely cure or substantially modify the course of the child's illness.

Religious conviction is never a defense for a refusal to provide medical care for a child (see, e.g., In the Matter of D.R., 20 P 3d 166, Okla Civil Appeals, 2001; *Hoang* v. *State*, 250 Ga App 403, 2001; AAP 1997d). For example, if a 3-year-old child of a Jehovah's Witness is in an automobile accident, needs a blood transfusion to which the parents object, and is expected to recover completely, a court order would be issued in any court in the country (*Jehovah's Witnesses of Washington* v. *King County Hospital*, 390 US 598, 1968). Similarly, if a child had acute appendicitis but his parents refused to consent to any medical care at all, a court order would be issued. When the need for life-saving treatment is urgent, a physician or hospital that provides such treatment without a court order and over parental objection will not be liable, as long as it is clear that there was no time to apply for and receive a court order (*HCA, Inc.* v. *Miller*, 36 SW 3d 187, Tex App 2000).

Failure to provide medical care to a child can be prosecuted as a criminal offense. Convictions of manslaughter and even murder (*Commonwealth of Pennsylvania* v. *Nixon*, 2000, 563 Pa 425, 761 A 2d 1151, 2000; *Commonwealth of Pennsylvania* v. *Barnhart*, 345 Pa Super 10, 497 A 2d 616, 1985) have been upheld when a child died without medical care. In these cases, the state must prove by "substantial medical evidence" that the illness or accident would not normally have been fatal if the child had been treated with usual and appropriate interventions.

When cure for a child's medical problem is unlikely or impossible, however, courts have been increasingly willing to allow parents to make decisions based on their subjective analyses of risks and benefits (*Newark* v. *Williams*, 588 A 2d 1108, Del 1991; *In the Matter of Matthews*, 225 A.D. 2d 142, 650 NYS 2d 373, 1996). If another physician can be found who agrees with the parents and testifies that she or he will assume responsibility for the care of the child after the original physicians declined to follow the parents' wishes, all courts will permit parents to remove their child to the other physician, even if the original physicians are convinced that the new physician's therapies are outside any accepted medical standard (*In re Hofbauer*, 47 NYS 2d 648, 419 NYS 2d 936, 393 NE 2d 1009, 1979). If a child's life is not *immediately* threatened, even if the underlying condition is desperately serious, most courts' longstanding practice is to refuse to order that high-risk therapies be given over parental objection (*In re Hudson*, 1955, 13 Wash 2d 673, 126 P 2d 765, 1942; *In re Seiferth*, 309 NY 80, 127 NE 2d 820, 1955).

It is one thing to treat a child in the hospital under court order when the child will then leave the hospital to return to normal life at home. It is quite another to obtain a court order to administer chemotherapy or other treatment over parental objections when the parents' cooperation is required to bring the child for continuing outpatient services. If their objections are sufficiently adamant, they can leave the state with the child (*In re Chad Green [In re: Custody of a Minor]*, 379 NE 2d 1053, 393 NE 2d 836, 1979). This raises the prospect that if a court order is obtained, the child will have to be either hospitalized during the entire period or removed under court order from his parents and placed in foster care. To inflict this on a family and a child at a time of suffering and perhaps impending death is something that should be considered only under the most extraordinary circumstances and when there are strong reasons to believe that the achievable goal is long-term remission or a potential cure.

In sum, a physician confronted with parents who, for whatever reason, are "uncooperative" may assume correctly that she or he can get a court order to treat the child. The ultimate question is whether such a step will, on balance, benefit the child. In many situations, it will not.

Parental Insistence on Treatment

The converse physician–parent conflict arises when the physician feels that further aggressive life-prolonging interventions for a dying child are futile or will cause suffering in excess of any potential benefit and the parents refuse to accept that decision (Paris et al., 1990). Some but not all of these conflicts arise when parents, for religious or other reasons, will not accept the concept of brain death.

If a patient (child or adult) is, by standard medical criteria, brain dead (see Chapter 1), no permission is required to pronounce the patient dead (see, e.g., *Lovato* v. *District Court*, 198 Colo 419, 601 P 2d 1072, 1979; *Alvarado by Alvarado* v. *New York City Health and Hospitals Corporation*, 145 Misc 2d 687, 547 NYS 2d 190, 1989). Even if the family objects, the physician may sign the death certificate and then remove the respirator (thus demonstrating that the patient was dead *before* life support was removed) (see, e.g., *Law* v. *Camp*, 116 F Supp 2d 295, 2000, 2001 WL 868354, CCA 2, July 27, 2001).

In some circumstances, however, physicians may find it advisable to obtain a court order before terminating life support over parental objections. One of these circumstances is when the child's condition is or may be the result of abuse inflicted by the parent (In re L.H.R., 253 Ga 439, 321 SE 2d 716, 1984; In re M.D., 758 A 2d 27, DC CA 2000.). When a parent will face a murder or manslaughter charge as soon as the child is pronounced dead, he or she will almost never consent to withdrawal of life support (AAP, 2000e). Since the circumstance of pronouncing the child dead will be the major issue in the parent's trial, it is important to have a clear record of the circumstances, including a judge's order to terminate life support—even if the child meets all criteria for brain death (*Truselo* v. *Carroll*, 2000 WL 33324536, Del Fam Ct 2000; In re Tabatha v. Ronda R., 252 Neb 687, 564 NW 2d 598, 252 Neb 864, 566 NW 2d 782, 255 Neb 818, 587 NW 2d 1909, 1998; In re Haymer, 115 Ill App 3d 349, 450 NE 2d 940, 1983; see also Massie, 1993; Fleming, 1999).

In most litigation involving parental insistence on treatment, however, the child is not brain dead but is in a persistent vegetative state. The physician feels that in the absence of any hope of recovery, continued maintenance of the patient on life support is a mistake. In contrast, the parents are simply thankful their child is "not dead" and refuse to allow termination of life support (see, e.g., *Velez v. Bethune*, 219 Ga App 679, 466 SE 32d 627, 1995; Moore, 1995). Even if they agree with the physician's judgment that there is no hope of improvement, they may take the position that if the child is not dead, he or she is still alive and should be treated. In one recent case (*Burks v. St. Joseph's Hospital*, 227 Wisc 2d 811, 596 NW 2d 391, 1999), a woman delivered a baby at 22 weeks of pregnancy. She was told (as she would be in virtually all hospitals in the country) that her 7 ounce daughter, even though she was breathing at birth, had no hope of survival. Although she asked that the baby be taken to the Newborn Special Care Unit, she was told that extensive efforts at resuscitation were inappropriate, and the baby died $2^1/_2$ hours later. She sued the hospital and the court held that she had a right to pursue the claim. Whether she will win and recover damages has not yet been determined.

The best known of case of this type was the case of Baby K, which has already been mentioned (In re Baby K., 16 F 3d 590, CCA 4, 1994; see also, In the Matter of Infant C., 1995 WL 1058596, Va. Cir November 17, 1995). Baby K was anencephalic but, for reasons still unclear, was put on a respirator in the delivery room. Her mother refused to permit a DNR order or removal of the respirator. She firmly believed that God would heal her child. Baby K was eventually discharged to a nursing facility that accepted babies. She was readmitted to the hospital several times for treatment of respiratory distress. Finally the hospital asked for an order from the court stating that it did not have to provide extraordinary medical treatment to this hopeless case. The court found that the federal Emergency Treatment and Active Labor Act, which requires any hospital to provide essential care to emergency admissions, applied to Baby K and the hospital could not refuse to treat her in the emergency department. The trial judge's decision was upheld when the hospital appealed to the United States Court of Appeals for the Fourth Circuit. Baby K finally died in the pediatric nursing home at age 14 months, still on full life support (Fletcher, 1997).

Thus, it is increasingly clear that before a physician may terminate life support on any patient, adult to newborn, when the parent or next of kin objects, she or he should assume that it is necessary to ask a court for an order. Refusal of such a request should not, however, come as a particular surprise (Massie, 1993). An ethics committee consultation may help mediate the issues and might persuade the parents to change their minds, particularly if the basic problem is the parents' lack of trust in the physician. Nonetheless, the findings of an ethics committee have no legal standing and cannot be used alone as the basis for termination of life support.

Parent–Child Conflict

Based on their experience, many physicians recognize that even very small children know when they are very sick. As discussed in Chapter 4, they are often far more aware of death than adults may realize.

Medical and nursing care of seriously ill children includes helping them to achieve a developmentally appropriate understanding of their illness and making sure that they know what to expect from tests and treatments. Their views should be taken seriously, but these views may or may not be the deciding factor in therapeutic decisionmaking.[15]

Preadolescent children are rarely, if ever, asked if they want the medical care their physician and parents decide is best for them. No one asks a 6-year-old if he wants an injection. He is told that he is going to get one and what it will feel like. (A child can still be offered choices such as which arm to use and can still be advised on what he or she can do to make it hurt less.)

For adolescents, the picture is more complicated. Under English common law, a minor was emancipated if he (not she) was a young man who was not subject to parental control or regulation. In all aspects of his life, he was considered to be a legal adult and could buy and sell property, sign contracts, get married, or do anything else adults could do.[16] The American legal system adopted the concept. In twenty-first century America, an emancipated minor is one who is married, is in the military (a much less frequent occurrence than it was when the age of majority was 21 instead of 18), or is self-supporting and living away from home. If a minor's marriage is dissolved, he or she remains emancipated. In addition to these categories of emancipated minors, many states have enacted statutes providing other contexts in which a minor (with or without a court order) is emancipated and, thus, whose parents have no further legal responsibilities for him or her.

---

[15] In distinguishing legal consent to treatment from a child's assent, the American Academy of Pediatrics (1995a, online, no page number) described the process of securing assent (consistent with the child's stage of development) as including at least these elements: "(1) helping the patient achieve a developmentally appropriate awareness of the nature of his or her condition; (2) telling the patient what he or she can expect with tests and treatment(s); (3) making a clinical assessment of the patient's understanding of the situation and the factors influencing how he or she is responding (including whether there is inappropriate pressure to accept testing or therapy); and (4) soliciting an expression of the patient's willingness to accept the proposed care." The AAP noted with respect to the last point that if, in fact, "the patient will have to receive medical care despite his or her objection, the patient should be told that fact and should not be deceived."

[16] At the time, women of any age could not own property or sign contracts, so there was no reason to consider emancipation for girls.

Adolescents now are being allowed to make decisions about their own medical care and other areas of their lives at a level that would have been astonishing 50 years ago (Holder, 1987; *Caldwell* v. *Bechtol,* 724 SW 2d 739, Tenn 1987; AAP, 1995a; Hartman et al., 2000). Beginning about 1950 with the epidemic of venereal diseases in adolescents, physicians realized that if a teenager knew that his or her parents would be contacted to provide consent for treatment, thus discovering what their son or daughter had been doing, the adolescent would forgo treatment, thus spreading the problem. As a result of physician influence, by the mid-1960s all states had enacted legislation permitting minors to be treated for venereal disease without parental notification, and today almost all states have similar laws allowing confidential treatment for drug and alcohol problems. At the time, some states began enacting minor treatment statutes giving a minor of a specified age (usually 16, but in some states as young as 14) the right to consent to any medical treatment on his or her own without parental consent.

Even in the absence of state statutes allowing minors to consent to treatment, it has been more than 40 years since a court awarded damages to parents against a physician who treated a child without their consent, as long as the adolescent patient gave a knowledgeable consent to the procedure. These court rulings have become known as the "mature minor" rule. The standard accepted by courts in virtually all states is that if a young person (14, 15, or older) understands the nature of the proposed treatment and its risks and expected benefits as well as an adult could, he or she may give consent. The maturity of the particular adolescent and the gravity of the illness must be factored into the assessment.

One might assume that if a patient may consent to treatment, then that patient may also refuse it. In fact, it is very unusual for a court in this country to allow an adolescent to refuse treatment that is clearly necessary (e.g., an appendectomy) even if it is not incontrovertibly life saving (see, e.g., Rosato, 1996; Skeels, 1990; Lonowski, 1995; Bidari, 1996; Penkower, 1996; Derish et al., 2000). In a few cases, all of which involve adolescent Jehovah's Witnesses and their refusal of blood transfusions, courts allowed adolescent patients to refuse transfusion based on a demonstration that they understood the nature of the illness, could articulate their own religious objections to the blood transfusion (i.e., were not merely reflecting parental pressure), and understood quite clearly the permanence of death. In at least one case involving a 16-year-old with leukemia, the child died (In re E.G., 133 Ill 2nd 98, 549 NE 2d 322, 1989; *Belcher* v. *Charleston Area Medical Center,* 188 W. Va 105, 422 SE 2d 827, 1992; Traugott and Alpers, 1997). Many more cases, however, have held in identical or similar circumstances that while the right to refuse treatment is available for any mentally competent adult, no such right exists for minors (*Novak* v. *Cobb*

County—Kennestone Hospital Authority, 849 F Supp 1559, DC Ga, 74 F 3d 1173, CCA 11 1996).

Except for West Virginia, states do not permit a minor, even if legally emancipated, to create a legally enforceable living will, durable power of attorney, or other statement that he or she would want treatment stopped in case of serious illness or accident (Hawkins, 1992).[17] This does not mean that the physician should neglect to find out what the child's views on continuing treatment may be if the long-term prognosis is not good (AAP, 2000g). Those views should still be taken into account when decisions are made (In re Chad Swan, 569 A 2d 1202, Maine 1990).

When parents and an adolescent patient disagree, the physician is the patient's, not the family's, advocate. If the prognosis is poor and the patient has "had enough," the physician is professionally obligated to do everything she or he can to persuade the parents to let the child's views control. Therapies that the physician considers inadvisable may not be required by distraught parents. On the other hand, if the prognosis is good but the patient does not want to continue therapy, the physician's responsibility is to understand and respond to the child's fears and help her or him through the treatment.

Parent–Parent Conflict

Although there may be instances in which parents are bitterly divided on the wisdom of continuing life-sustaining treatment for a child who is likely to die, the committee located only one case on the question. A terminally ill 13-year-old girl was in a coma. Her mother agreed with her physicians that a DNR order was the appropriate next step. Her father adamantly disagreed and wanted her treated as aggressively as possible. The hospital turned to the court for guidance, and the trial court and state supreme court each held that both parents had to agree before a DNR order could be written (In Re Jane Doe, 262 Ga 389, 418 SE 2d 3, 1992).

In cases of this sort, the parent who wishes the child to continue "living" is likely to be upheld by a court. If the parents are divorced, the legal custodian is likely to prevail in such a conflict (*Durfee* v. *Durfee,* 87 NYS 2d 275 NY 1949).

---

[17]In 2000, West Virginia passed the Health Care Decisions Act (Annotated Code of West Virginia, Chapter 16, Article 30, Section 3(b)), which defines an adult, for purposes of health care decisionmaking including advance directives, as "a person who is eighteen years of age or older, an emancipated minor who has been established as such pursuant to [other laws], or a mature minor." A mature minor is "a person less than eighteen years of age who has been determined by a qualified physician, a qualified psychologist or an advanced practice nurse in collaboration with a physician to have the capacity to make health care decisions."

Children Who Are Wards of the State

State officials must approve medical care provided to children who are wards of the state, for example, children in foster care or correctional facilities. State officials and policies, which are not always in writing, determine whether health care providers can obtain consent for measures such as DNR orders or removal of mechanical ventilators. Although committee members had considerable experience with state refusals to grant consent for such measures, written information on policies and their application is very limited. This leaves physicians in a difficult position and potentially encourages substandard care and preventable suffering.

The Newborn with a Correctable Defect or Extreme Prematurity

The care of newborns with severe handicaps or extreme prematurity became a political issue during the 1980s following the well-publicized case of a baby with Down syndrome and a tracheoesophageal fistula who died because his parents refused to consent to surgery. An anonymous person tried to get a court to order surgery, but the local juvenile court held that the baby's parents had the right to make the decision. The Indiana Supreme Court concurred, and the baby died while an appeal to the United States Supreme Court was being sought.

The Department of Health and Human Services (HHS) then issued regulations requiring treatment of all handicapped infants except those who would inevitably die of their irreparable conditions (Shapiro, 1984). These regulations applied only to children with birth defects who had not yet had their first birthday. They did not apply, for example, to a healthy newborn severely injured in an automobile accident on the way home from the hospital or to a 13-month-old child with birth defects. The regulations were struck down, republished, and finally declared unconstitutional by the United States Supreme Court in 1986 (*Bowen* v. *American Hospital Association*, 476 US 610, 1986). In the meantime, however, the American Academy of Pediatrics and HHS reached agreement on regulations requiring any state seeking federal funds for child abuse programs to agree to enact state regulations to require that handicapped infants be treated except in certain specific circumstances. Those circumstances are that the infant was irreversibly comatose, the treatment would be "inhumane," the treatment would be "futile," or the provision of treatment would merely prolong the infant's dying (Child Abuse Amendments of 1984, P.L. 98-457).

Since the 1980s, the federal government has not intervened on behalf of any allegedly neglected newborn. As was the case before the "Baby Doe" regulations, state courts have dealt with conflicts arising when physicians wish to override a parent's decision to withdraw a treatment from a baby

(Stahlman, 1990). The federal investigations and rules may have, at least for a while, made neonatologists more fearful of forgoing life-sustaining interventions that they truly believed to be unwise (Kopelman et al., 1988).

CONCLUSION

High-profile litigation, regulations, and legislation about decisions at the end of life are uncommon but may create anxiety and fear among clinicians that have the potential to distort the way physicians inform and counsel patients and families (see, e.g., Kopelman et al., 1988). Some of this anxiety and fear is based on misunderstandings of statutes, regulations, and judicial decisions, although some may also be based on excessive caution on the part of hospital or other legal counsel and management. Efforts by professional societies, health professions educators, and organizations to improve end-of-life care may help correct erroneous views and overcome undue caution. These groups may also help to promote wider discussion and evaluation of strategies for preventing, resolving, and managing conflicts about care for dying patients.

Not all conflicts can be avoided, but they can be handled in ways that increase or decrease the potential for damage to the involved parties. Strategies include developing evidence- and consensus-based guidelines for care, improving communication skills, fostering sensitivity to cultural differences, and developing organizational procedures for identifying and defusing potential conflicts and promoting trust. Although the emphasis of these strategies will often be on physicians and parents as decisionmakers, as recommended in Chapter 4, children should be involved in discussions about their care consistent with each child's intellectual and emotional maturity and preferences and with sensitivity to family cultural background and values.

The next chapter discusses directions for improving health professions education in palliative, end-of-life, and bereavement care. It notes that education in these issues is often restricted to ethical concerns and argues that competence in palliative and end-of-life care cannot be achieved without guided clinical experience and training that is backed by a good understanding of available scientific evidence.

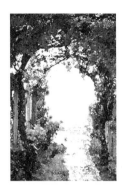

CHAPTER 9

EDUCATING HEALTH
CARE PROFESSIONALS

*The medical student population is probably the one that on a
daily basis, offends parents the most. . . . I have been vocal with
residents, like this person needs 101 in how to work with a parent.
. . . But there is no real formal process set up for that feedback.*
Tina Heyl-Martineau, parent, 2001

Whether the issue is insensitivity to feelings and emotions, inattention
to pain and other symptoms, or inadequate information, children and families suffer when they encounter pediatricians and other professionals who
are ill-prepared to offer them competent, consistent, and compassionate
palliative, end-of-life, and bereavement care. Although education alone cannot ensure such care, undergraduate, graduate, and continuing health professions education is necessary to provide an essential foundation of scientific knowledge, ethical understanding, and technical and interpersonal
skills.

Even for medical conditions that are invariably or often fatal, the focus
of classroom lectures, clinical rotations, and textbooks is almost exclusively
on the pathophysiology of disease and the conventional or experimental
interventions that might prolong life—often with little regard for the likelihood of success and with little attention to the burdens experienced by
dying patients and their families. In one recent survey of pediatric
oncologists, respondents reported that the most common way they learned
about end-of-life care was "trial and error" (Hilden et al., 2001a). Although a substantial fraction of children diagnosed with cancer die, only 10
percent of the pediatric oncologists reported having taken a formal course

in end-of-life care, and only 2 percent reported a rotation in a palliative care or hospice service. Unstructured and unguided learning by experience puts patients and families at risk of much preventable suffering.

Most efforts to improve education in palliative, end-of-life, and bereavement care, not surprisingly, have emphasized older adults. Recently, however, several educational initiatives have focused on children who die and their families. For example, a new text on palliative nursing includes chapters on pediatric care (Ferrell and Coyle, 2001), and succeeding editions of the major text on palliative medicine have been enriched by discussions of care for children who die (Doyle et al., 1998). A recent manual on palliative medicine for psychiatrists also includes chapters on pediatric care (Chochinov and Breitbart, 2000). A series of self-study programs developed by the American Academy of Hospice and Palliative Medicine will include a monograph on pediatric care. The National Hospice and Palliative Care Organization and the Children's International Project on Palliative/Hospice Services are also developing educational materials.

The 1997 Institute of Medicine (IOM) report on end-of life care included an extensive examination of health professions education. This chapter draws on that discussion, much of which applies generally to the education of pediatricians and other professionals who care for children who die and their families. It also draws on other pediatric-specific sources, including Appendix G. The rest of this chapter considers

- basic elements of competence-building education in pediatric palliative and end-of-life care,
- deficiencies in current professional education in palliative and end-of-life care,
- responses to those deficiencies, and
- directions for further changes in health professions education.

The committee recognizes that educational reforms, albeit a commonly urged strategy for changing clinicians' attitudes and practices, are often difficult to achieve and that documentation of their success (especially over the long-term) in achieving desired objectives is often sparse. If the rewards for clinicians—financial, professional, and organizational—are not supportive of these objectives, then educational changes may be more symbolic than consequential. Educational reform is certainly not "the" solution to deficits in palliative and end-of-life care and might sometimes distract from the pursuit of other, potentially more important changes. Nonetheless, the objectives and information emphasized in health professions education are important symbols of what the professions should value. Educational reforms—and persistence in seeking and evaluating such reform—are one necessary element in a comprehensive strategy for improving palliative, end-of-life, and bereavement care as outlined elsewhere in this report.

BASICS OF HEALTH PROFESSIONS EDUCATION FOR PEDIATRIC PALLIATIVE AND END-OF-LIFE CARE

The committee believes that educational strategies to improve palliative and end-of-life care should begin with the early stages of a health professional's education, intensify and gain focus during more specialized training, and then provide reinforcement and updating as needed through-out a professional's career. At each stage, the aim should be, in individual terms, to produce the foundation of knowledge, skill, and attitudes appropriate to a professional's or future professional's role in the health care system and, in social terms, to generate a sufficient level and range of medical, nursing, and other expertise to meet diverse patient and family needs. Thus, educational strategies should include elements suitable for

- beginning students of medicine, nursing, social work, and other fields;
- medical residents in different specialties and fellows in different subspecialties;
- psychologists, social workers, and others in relevant graduate or advanced study programs;
- practicing generalist and specialist professionals in hospitals, hospices, and other settings; and
- paramedics, law enforcement personnel, staff of medical examiners' offices, and others who respond to sudden or traumatic deaths or are involved with survivors of such deaths.

In pediatric medicine, even though a general pediatrician will usually refer children with life-threatening medical problems to specialists, he or she may continue to care for the child, for example, after a disease-related treatment regimen concludes or after a child returns home following treatment at a distant center. He or she may also care for the child's siblings and, generally, may be a trusted resource for a family even after a child has been referred or died. Undergraduate and graduate medical education should prepare general pediatricians for these roles. Clinicians who specialize in pediatric critical care or oncology should be more intensively prepared for their extensive involvement with seriously ill or injured children and their families.

Because the number of child deaths is very small compared to the number of adult deaths, attention to end-of-life issues in pediatric education may seem peripheral to some, especially given the competition for time in the medical curriculum. This committee acknowledges the pressures on educators to add a long list of new topics—ranging from attention-deficit and hyperactivity disorder to the ethics of genetic screening—to an already crowded curriculum. It believes, however, that strengthening education in end-of-life care will not impose an undue burden. As argued by an earlier group (IOM, 1997, p. 212):

> First, palliative care is not a special interest issue; its principles of whole-patient care and teamwork provide a model for many other areas. Second, curriculum change need not be just an expensive addition but can also be an enrichment of established educational content and formats. Third, the use of existing program models and sharing of information can reduce the curriculum development burden on any single school. Fourth, the need to look beyond the hospital setting for educational opportunities is not unique to end-of-life care, but can be considered as part of a more general effort to develop non-hospital arrangements for improved training in primary care, chronic care, and outpatient care.

Moreover, many of the concepts, principles, and research findings that guide education for professionals who care for adults are broadly relevant to the education of those who care for children and their families. Some adaptations in educational goals and content will, however, be necessary to reflect the special needs of infants, children, and adolescents with life-threatening illnesses. For example, education in pain assessment, prevention, and management will have to consider the particular challenges of assessing symptoms in infants and preverbal children and in prescribing analgesic medications given the frequent lack of research-based information on doses for children at different developmental stages.

The development of a group of specialists in pediatric palliative care clearly has begun, often with support from the larger group of palliative care specialists who focus on adult care. These pediatric palliative care specialists are already helping to focus the attention of other clinicians, educators, professional societies, research funders, managers, and policymakers on strengthening educational and organizational resources for pediatric palliative care and enlarging the scientific foundation for that care. Consistent with the 1997 IOM report, this committee strongly supports the continued evolution of palliative care "as a defined and accepted area of teaching, research, and patient care expertise" (IOM, 1997, p.227).

At any level, professional competence has intellectual, interpersonal, and moral elements (Papadatou, 1997; Epstein and Hundert, 2002). It evolves as a professional accumulates training and experience and develops the capacity to integrate knowledge and awareness gained in varied clinical, organizational, and social contexts. Box 9.1 lists a set of basic competencies in four areas: (1) scientific and clinical knowledge; (2) interpersonal and other skills; (3) ethical and professional principles of care; and (4) organiza-

BOX 9.1
Preparing Health Care Professionals to Provide Palliative, End-of-Life, and Bereavement Care to Children and Families

Scientific and clinical knowledge and skills, including the following:

- Learning the biological mechanisms of end-stage medical conditions as manifested in infants, children, and adolescents
- Understanding the pathophysiology of pain and other physical and emotional symptoms as it interacts with children's physiologic development and medical condition
- Developing appropriate expertise and skill in the pharmacology of symptom management in children, taking advantage of advances in pediatric drug research and labeling
- Acquiring appropriate knowledge and skill in nonpharmacological symptom management, including complementary and alternative medicine and behavioral strategies
- Understanding the tools for assessing patient symptoms, status, quality of life, and prognosis that have been developed or adapted for children at different developmental stages
- Recognizing when consultation with palliative care specialists is appropriate
- Understanding the epidemiology of death in childhood
- Learning clinical indications for and limits of life-sustaining treatments

Interpersonal skills and attitudes, including the following:

- Listening to child patients, families, and other members of the health care team
- Conveying difficult news to children and their families
- Providing clear, timely, relevant information and guidance on prognosis and options
- Understanding and managing child and family responses to a child's life-threatening illness, including anticipatory grief and bereavement
- Sharing goal setting and decisionmaking with the care team, including family members

tional skills to help patients and families navigate the health care system. In general, the list is oriented toward pediatricians as those most broadly accountable for patient and family care. Given the range of professionals involved and skills needed, no single set of competencies in pediatric palliative and end-of-life care can comprehend all relevant issues.

Beyond the basics, education must prepare clinicians who specialize in care for children with life-threatening medical problems for the special clinical, psychological, and other challenges of such care. These challenges, in particular, include the risk of "burnout" and other emotional problems

- Developing skills in avoiding and resolving conflicts involving patients, family members, and other members of the health care team
- Cultivating empathy, compassion, humility, and altruism
- Developing sensitivity to religious, cultural, and other differences among children and families and among professionals and relevant others
- Recognizing and understanding one's own feelings and anxieties about the death of a child

Ethical and professional principles, including the following:

- Acting as a role model of clinical proficiency, integrity, and compassion
- Determining and respecting child and family preferences, taking into account children's stage of development and legal requirements
- Learning principles of pediatric palliative and end-of-life care, including advance care planning
- Understanding societal and population interests and resources
- Balancing competing objectives or principles
- Being alert to personal and organizational conflicts of interests

Organizational knowledge and skills, including the following:

- Developing and sustaining effective professional teamwork
- Identifying and mobilizing supportive resources (e.g., hospice, school, and other community-based assistance), including resources for children with special health care needs
- Understanding and managing relevant rules and procedures set by health care organizations, insurers, and government units (e.g., medical examiner's office, social welfare agencies)
- Protecting children and their families from harmful rules and procedures
- Assessing and managing care options, settings, and transitions
- Making effective use of existing financial resources and cultivating new funding sources

SOURCE: Adapted from IOM, 1997, with additional information from Appendix G.

that may arise after intensive, day-to-day care of children who die and their families.

Hospices, in particular, have recognized the need for strategies to help professionals cope with the stresses of end-of-life care (see, e.g., Harper, 1977, 1993; Dean, 1998; Sumner, 2001). Some of their strategies focus on organizational policies and environments (e.g., assigning shared responsibility for care, ensuring emotional support and empathy from administrative staff and coworkers). Other strategies emphasize coping mechanisms as part of initial training and continuing education programs.

CURRENT STATUS OF PROFESSIONAL PREPARATION IN PALLIATIVE AND END-OF-LIFE CARE FOR CHILDREN AND THEIR FAMILIES

Despite an increasing list of educational programs that incorporate or focus on palliative and end-of-life care, surveys and other assessments continue to reveal shortfalls in the preparation of health professionals to care for adults and children who die and their families. These shortfalls characterize undergraduate, graduate, and continuing education. Most assessments have focused on physician education, but nursing and social work education appears to show a similar pattern of inattention.

The major—and not unexpected—exception to the pattern of inattention involves on-the-job and continuing education for the many different professionals who provide hospice care. Hospices also offer training both for volunteers and for family members who provide physical care to dying loved ones.

Undergraduate Medical Education

After discussing this . . . [the attending physician] casually told the intern and myself to tell the patient she had end-stage cancer, that we would be doing tests to find the source, and that was all we could do for her. I could not believe it. Finally I understood the difference between knowing and understanding.

Fourth-year medical student (Wear, 2002, p. 272)

This period in the education of physicians involves profound processes of professional socialization that affect attitudes and practices throughout their professional life. By the time medical students end their fourth year, they will have been directly involved with hospitalized patients, typically with little preparation for the interpersonal aspects of caring for gravely ill individuals and their families. One educator's survey of fourth-year medical students suggested that students sometimes became involved with dying patients as a result of an attending or resident physician's discomfort or lack of concern. The disbelieving student quoted above offered one example of such involvement. Another student reported that he felt his inept and unguided effort to discuss a patient's preferences for resuscitation "doomed" the patient to a terrible, prolonged death. Although students knew that textbooks and lectures could not substitute for direct involvement with real patients, this kind of "sink-or-swim" experience was deeply troubling and not constructive (Wear, 2002). The discussion below has to be understood in this context. (For other personal accounts, see the physician narratives published by the American Board of Internal Medicine [ABIM, 1996b].)

One review of the literature on training for end-of-life care in medical education from 1980 to 1995 concluded that even though most medical schools appeared to include some formal instruction in the topic, "there is considerable evidence that current training is inadequate, most strikingly in the clinical years" (Billings and Block, 1997; see also Barnard et al., 1999). Several subsequent surveys have documented continued deficiencies in medical school and residency programs.

For example, results from the 1997–1998 survey of medical schools by the Liaison Committee on Medical Education (LCME) indicated that one-third of the schools reported no required instruction in at least one of three key topics (death and dying, pain management, palliative care), and half offered no elective courses related to end-of-life issues (Barzansky et al., 1999).[1] Most schools reported that they covered these issues in their basic curriculum. Only 4 of 125 medical schools reported that a course in death and dying was required. The next LCME survey (1998–1999) indicated that one-fifth of medical schools required no experience in home hospice or inpatient palliative care, and one-fifth did not even provide the opportunity for such experience on an elective basis (Barzansky et al., 1999). In principle, students could seek some experience through volunteer activities, for example, with children's hospitals, hospices, or camps for children with advanced illness, but only the most aware and dedicated are likely to do so. Another challenge in medical education is that students in their last undergraduate year often are already thinking about specialization.

The LCME surveys give only the most general picture of medical school instruction in end-of-life care. Coverage of end-of-life issues in the basic curriculum might involve no more than a single lecture or a set of readings. The lecture or readings might or might not reflect the clinical, professional, and other principles of palliative and end-of-life care endorsed in this and similar reports. As discussed further below, many opportunities exist to use end-of-life care or questions to illustrate more general themes related to compassion, humanism, ethics, patient- and family-centered care, behavioral interventions, and many other topics. Such an effort to diffuse palliative and end-of-life topics more broadly in the curriculum would, however, take creativity and persistence.

---

[1]The LCME, which is supported by the American Medical Association and the American Association of Medical Colleges, accredits medical schools.

Graduate Medical Education

Results from the American Medical Association's (AMA's) 1997–1998 survey of residency programs showed considerable variability in their attention to end-of-life issues, not unexpected given the difference in clinical focus of various specialties (Barzansky et al., 1999). Almost all critical care residency programs reported some kind of structured curriculum in end-of-life care as did more than 90 percent of programs in family practice and internal medicine. Percentages were lower—between 60 and 70 percent—for programs in pediatrics, obstetrics–gynecology, psychiatry, and surgery. A more recent review by Weissman and Block (2002) reported that most surgical residency requirements were limited to ethics. For the 46 specialties reviewed, the most common requirements related to ethics (25 specialties) and psychosocial care (22). Only five mentioned clinical experiences.

In Appendix G, Himelstein and Kane report on a recent survey of pediatric residency program directors and pediatric residents in training. In contrast to the routine annual surveys by the LCME and AMA, this survey generated a low response rate from program directors (22 percent) and residents (42 percent), so the results may not be generalizable. Although 62 percent of respondents reported that their residents were involved in end-of-life situations, only 42 percent indicated that their residents received direct education in palliative care. Only one program director reported that hospice care was a scheduled resident rotation, and one-quarter of respondents thought that their program included no experts in palliative care. Virtually all responding residents in training indicated that they had been involved in end-of-life care for at least one child, and 86 percent said that they had been actively involved. Active involvement by a resident does not necessarily mean that his or her performance was guided or assessed. An earlier survey of medical residents found that one-third said that they had never been observed in a discussion with a patient about a do-not-resuscitate (DNR) order and most had only been observed once or twice (Tulsky et al., 1996).

As noted elsewhere, arranging clinical experiences involves a number of challenges (IOM, 1997). One is to provide adequate oversight, guidance, and feedback and thereby limit experiences that are little more than unstructured observation of clinicians and unguided interactions with patients. Maintaining such oversight and guidance is especially difficult as clinical experiences increase and trainees move into the community.

Nursing, Social Work, and Other Professionals

The committee located no detailed assessment of the inclusion of palliative care or end-of-life content in nursing, social work, or other health professions curricula. The American Association for Collegiate Nursing has concluded that "end-of-life education and training is inconsistent at best and sometimes completely neglected within nursing curricula" (AACN, 1998). The American Psychological Association similarly concluded that no systematic efforts have been undertaken to educate psychologists about end-of-life issues. The organization now encourages psychologists to obtain training in ethics as applied to end-of-life decisions and care and endorses "psychologists' acquisition of competencies with respect to end-of-life issues, including mastery of the literature on dying and death and sensitivity to diversity dimensions that affect end-of-life experiences" (APA, 2001a, no page).

Based on their review of program requirements, Himelstein and Kane (Appendix G) identified no structured training in palliative care or end-of-life care for clinical social workers. In general, however, educational requirements for social work are supportive of the approach to palliative and end-of-life care presented in this report. With private foundation funding, several social work educators are developing educational materials and programs to strengthen social workers' formal preparation to support people who are dying and to assist their families (PDIA, 2001a,b).

Various groups, including individual religious organizations, set standards for ministers, priests, rabbis, and others involved in pastoral care. As generally described in Appendix G, these requirements focus on knowledge, attitudes, and behaviors that are consistent with the principles of palliative care, but the committee located no formal assessments of these requirements, their implementation, or their effectiveness.

Professionals with varied backgrounds provide bereavement care, and the field is still evolving. Several organizations offer training and certification, but as yet, no generally accepted national standards for training exist. The National Hospice and Palliative Care Organization (specifically, its section for bereavement professionals) is collaborating with the National Council of Hospice and Palliative Professionals to develop guidelines for hospice bereavement care. The guidelines are expected to discuss, among other topics, education for bereavement care providers (Personal communication cited in Appendix G from Barbara Bouton, Bridges Center, Louisville, Kentucky).

In addition to training their own new and established staff, many hospices have education programs for community health care providers. Some hospices offer rotations or other experiences for medical students and other health professionals in training. For example, in a recent survey of approximately 4,000 hospices, about 10 percent reported training for pharmacists, who can be a valuable resource for professionals treating adults and children with symptoms of advanced disease (Herndon et al., 2001).

Appendix G lists the organizations responsible for setting accreditation, licensure, and similar standards for other professionals including social workers, child-life specialists, and clergy. It also reports what the authors found on organizational Web sites and through personal conversations regarding inclusion of material about palliative and end-of-life care, including care for children. For the most part, coverage was slight to nonexistent. An in-depth survey might uncover more, but the committee suspects that the basic conclusion would be the same: most educational programs and resources ignore the end of life.

Health Professions Textbooks

Medical textbooks have traditionally paid little attention to the description or management of either the end stages of diseases such as cancer and heart disease or the symptoms and distress commonly experienced by gravely ill or dying patients. One study of four widely used general medical textbooks concluded that they had little that was helpful to say about end-of-life care and that discussions of specific diseases usually dealt with "only prognostication and medical treatments to alter the course of the disease" (Carron et al., 1999, p. 82). A more comprehensive review of 50 medical textbooks likewise concluded that top-selling medical specialty textbooks "generally offered little helpful information on caring for patients at the end of life" and that discussions of specific disease had "no or minimal end-of-life care content" (Rabow et al., 2000, p. 771). A separate investigation of four leading surgical textbooks concluded that "disease epidemiology, prognosis/prevention, progression, and medical interventions were generally well discussed in all textbooks . . . [but] little helpful information was provided [about] breaking bad news/advanced care planning, mode of death, treatment decision-making, effect on family/surgeon, and symptom management" (Easson et al., 2001. p.34).

A similar analysis of the content of 50 leading nursing textbooks found that pain was the most commonly discussed topic related to end-of-life care, but such discussion comprised less than one-half of 1 percent of the text content (counted by pages) (Ferrell et al., 2000). The reviewers also found that the discussion of pain was often deficient in scope and sometimes inaccurate. A similar survey of social work textbooks is planned (PDIA, 2001a,b).

The committee found no similar, systematic assessments of pediatric textbooks. However, editors of one text have begun to include more information on end-of-life issues and palliative care (Behrman et al., 2000). Still, in this and other texts, the sections on many conditions that are usually or often fatal include little or no discussion of the end stage of the disease or attention (directly or by cross-reference) to the care of dying patients and their families.

INITIATIVES TO IMPROVE EDUCATION FOR PEDIATRIC PALLIATIVE AND END-OF-LIFE CARE

General

Changing health professions education is not easy. Deans of health professional schools, department chairs, residency program directors, certification and accreditation bodies, textbook authors, and other leaders face an avalanche of demands for new topics or perspectives to be included in curricula, residency program requirements, and other elements of health professions education. Academic medical centers and medical, nursing, and other health professions schools or programs also face financial pressures, particularly when state governments are trimming health and education budgets.

Change often requires a years-long process of developing, reviewing, ratifying, and implementing new educational requirements or methods. For example, a change in residency requirements usually involves years of preparation, discussion, negotiation, and review before adoption, which is then followed by more time to allow implementation before programs are assessed for compliance. Changing course offerings and requirements in a medical or nursing school, particularly adding a requirement, is often a highly political process as different disciplines compete for priority in an already overloaded curriculum. Thus, those promoting educational reforms may also pursue less formal strategies such as persuading individual instructors to include palliative care issues as illustrations in existing courses.

Efforts to improve the education of health professionals in palliative and end-of-life care can take several forms. They can include actions to

- improve curricula, clinical experiences, or resources (e.g., faculty preparation) for single educational institutions or programs or for consortia of institutions;
- set curriculum or other standards for a category of educational institutions, programs, or professionals;
- develop faculty expertise and other educational resources, including textbooks and Internet sites; and
- expand educational opportunities available to practicing professionals.

Some initiatives focus on the development of materials or models that have general application across institutions, for example, standards for educational programs or requirements for licensure. The Robert Wood Johnson Foundation has supported work by the National Board of Medical Examiners (which administers the physician licensing examination that is an element in state licensure requirements) to develop examination questions on end-of-life care (RWJF, 2001). Coverage of palliative care and end-of-life issues in licensure examinations is intended to reinforce curriculum standards.

The Residency Review Committee for Pediatrics, a subcommittee of the Accreditation Council for Graduate Medical Education, establishes requirements for the more than 200 pediatric residency programs. Box 9.2 lists requirements that specifically mention terminal conditions, death, some aspect of symptom management, or decisions about life-sustaining medical interventions. Other, generally relevant requirements include those relating to communication and interpersonal skills, team care for chronic or complex conditions, cultural dimensions of care, and quality assessment and improvement. The list mentions pain management but not quality of life or the symptoms other than pain that are common consequences of many life-threatening medical conditions or their treatment.

Recently, some pediatric subspecialties—emergency medicine, hematology–oncology, and neurology—have added provisions related to palliative or end-of-life care (also shown in Box 9.2). The specifics vary. Although subspecialty programs are supposed to cover skills related to "complications of death," residency requirements for some subspecialties that care for significant numbers of children who die—notably neonatalogy, pediatric critical care, and pediatric pulmonary medicine—are silent on palliative and end-of-life care. Requirements for family medicine are also relevant. They refer to integration of "end-of-life issues" into the educational experience (ACGME, 2000).

Some states have acted to encourage attention to end-of-life issues in health professions education. For example, California added training in end-of-life care and pain management to the requirements for candidates for medical licensure, effective June 1, 2000 (Medical Board of California, 2000). In New York, a voluntary statewide effort is attempting to improve coverage of palliative and end-of-life care in the medical curriculum. One element of that effort has been the development of the Palliative Care Assessment Tool, which is intended to help medical schools in New York state assess and strengthen their curricula (Abele Meekin et al., 2000).

The creation of such general standards for education programs can provide a broad stimulus for change. Nonetheless, support for education in palliative and end-of-life care still has to be mobilized on an institution-by-institution or organization-by-organization basis.

Educational Strategies and Tools to Improve Palliative, End-of-Life, and Bereavement Care

Integration and Illustration

Ethics courses or course segments offer many opportunities for adult or pediatric end-of-life issues to be raised, for example, informed consent, double-effect decisionmaking, rationing, and truth telling. The humanities, which have become a more visible element of health professions education in recent years (see, e.g., Charon et al., 1995; Charon, 2001; Skelton et al., 2001), likewise provide rich opportunities to consider the human meaning of serious illness, suffering, and death.

Competence in palliative and end-of-life care cannot, however, be achieved if these topics are isolated in ethics and humanities seminars. Scientific education and clinical training are also necessary in many areas. These include understanding the pathophysiology and natural history of life-threatening medical conditions; determining diagnosis and prognosis; assessing, preventing, and managing physical and mental symptoms of advanced disease; evaluating the potential benefits and burdens of pharmacological, behavioral, and other treatment options; and understanding how children's developmental stage may affect pathophysiology, diagnosis, prognosis, symptoms, and treatments.

More generally, a basic principle of education is repetition and reinforcement of—not one-time exposure to—important concepts. To use an analogy, "You give the immunization in the first year of medical school, but then you've got to boost them at two, and then you've got to boost them again at four and at six."

To this end, many opportunities exist to use palliative care and end-of-life issues as powerful illustrations in teaching other concepts, principles, and techniques during the didactic and clinical components of undergraduate medical education and the similar stages of nursing and other health professions education. One advantage of an "illustrative" strategy is that it is less threatening to established interests than changes in requirements. Also, educators are often interested in finding compelling and challenging examples and teaching materials for lectures, small-group discussions, and other experiences. For resident physicians, end-of-life issues can be considered in mortality and morbidity conferences and similar sessions based on the circumstances of actual patients. With educational materials increasingly available through the Internet, the traditional content constraints related to textbook selection and library resources are less of an impediment to curricular enrichment than in the past.

BOX 9.2
Program Requirements for Residency Education

Common Residency Program Requirements (February 2002)

Programs must prepare residents to demonstrate competence in six areas:

- Patient care that is compassionate, appropriate, and effective for the treatment of health problems and the promotion of health;
- Medical knowledge about established and evolving biomedical, clinical, and cognate (e.g., epidemiological and social–behavioral) sciences and the application of this knowledge to patient care;
- Practice-based learning and improvement that involves investigation and evaluation of their own patient care, appraisal and assimilation of scientific evidence, and improvements in patient care;
- Interpersonal and communication skills that result in effective information exchange and collaboration with patients, their families, and other health professionals;
- Professionalism, as manifested through a commitment to carrying out professional responsibilities, adherence to ethical principles, and sensitivity to a diverse patient population; and
- Systems-based practice, as manifested by actions that demonstrate an awareness of and responsiveness to the larger context and system of health care and the ability to effectively call on system resources to provide care that is of optimal value.

Pediatric Residency Program Requirements That Mention Death, Terminal Conditions, or Palliative Care (September 2000)

Programs must provide instruction that enables residents to develop skills related to

- Impact of chronic diseases, terminal conditions, and death on patients and their families (behavioral developmental pediatrics);
- Pain management (procedural skills); and
- Relationship of the physician to patients, e.g., initiating and discontinuing the treatment relationship, confidentiality, consent, and issues of life-sustaining treatments (additional curricular requirements, medical ethics).

Techniques and Tools

Beyond lectures, an array of education techniques and tools exists to help health professionals develop competence in clinical care, including its psychosocial, ethical, and cultural dimensions. Common goals include improving patient–physician communication, encouraging teamwork among health professionals, and extending students' experiences into physician office, nursing home, home, and other community settings. Many tools and

Residency Program Requirements for Subspecialties of Pediatrics: General (July 2000)

This curriculum should include the pathophysiology of disease, reviews of recent advances in clinical medicine and biomedical research, conferences dealing with complications and death, as well as instruction in the scientific, ethical, and legal implications of confidentiality and of informed consent (education program, curriculum).

Residency Program Requirements for Child Neurology (February 1999)

The resident must receive instruction in appropriate and compassionate methods of terminal palliative care, including adequate pain relief, and psychosocial support and counseling for patients and family members about these issues (education program, clinical teaching).

Residency Program Requirements for Pediatric Emergency Medicine (June 1998)

There must be an emphasis on developing a compassionate understanding of the stress associated with sudden illness, injury, and death so that the resident may be responsive to the emotional needs of the patients, their families, and the staff of the emergency department. Discussion and appreciation of the many ethical issues involved in pediatric emergency medicine should be part of the educational program (curriculum).

Residency Program Requirements for Pediatric Hematology–Oncology (September 1999)

The subspecialty resident should participate in the activities of the tumor board and in the provision of comprehensive care to the child with cancer and should have experience in support of the patient, family, and staff in dealing with terminal illness. Residents should be guided in the development of skills in communication and counseling, including the recognition and management of psychosocial problems in pediatric patients (education program, clinical experience).

SOURCE: Accreditation Council on Graduate Medical Education (http://www.acgme.org).

techniques have the additional goals of improving the effectiveness of education by engaging students more directly in the learning process, strengthening problem-solving and reasoning skills, increasing the connections between scientific knowledge and clinical practice, and better preparing students for lifelong learning.

Evaluations of the strategies summarized here and in Appendix G, while often promising, are limited, especially in the area of palliative care.

Much is undertaken on the basis of experience and logic. Chapter 10 discusses directions for research to build the knowledge base for effective education in pediatric palliative care.

Patients and Families as Teachers

> *A social worker raised the astounding idea that instead of using actors or social workers, why not have standardized parents be actual parents, who went through the same training about giving feedback [to residents]?*
>
> Deborah Dokken, parent, 2001

At the Lucile Packard Children's Hospital, a six-session seminar in pediatric palliative care for first-year pediatric residents began in July 2001. The seminar runs continuously with the goal of having every resident rotate through and complete the course. During one of the six sessions, volunteer parents who have lost a child talk to the group about their experiences. As one family participant attested: "Now there is some emotion. There is a face. I think they realize their actions stay with these people for their lifetime" (Conlon, G., 2001). In a mentor session, a senior faculty member discusses with the group his or her experience working with children who die and their families. In other sessions, residents discuss their own professional and personal experiences with death and learn about symptom management, spiritual and cross-cultural aspects of care, and practical issues such as death certificates and coroner notification. (The needs assessment undertaken as part of the development of this course is described in Contro et al., 2002.)

One frequently cited effort to strengthen the medical school curriculum is Harvard University Medical School's elective course in "Living with Life-Threatening Illness" (Billings and Block, 1997; Block and Billings, 1998).[2] The approach is to pair students with volunteer patients (sometimes including children) who have a life-threatening medical problem and then use that ongoing relationship as the focus of the course's examination of issues in palliative and end-of-life care. A video and educational guide developed by the Education Development Center, which examines the experiences of students enrolled in the class over a two-year period, is part of an effort to encourage other schools to develop similar programs (Romer and Solomon, 2000). Earlier, Mermann and colleagues (1991) pioneered a similar course at Yale, but that course is no longer taught.

---

[2]A range of materials was developed in support of this course by its faculty (Billings and Block, 1997).

Simulated or Standardized Patients or Parents   Simulated patients are a well-accepted educational and assessment tool. Recently, the Federation of State Medical Boards and the National Board of Medical Examiners, which jointly administer the national licensing examination for physicians, announced that a clinical skills examination including standardized patients would be added to the examination (FSMB, 2002).

Use of standardized patients is more challenging in pediatric than in adult settings. Lane and colleagues, however, describe the use of child standardized patients in an evaluation of a pediatric clinical skills assessment tool and reported that their use proved feasible for the evaluators, enjoyable for the children, and acceptable to the children's real and standardized parents (Lane et al., 1999). Educators might, however, be hesitant to use child actors or volunteers to portray gravely ill or dying children. If their use was part of research to evaluate the strategy, an institutional review board, which must approve most human research, might object.

Use of standardized family members presents fewer complications (see generally Clay et al., 2000). In a project exploring ways to increase organ donation, Williams and colleagues have studied the standardized families, in this case, people trained to behave as family members being confronted with bad news, decisions about end-of-life care, and requests for organ donation (Williams et al., 2001b; 2002). These sessions were intended to improve the communication skills of physicians, nurses, clergy, and transplant coordinators participating as a team The standardized families did not operate from explicit scripts and the sessions could be interrupted to discuss and even restart "problem" conversations. The families, trainers, and other participants provided feedback. The rate of consent to organ donation requests rose from 25 percent before to 75 percent after the intervention but then fell back with staff turnover (Personal communication, Michael Williams, M.D., Johns Hopkins Medical Institutions, March 11, 2002). The researchers are still preparing their final report and are seeking another grant to study the strategy in two to four community hospitals.

In another project, researchers at George Washington University videotaped and evaluated skills of pediatric residents and emergency department fellows in communicating news of a child's death to standardized parents and then provided feedback to the residents and fellows (Greenberg et al., 1999). During a similar exercise several weeks later, the researchers found improvements in information and counseling skills.

Hospice and Inpatient Palliative Care Experiences   As noted earlier, some hospices offer educational programs not only to their own staffs and volunteers but also to health professions students and community providers. Gomez (1996) described one inpatient hospice program that was linked to a community-based home hospice program. It offered educational experiences for residents, medical students, and nurses. As described above, a survey of directors of pediatric residency programs suggests that such experiences are rare, even for clinicians who routinely care for children who die.

Mentors and Role Models   One objective of developing a cadre of palliative care specialists is to provide established clinicians and clinicians-in-training with role models and mentors. Mentoring implies a more directed effort to teach and counsel a particular individual rather than to teach by example in group situations such as clinical rounds for medical residents and other trainees. Examples of mentoring strategies (as part of broader educational programs) include matching medical students with community-based physicians known for their attention to spiritual issues in practice and matching first- and third-year medical students to work with chaplain mentors in sessions with patients.[3]

In a controlled trial of an ethics education program, Sulmasy and colleagues (1995) compared groups of house officers, one that received lectures and another that received a more extensive intervention that included a physician ethicist as role model who participated in clinical rounds where he raised ethical questions about patients' care. The trial also included two control groups. Those in the extensive intervention group showed more confidence on procedural issues and noted more concurrent care concerns (e.g., pain management) associated with DNR orders.

Faculty Development   Among other goals, a broad initiative to improve end-of-life care in Department of Veterans Affairs (VA) hospitals has aimed to increase the number of "faculty leaders and innovators" in the field and to develop curricula for the VA's internal medicine residency programs (http://www.va.gov/oaa/flp/docFLPFactSheet.asp). The VA does not care for children and no equivalent care system exists for children. Nonetheless, this initiative has an evaluation component that may generate lessons useful for other faculty development efforts.

Projects at Harvard and Stanford also aim at faculty development. In addition to covering palliative care principles and practice, Harvard's program for nursing and medical educators (Harvard Medical School, 2002, http://www.hms.harvard.edu/cdi/pallcare/program.html) examines oppor-

---

[3]These examples are included in short descriptions of programs that received awards for education in spirituality and medicine from the George Washington Institute for Spirituality and Health, George Washington University Medical School (http://www.gwish.org/courses/id44.htm). Systematic evaluations of program effects were not described.

tunities and challenges in palliative care education and program development. A one-month program at Stanford aims to provide participants "with background knowledge and seminar leadership skills required to deliver a series of eight 2-hour seminars to their colleagues and to residents at their home institutions" (Stanford Faculty Development Center, 2002, http:// www.stanford.edu/group/SFDP/progeol.html). Again, these programs focus on adult care.

Continuing Education   Other important initiatives focus on continuing education for physicians and nurses. The Education for Physicians on End-of-Life Care (EPEC) Project (with leadership from the American Medical Association's Institute for Ethics) has developed an education package that includes a mix of didactic sessions, videotape presentations, interactive discussions, and practical exercises (Emanuel et al., 1999). The Decisions Near the End of Life program, which has been used by interdisciplinary leadership teams in more than 230 institutions, includes a series of case-based seminars on ethical issues in end-of-life care (Solomon et al., 1997). Neither of these initiatives focuses on care for children and their families but both recognize the need for age-appropriate care. Both also have a "train-the-trainer" strategy with the objective of more broadly disseminating the resources for education in end-of-life care. The EPEC trainer's guide includes a module on the evaluation of training sessions.

A similar initiative for nurses is the End-of-Life Nursing Education Consortium (ELNEC), a partnership of the American Association of Colleges of Nursing and the City of Hope National Medical Center. The initiative focuses specifically on preparing nurse educators to bring education in end-of-life care to nursing schools and continuing education programs in a variety of settings (AACN, 2002). A pediatric version of ELNEC has been pilot tested (Personal communication, Betty Ferrell, Ph.D., City of Hope Medical Center, July 8, 2002). Other pediatric materials are being developed as part of Initiative for Pediatric Palliative Care described in Chapter 1.

As noted in the introduction to this chapter, major textbooks on palliative medicine, nursing, and psychiatry now include chapters on pediatrics, and a self-study program on pediatric palliative care and other education materials should be available soon. In addition to these resources, other resources include several books and similar materials that discuss concepts, principles, and practical aspects of palliative and end-of-life care for children and their families (see, e.g., Goldman, 1999, ChIPPS, 2001; Armstrong-Dailey and Zarbock, 2001).

DIRECTIONS FOR EDUCATORS

The goal of professional education in palliative, end-of-life, and bereavement care is to build the competence of physicians, nurses, and others who care for people with fatal or potentially fatal medical conditions. Education cannot, however, ensure competent practice. As discussed throughout this report, that requires organizational environments, professional culture, financing policies, and laws and regulations that reward—or at least do not discourage—such practice. Nonetheless, undergraduate, graduate, and continuing health professions education must provide the basic knowledge, skills, and attitudes required for competent practice.

Effective and compassionate care for children with life-threatening medical problems and their families will typically involve a range of health professionals as described in Chapter 5. Thus, education strategies must not only be appropriate to each profession's role but also prepare professionals to work effectively in teams. Further, although educational programs will typically focus on pediatricians and other child health specialists, training is also important for others (e.g., emergency first responders) who are commonly involved in the care of children with life-threatening medical problems or have contacts with family members (e.g., police officers investigating an infant death at home).

Recommendation: Medical, nursing, and other health professions schools or programs should collaborate with professional societies to improve the care provided to seriously ill and injured children by creating and testing curricula and experiences that

- **prepare all health care professionals who work with children and families to have relevant basic competence in palliative, end-of-life, and bereavement care;**
- **prepare specialists, subspecialists, and others who routinely care for children with life-threatening conditions to have advanced competence in the technical and psychosocial aspects of palliative, end-of-life, and bereavement care in their respective fields; and**
- **prepare a group of pediatric palliative care specialists to take lead responsibility for acting as clinical role models, educating other professionals, and conducting research that extends the knowledge base for palliative, end-of-life, and bereavement care.**

Many efforts to improve care for adults and children who die emphasize communication, ethical concerns, and similar issues. The studies reviewed earlier in this report underscore that education in palliative and end-of-life care must also respond to deficiencies in symptom management and other clinical care that permit needless suffering at the end of life. Overall, educators, like clinicians, must be held accountable for the kind of patient care they honor, as evidenced in the curricula, requirements, and experiences they provide for health professionals in training.

No single educational strategy or format will be sufficient to prepare professionals for the intellectual, emotional, cultural, and practical challenges of providing palliative, end-of-life, and bereavement care to children and their families. Likewise, varied incentives will be needed to reinforce educational initiatives including residency program requirements and inclusion of questions in licensure and certification examinations.

> **Recommendation: To provide instruction and experiences appropriate for all health care professionals who care for children, experts in general and specialty fields of pediatric health care and education should collaborate with experts in adult and pediatric palliative care and education to develop and implement**

> • **model curricula that provide a basic foundation of knowledge about palliative, end-of-life, and bereavement care that is appropriate for undergraduate health professions education in areas including but not limited to medicine, nursing, social work, psychology, and pastoral care;**
> • **residency program requirements that provide more extensive preparation as appropriate for each category of pediatric specialists and subspecialists who care for children with life-threatening medical conditions;**
> • **pediatric palliative care fellowships and similar training opportunities;**
> • **introductory and advanced continuing education programs and requirements for both generalist and specialist pediatric professionals; and**
> • **practical, fundable strategies to evaluate selected techniques or tools for educating health professionals in palliative, end-of-life, and bereavement care.**

The committee believes that these strategies for health professions education, if implemented and sustained, will be broadly beneficial. That is, they should reduce the suffering experienced by children who survive as well as children who die, and they should improve the support provided to all families who confront a child's serious medical problem or death. To confirm this expectation and refine strategies, educational programs and tools will require evaluation to determine whether they are changing knowledge, attitudes, and behaviors, ideally over the longer term as well as in the short term.

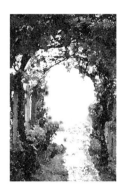

CHAPTER 10

DIRECTIONS FOR RESEARCH

Awful as it was, I was given a gift of experience. If I can use it [in research] to help someone else, it makes [my daughter's] life mean something still.

Bereaved parent (Contro, 2002, p.15)

Among the most common phrases in this report are "research is limited" and "systematic data are not available." Clinicians and parents must often make decisions about the care of children with little guidance from clinical or health services research that documents the potential burdens as well as the potential benefits of medical interventions. For example, parents of infants born more than 14 weeks prematurely are faced with urgent decisions about the extent of life support that they wish for their infant. They frequently must confront unanswerable questions and make their best guesses about what to do with the help and support of neonatolgists and nurses who must often, in turn, rely on their own experience and judgment with limited scientific knowledge to guide them. Neonatologists generally lack validated predictors of very premature infants' risk of death or long-term morbidity, although both outcomes are frequent.

The knowledge base for organizational and policy decisions is likewise limited. For example, organizations considering the creation of a pediatric palliative care program have little research on which to base decisions about services, staffing, outreach, budgets, and similar matters. What information is available relies heavily on descriptive case studies of adult programs. Funding for comparative health services research to test different approaches to organizing adult or pediatric palliative care is minuscule

350

compared to the funding available for clinical research. Even when hospices and hospitals undertake data-intensive internal studies (e.g., for quality improvement projects), they often lack the resources and motivation to produce analyses that meet peer-review standards for publication and wider dissemination.

Researchers, clinicians, and policymakers have recognized shortfalls in clinical research involving palliative and end-of-life care for children and have taken steps to encourage and guide such research, some of which are described later in this chapter. The remainder of this chapter

- briefly reviews initiatives to encourage pediatric research in general and in palliative and end-of-life care specifically;
- describes directions for clinical, health services, and educational research to guide improvements in palliative, end-of-life, and bereavement care for children and their families;
- summarizes the practical challenges of undertaking pediatric research; and
- reviews ethical and legal questions raised by research involving children.

Lessons learned from the kinds of research recommended here should help inform and improve the care of children who survive as well as children who die. It should likewise help all families who experience a child's serious or fatal medical problem.

INITIATIVES TO ENCOURAGE PEDIATRIC RESEARCH

General

Federal policymakers have taken steps to encourage certain kinds of pediatric research. In 1998, following directions from Congress in 1995, the National Institutes of Health (NIH) issued policies and guidelines for including children as research participants (NIH, 1998). Under the policy, children are to be included in all such research funded by the NIH unless their exclusion is justified on scientific or ethical grounds. Exclusion would, for example, be justified when a medical problem does not affect children. For some medical conditions, children's developmental characteristics might suggest the need for a separate, child-only study.

Legislative conference language accompanying the legislation encouraged but did not require the NIH to establish pediatric research priorities (NIH, 1998). The organization has not developed an overall set of priorities, although some individual institutes have developed priorities for certain clinical problems or services including kidney disease (NIDDK, 2001),

HIV/AIDS (NIH, 2001a), and emergency medical services (NIH, 2001b). The priority-setting activity related to emergency services was stimulated in part by recognition that more needed to be done to implement the research recommendations in the 1993 Institute of Medicine (IOM) report on emergency medical services for children (IOM, 1993).

In 2000, the Children's Health Act (P.L. 106-310), among its other provisions, created a pediatric research initiative to increase NIH support for research on diseases, disorders, and other conditions in children. The legislation also supported the training of more pediatric researchers to conduct basic and clinical research. Earlier, the Food and Drug Administration Modernization Act of 1997 (P.L. 105-115) provided incentives for pharmaceutical companies to test drugs in children, and Congress renewed that legislation with slight modifications late in 2001 (Best Pharmaceuticals for Children Act, P.L.107-109). Companies that undertake studies on their products' effects on children get six months of exclusive marketing rights for the drugs in return.[1] (A later section of this chapter describes provisions in this and other legislation and regulation related to protection of child participants in such studies.) In addition to the pediatric exclusivity provision, the Food and Drug Administration (FDA) issued regulations in 1998 that allow it to require drug companies to undertake pediatric testing for certain drugs likely to be used in children (63 Fed. Reg. 66632, December 2, 1998, effective April 1, 1999).[2]

In May 2001, the FDA published an updated list of priorities for pediatric drug research that included more than 425 drugs or drug uses (FDA,

---

[1]Federal regulations requiring pediatric studies of certain drug and biologic products were proposed in 1997 and issued in final form in 1998 (http://www.fda.gov/ohrms/dockets/98fr/ 120298c.txt). In 2002, the government announced that it would suspend these rules for two years pending study of the need for them (Connolly, 2002); a month later, it reversed that decision (Kaufman and Connolly, 2002; Landa, 2002). Unlike the legislation, the regulations also cover biologics (e.g., vaccines, blood products, gene therapy products, HIV and hepatitis tests, innovative therapies for diseases such as cancer and arthritis).

[2]In a set of questions and answers about the rule, the FDA has stated (emphasis in the original deleted): "Under the rule, FDA has the authority to require pediatric studies on a drug product for the product's approved indications if there is substantial use in the pediatric population or the product would provide a meaningful therapeutic benefit—and the absence of adequate labeling could pose significant risk (see 21 CFR 201.23(a)). At this time, however, FDA will not require studies of approved drugs except if approved by the Center Director. Instead, FDA will seek to have manufacturers voluntarily submit studies for marketed drugs under the incentives provided by [the legislation] (see 63 FR 66634 Sec II). For those drugs in which voluntary measures fail to obtain necessary pediatric studies, FDA will consider requiring studies" (http://www.fda.gov/cder/pediatric/faqs.htm#the "Rule"; last update: March 8, 2001).

2001b). Of these, about two dozen uses might relate to symptoms of life-threatening illnesses.

In a report on the pediatric exclusivity provisions, the General Accounting Office noted that when the legislation was passed, approximately 70 to 80 percent of drugs were not adequately labeled for use with children. Since then, pediatric drug research has increased substantially and has provided "new and useful information about whether and how drugs work in children" (USGAO, 2001b, p. 6). According to a recent FDA report to Congress, "the pediatric exclusivity has done more to generate clinical studies and useful prescribing information for the pediatric population than any other regulatory or legislative process to date" (FDA, 2001c, p. ii). The FDA report also noted continuing problems in some areas including the irrelevance of exclusivity provisions to certain old, "off-patent" antibiotics and other drugs and to drugs with low volumes of sales ("orphan drugs"). Another problem has been inadequate incentives for studies in neonates and very young children that must follow studies conducted on older children. In addition, following the completion of studies, manufacturers have sometimes been slow to change drug labeling to reflect the results.

The 2001 legislation renewing "pediatric exclusivity" included provisions to encourage timely changes in drug labeling to reflect new research results. It also established an Office of Pediatric Therapeutics within the FDA to coordinate the agency's activities related to children and pediatric practice and provided for the NIH-based Foundation for the National Institutes of Health (formerly the Foundation for Biomedical Research) to collect funds to support pediatric drug research.

Pediatric Palliative and End-of-Life Care

Research to support improvements in palliative, end-of-life, and bereavement care for children and their families constitutes only a tiny fraction of research involving children. Likewise, research involving children and their families occupies a small niche in the world of research on palliative and end-of-life care, which itself is small in comparison to other areas of clinical and health services research.

Some units of the National Institutes of Health are supporting or show a potential willingness to support relevant research (NINR et al., 1997). For example, in soliciting research proposals on emergency medical services for children, the National Institute of Child Health and Development (NICHD) identified the need for research on the biobehavioral aspects of pain, stress, and coping with illness or injury in situations of emergency care (NIH, 2000b). The National Institute of Mental Health suggested research on aspects of emergency medical services delivery (e.g., medical staff communication style, follow-up care) that could potentially identify processes of emergency care that positively or negatively affect the experience of families whose children die.

In addition, as discussed elsewhere in this report and in Appendix H, the Center for Medicare and Medicaid Services (CMS) is funding several demonstration projects that are intended to provide information about the development, operation, effectiveness, and costs of comprehensive programs of palliative care for children and families from the time of diagnosis through bereavement. Although the evaluation designs do not involve controlled comparisons, the evaluations should provide considerable descriptive and analytic detail about the structure of palliative care programs, populations served, and costs.

Foundation-supported studies have been and continue to be particularly important in extending the knowledge base for adult and pediatric palliative, end-of-life, and bereavement care. Two pediatric programs are among 22 projects funded by the Robert Wood Johnson Foundation to test creative strategies for improving palliative care (Promoting Excellence, 2001). One, led by Children's Hospital and Regional Medical Center of Seattle involves the state health department and regional Blue Cross Blue Shield plans in developing innovative ways to extend health plan coverage for palliative care during a child's life-threatening illness. (See also Chapter 7.) The other, led by SSM Cardinal Glennon Children's Hospital in St. Louis, involves support for a statewide network of health care providers ready to care for children at home. The hospital is developing a palliative care consult program to provide 24-hour consultative services, with a palliative care team to educate physicians, hospice providers, and community hospital staff.

Another example of a privately funded initiative is the already-cited project supported by the Nathan Cummings Foundation and the Open Society Institute that is led by the Education Development Center of Boston (Solomon et al., 2001a). It involves eight children's hospitals (Children's Hospital/Dana-Farber Cancer Institute, Boston; Children's Hospital of Philadelphia; Children's Hospital and Health Center of San Diego; Johns Hopkins Children's Center; Children's Mercy Hospital, Kansas City; Lucile Packard Children's Hospital, Stanford University Medical Center; University of California, San Francisco Children's Hospital; and Vanderbilt Children's Hospital). This project has examined clinicians' and parents' perspectives on palliative care and is developing quality improvement models and educational materials to support improvements in care for children with a range of life-threatening medical problems and their families.

Another project involving support from multiple private foundations (including Soros and the Charitable Leadership Foundation) is the Pediatric Advanced Illness Coordinated Care (PAICC) initiative that was discussed in Chapter 6. This effort, being led by the Center for Advanced Illness Coordinated Care of Albany, New York, is now developing, evaluating, and refining a standardized model of communication and care coordination in five institutions (Himelstein et al., 2002; Hilden and Tobin, 2002).

DIRECTIONS FOR FUTURE RESEARCH

General

Throughout its work, the committee has been hampered by the lack of basic descriptive information about death in childhood as well as scant research testing the effectiveness of clinical interventions and organizational processes and structures in providing palliative, end-of-life, and bereavement care that meets the needs of seriously ill or injured children and their families. Studies reviewed by the committee in Chapter 3 describe deficits in care received by children who die and their families. Unfortunately, available research leaves much that is unclear about the extent and causes of shortfalls in care, the number and kinds of children and families who could benefit from palliative and end-of-life care, and the effectiveness of specific strategies to improve the delivery and financing of this care.

Recommendation: The National Center for Health Statistics, the National Institutes of Health, and other relevant public and private organizations, including philanthropic organizations, should collaborate to improve the collection of descriptive data—epidemiological, clinical, organizational, and financial—to guide the provision, funding, and evaluation of palliative, end-of-life, and bereavement care for children and families.

In the 2001 report *Improving Palliative Care for Cancer* (IOM, 2001c), the IOM's National Cancer Policy Board included two recommendations aimed at stimulating palliative care research in designated "centers of excellence" and encouraging such centers to take a lead role as agents of national policy in promoting palliative care. The Board also recommended that the National Cancer Institute (NCI) should add the requirement of research in palliative care and symptom control for an institution's designation as a "comprehensive cancer center." The research activities suggested for such centers included the following:

• formal testing and evaluation of new and existing practice guidelines for palliative and end-of-life care;
• pilot testing of "quality indicators" for assessing end-of-life care at the level of the patient and the institution;
• uncovering the determinants of disparities in access to care by

minority populations and developing specific programs and initiatives to increase access; and

• providing clinical and research training fellowships in medical and surgical oncology in end-of-life care for adult and pediatric patients.

This general strategy should also prove productive in stimulating palliative, end-of-life, and bereavement care research involving children and their families. While by no means discouraging research in other institutions, the committee encourages initiatives that build on federally funded pediatric centers, networks, and similar structures.

Recommendation: Units of the National Institutes of Health and other organizations that fund pediatric oncology, neonatal, and similar clinical and research centers or networks should define priorities for research in pediatric palliative, end-of-life, and bereavement care. Research should focus on care for infants, children, adolescents, and their families, including siblings, and should cover care from the time of diagnosis through death and bereavement. Priorities for research include but are not limited to the effectiveness of

• **clinical interventions including symptom management;**
• **methods for improving communication and decisionmaking;**
• **innovative arrangements for delivering, coordinating, and evaluating care, including interdisciplinary care teams and quality improvement strategies, and**
• **different approaches to bereavement care.**

By organizing multiple sites to investigate a common problem using a common methodology, this strategy should increase the number of children involved in studies and increase the credibility of the findings. It should also stimulate the development of investigator expertise in pediatric palliative care research, encourage the formulation and successful completion of more high-quality research projects, and promote attention to palliative care, end-of-life, and bereavement issues in both pediatric clinical trials and regular patient care. By involving designated institutional participants in collaborative research, a "centers" strategy should also encourage tests of organizational interventions (e.g., random assignment of institutions to test innovations in information systems, training, staffing, or conflict management). The results should benefit children who survive, children who die, and the families of both groups.

The committee recognizes that the infrastructure for biomedical and clinical research varies considerably for different diseases, disorders, and other medical conditions affecting children. For example, the Children's

Oncology Group (COG), supported by the NCI, involves nearly 240 centers (COG, 2001), whereas the Neonatal Research Network funded by the National Institute of Child Health and Development (NICHD) includes approximately a dozen centers (NICHD, 2000; see also http:// neonatal.rti.org). Given differences in the research infrastructure and in the conditions that bring death to children, the specific incentives and mechanisms for a center- or network-focused research strategy will have to be flexible and creative. Although the recommendation focuses on NIH-funded centers and networks, philanthropic foundations and other private organizations can also participate in supporting creative projects that are based on these networks but are not limited to NIH priorities.

Flexibility and creativity on the part of both research sponsors and investigators will also be required to extend research earlier into the period following the diagnosis of a life-threatening problem and later into the period of bereavement experienced by the families of so many children with grave medical problems who participate in clinical research. If researchers focus on earlier stages in the trajectory of fatal and potentially fatal conditions, they may be able to increase the number of children participating in research on certain aspects of palliative care (e.g., effective symptom management). They may also be able to develop a fuller understanding of the symptoms and distress associated with serious illnesses (and their treatments) and the benefits and challenges of incorporating aspects of palliative care earlier in the course of a life-threatening condition.

In proposing directions for research to improve pediatric palliative and end-of-life care, the committee tried to focus on the gaps in the knowledge base needed to put the principles set forth in Chapter 1 into practice and to implement the recommendations listed in subsequent chapters. The discussion below focuses on several specific areas for further research including quality of life, symptom measurement and management, bereavement, education, and models for delivering and financing palliative, end-of-life, and bereavement care. At a more general level, a comprehensive research agenda for pediatric palliative, end-of-life, and bereavement care should consider

- the needs of infants, children, and adolescents and developmentally appropriate care strategies;
- a range of causes and trajectories of death including sudden, unexpected deaths, deaths from progressive chronic conditions, and deaths from conditions diagnosed prenatally;
- the effects of uncertainty in diagnosis, prognosis, and treatment on communication with children and families, establishment of care goals and care plans, decisions about interventions, preparation for death, and family perspectives and emotions after death;
- the needs of parents, siblings, and other family members;

- the roles and relationships of different health care professionals and other personnel who are involved with children who may die or who have died and their families;
- the range of care settings and organizations that are involved with children who may die or have died and their families (e.g., emergency first-response units, emergency departments, intensive care units, other inpatient units, hospices, home health agencies, and medical examiners' offices);
- the contribution of family, provider, and other factors to timely or delayed recognition that death is near and to differences in family and physician assessments of prognosis and care options;
- the reports of children and families about their specific experiences with care (preferably concurrent with care rather than after the child's death), not just their global assessments of satisfaction with care;
- the experiences of children and families outside the health care system, including with schools;
- the psychological effects on professionals of caring for children who die and the consequences for their ability to care for children and parents; and
- methods and processes for improving communication and preventing or resolving conflicts among clinicians, patients, and family members.

Much of the research suggested in this chapter is descriptive and qualitative. It involves epidemiological, methodological, behavioral, organizational, and policy studies as well as clinical research. Controlled research strategies, including randomized clinical trials and careful case-control studies, should be encouraged. Such approaches will, however, often be difficult given the small numbers of children who die and the charged emotional circumstances surrounding a child's life threatening illness or injury. Even for relatively narrow clinical questions (e.g., comparison of one pain management regimen versus another), randomized trials are relatively uncommon. Qualitative studies have an important role to play in describing the experiences, perspectives, and values of patients, family members, and caregivers (see, e.g., Sackett and Wennberg, 1997). In devising suitable research strategies, researchers will need to combine creativity, flexibility, and sensitivity both to patient and family burdens and anxieties.

Each research topic suggested here presents different methodological challenges. In general, researchers may encounter problems in defining and recruiting sufficient numbers of research participants, collecting information about subjective experiences from individuals who may be physically or emotionally limited in their ability or willingness to respond to questions, identifying necessary information in medical or other records, and defining measures relevant to patient and family experiences at different stages of life-threatening medical experiences. Epidemiologic and health services research may have to rely on data that is years old by the time it is released. Researchers may also encounter difficulties in getting research approved by Institutional Review Boards, a topic that warrants investigation in its own right.

Research Directions: Quality of Life for Children and Families

To identify practices that affect the quality of life experienced by a child with a life-threatening medical problem requires measurement tools that can reliably and validly reflect the child's experience, particularly when the problem has reached an advanced stage and death is expected or possible in the foreseeable future. Appendix C identifies some of the limitations of current measurement tools (especially those intended for well children) and the complexities of developing better ones. Although improvements in measures relevant for pediatric palliative and end-of-life care can build in a general way on measurement strategies used for adults, much of the work needed will have to be specific to infants, children, and adolescents. Box 10.1 summarizes some important directions for such work.

As discussed in Appendix C, existing pediatric quality-of-life instruments may be generic in nature or they may be disease and condition specific. Either way, such instruments are designed primarily for well or chronically ill children and adolescents. They include items that measure function, problems with physical activities, emotional concerns, cognitive abilities to concentrate on and complete school tasks, and concerns with certain symptoms. Many of these items may not be relevant for a child with advanced illness. The instruments may also overlook some issues, for example, spiritual or existential concerns. In addition, completing an instrument intended for healthier children may be unduly burdensome for a seriously ill child.

BOX 10.1
Directions for Research on Quality-of-Life Measures for Children and Families

- Identify domains of quality of life relevant for children with advanced illness and for their family members.
- Investigate the importance of different domains of quality of life for children and for family members, including how their importance may vary over time.
- Assess the need to adapt measurement instruments to reflect differences in the ill child's stage of development, the nature of the illness, and other child and family characteristics.
- Evaluate the degree and nature of agreement or disagreement between child self-reports and proxy reports by parents or others.

Some instruments also exist to assess quality of life for parents of children who are seriously ill. These focus primarily on elements of caregiver burden and may only incompletely capture the quality of life of the parent of a dying child. The committee is aware of no instruments that assess quality of life for siblings of seriously ill children.

One task for methodologists is to identify specific domains (e.g., physical, spiritual) of quality of life that are relevant for a child with advanced illness. Another task is to determine whether the importance of a domain changes over time as an illness progresses. Methodologists will also have to consider the influence of development stage, culture, and context (e.g., sites of care, nature of the illness, family circumstances) both in the design of instruments and in their application. For example, an instrument may require different formats for young children and adolescents.

Interventions directed toward improving or at least maintaining a dying child's quality of life could also improve the quality of life of family members who suffer with the child. Likewise, interventions to help parents, siblings, and other family members could benefit the ill child. Researchers designing interventions to protect and improve the quality of life of children with advanced illness and their families should consider how they might evaluate these "spillover" effects.

When possible, obtaining the dying child's own report of his or her quality of life is preferred. It may not, however, be possible to identify definitively when a child is dying until illness is far advanced. Also, given the uncertainties associated with predicting time of death, death may come earlier than expected. Thus, some dying children will not be capable of providing self-reports, and the report of a parent or other proxy or surrogate may be necessary. Studies comparing children's self-reports with reports from parents or professionals tend to show low to moderate agreement in ratings of symptoms or other aspects of quality of life (see Appendix C). Comparisons have not been completed for dying children and their parents or health care providers. Another question may arise when dying children experience changes in health care setting (e.g., home to hospital, distant medical center to community hospital) or health care provider (e.g., pediatric oncologist to generalist pediatrician or hospice professional). How such changes might affect proxy reports, especially those of health care professionals, is unknown.

Comparisons of child self-reports and proxy reports will be challenging in the context of a child's advanced illness and will require great sensitivity. Nonetheless, it is important to get a better sense of the degree and nature of agreement or disagreement between the two and of the factors that might increase or diminish agreement (e.g., child's development stage, family culture, location and continuity of end-of-life care). If parents or other proxies tend to overestimate, underestimate, or otherwise misperceive the quality of life experienced by their children, their reports may misdirect efforts to improve care.

Research Directions: Physical and Psychological Symptoms of Serious Diseases and Their Treatments

In 1997, another IOM committee argued that pain research, which has achieved considerable success in illuminating the pathophysiology of pain and developing effective interventions, should be considered as a model for other areas of symptom research. It urged interaction between basic scientists and clinical investigators to direct new intellectual energy to research on significant end-of-life symptoms including fatigue, shortness of breath, nausea, confusion, anxiety, and depression.

This committee agrees with its predecessor that many features of the pain research strategy can be productively generalized to other symptom areas. These features include the following:

• building the neuroscience base for understanding symptoms, for example, continuing to investigate the role of symptom-inhibiting neurotransmitters and receptor-specific opioids that avoid some unwanted opioid side effects;

• encouraging the development and use of more precise descriptive terminology and classification schemes for symptoms to provide a "common language" for researchers;

• continuing the development, testing, and refinement of standard tools for assessing symptoms including their "felt" burden;

• studying the prevalence and severity of symptoms by physiological source or mechanism, medical condition, developmental stage, and other relevant characteristics; and

• investigating potential therapies based on better understanding of both the pathophysiology of symptoms and the patient's reported or observed experience of symptoms.

Research on symptoms has been constrained by numerous factors that have historically limited other pediatric research: small numbers, ethical constraints, complexities associated with outcomes measurement, and lack of financial incentives for the pharmaceutical industry (until recently). The limited research that has been performed has primarily concerned pain management, often in oncology patients only. Problems such as nausea, fatigue, sedation, shivering, anxiety and agitation, depression, seizures, spasticity, constipation and diarrhea, dyspnea, dysphagia, anorexia and cachexia, and dermatologic manifestations of disease and treatment (e.g., itching, mouth ulcers) require attention as well.

Further, although both children and adults have benefited from progress in pain research, many areas for investigation remain in this arena, including identifying the reasons for the underuse of effective therapies to prevent or relieve pain and devising interventions to increase appropriate use of these therapies. The American Academy of Pediatrics (AAP) recently noted the lack of research on the management of pain in newborns with conditions associated with extensive tissue damage or recurrent or chronic pain (e.g., necrotizing enterocolitis, meningitis) (AAP, 2000a). It also noted that the benefits and harms of sedatives and other agents to manage apparent anxiety in neonates have been little studied. Research directions for several areas related to the prevention and relief of pain and other symptoms are summarized in Box 10.2.

BOX 10.2
Directions for Research on Assessment and
Management of Symptoms

• Document the prevalence and incidence of children's physical symptoms, in addition to pain, that are associated with life-threatening illnesses or their treatment.
• Document the prevalence and intensity of psychological symptoms in children diagnosed with a life-threatening medical condition.
• Develop instruments to measure pain in selected pediatric populations (e.g., pre- or nonverbal children) and to measure other symptoms in all pediatric populations.
• Develop, refine, and evaluate pharmacologic and other strategies for the effective prevention and treatment of pain and other symptoms in children, including nausea, fatigue, sedation, depression, spasticity, anxiety, and anorexia with priority on the following:
—Developmental pharmacology
—Guidelines for use of different interventions
—Side-effect management
—Long-term effects on the developing organism
—Novel routes of administration
—Procedural sedation and analgesia
—Behavioral techniques
• Evaluate the effects of strategies to prevent or relieve symptoms on children's quality of life, length of life, and hospital use (e.g., length of stay, rehospitalization rates), and on family functioning and well being.
• Document the effectiveness of alternative and complementary medicine techniques in alleviating symptoms.

Prevalence and Intensity of Symptoms in Children and Families

The prevalence and intensity of physical and psychological symptoms in children, especially symptoms other than pain, is inadequately documented. In particular, the extent and severity of psychological symptoms in children with life-threatening illness—and their parents and siblings—are unknown and probably significantly underappreciated. Depression, anxiety, posttraumatic stress disorder (PTSD), and other psychological and behavioral symptoms can significantly reduce the quality of life for children and their families. They can also compromise the ability of children and families to adhere to treatment regimens.

In addition to experiencing symptoms associated with their medical condition, many children with a life-threatening illness face a barrage of painful or uncomfortable procedures (e.g., aspiration of bone marrow or spinal fluid, drawing of blood, injections of diagnostic or therapeutic agents) that may not be necessary for adequate diagnosis and treatment. Painful or distressing procedures, including demanding chemotherapy or mechanical ventilation, often continue when children are nearing death. Stopping certain life-sustaining interventions for a dying child, for example, mechanical ventilation, can involve physical and emotional distress. Research should investigate the prevalence and intensity of treatment-related distress in children with different medical conditions as well as ways to prevent or relieve it.

Measuring symptoms in infants is a particular challenge. As discussed in Chapter 4 and early in this chapter, pain in infants was not recognized or taken seriously until fairly recently. Now, pediatric researchers are attempting to measure pain, stress, and more generally, distress or comfort in these populations using systematic clinical observations and physiological indicators (see, generally, Schecter et al., 1993; Taddio and Ohlson, 1997; Ballantyne et al., 1999; Stevens et al., 2001).

Measurement of Symptoms

Adequate measurement is the cornerstone of adequate treatment. Without the ability to quantify a clinical problem, it is often impossible to determine if interventions have been effective at ameliorating it. Although many developmentally appropriate instruments are available for most pediatric pain management situations, no uniformly accepted instruments exist for certain subpopulations such as children who are developmentally delayed or intubated. In addition, for symptoms other than pain, easy-to-use, reliable assessment tools are scarce. Treatment of fatigue, shortness of breath, drug-related sedation, spasticity, nausea and other more generalized suffering would all benefit from more uniform, quantified, and validated measurement strategies.

Management of Symptoms

In addition to better documenting the prevalence and intensity of psychological symptoms, research is also needed to refine and compare interventions appropriate for children of different ages and at different stages of a life-threatening medical condition. These interventions include individual psychotherapy, group support, and psychotropic medications.

Most of the pharmacologic agents used for physical and psychological symptoms have not been adequately studied in children. Despite recent incentives for drug research involving children, the developmental pharmacokinetic profile in children of many existing drugs is still unknown and must be established to allow and guide their "on-label" use. Then, evidence-based guidelines can be developed for selecting patients for different drug regimens, escalating or tapering off doses, and managing side effects. Although the negative long-term impact of unrelieved symptoms such as pain is well established, the long-term effects of opioids and other drugs used to ameliorate pain have yet to be established for children with serious, chronic problems that persist for months or years.

To reduce children's discomfort during the administration of medications and to encourage cooperation with uncomfortable treatment regimens, novel routes of drug administration, including transdermal, transmucosal, and regional approaches, must be further developed in addition to better-tasting formulations of existing, orally administered drugs (AAP, 1997a). Development of new agents such as long-acting (e.g., days long) local anesthetics for children experiencing post-operative pain and better treatments for neuropathic and bone pain would also reduce the burden of suffering for many children.

In general, more research is needed both to develop better sedation and analgesic regimens and nonpharmacologic strategies for preventing and relieving procedural pain and to verify the safety and effectiveness of existing regimens. Although not an issue of procedure management per se, the efficacy of intensive, controlled sedation to relieve intractable pain, seizures, or other distress at the end of life also requires continued investigation. Such research is important regardless of one's position on the use of such sedation when a side effect may be hastened death, although that result appears to be uncommon (see Chapters 5 and 8).

As discussed earlier in this report, pain management programs are now a requirement for hospital accreditation and an increasing focus of quality assessment initiatives (JCAHO, 2001). Careful documentation and analysis of sedation failures can improve the quality of care in an institution and also improve the evidence base overall for effective pain management.

Impact of Symptom Control

Documentation of the impact of symptom control on children and families may promote a wider understanding and appreciation of its benefits among patients, families, and clinicians. Even today, some families may believe that severe pain and other physical distress are inevitable and must simply be endured because nothing can be done about them. Likewise, not all clinicians are aware of shortfalls in the management of pain and other symptoms or not all are knowledgeable about the impact on child and family quality of life of proven strategies for relieving symptoms.

Hospital, hospice, and insurance managers may be influenced if further research supports suggestions that better symptom control may shorten hospital stays and reduce rehospitalizations. Given the high cost of certain medications for pain and other symptoms, such evidence may also encourage rethinking of hospice reimbursements so that the appropriate use of highly effective but costly medications is not discouraged.

Complementary Medicine

What are termed "complementary" or "alternative" therapeutic approaches[3] such as acupuncture, massage, therapeutic touch, and aromatherapy may play a significant role in future symptom management. Most of these techniques are noninvasive, and some may be pleasurable for healthy and ill individuals alike. This makes them attractive to children and families facing pharmacological regimens with distressing side effects. The efficacy and acceptability of these techniques for children, especially those with life-threatening illnesses, has not been sufficiently studied to allow routine recommendation of their use. Research in this area could give children and their families, as well as providers, a new array of documented, effective treatment options. Credible research could also alert families to therapies that do not meet the claims made for them.

The benefits of cognitive and behavioral techniques are already well established in the area of pain management (see, e.g., Schechter et al.,

---

[3]As described by the NIH's National Center for Complementary and Alternative Medicine (NCCAM), complementary and alternative medicine (CAM) "covers a broad range of healing philosophies, approaches, and therapies. Generally, it is defined as those treatments and health care practices not taught widely in medical schools, not generally used in hospitals, and not usually reimbursed by medical insurance companies. . . . People use these treatments and therapies in a variety of ways. Therapies are used alone (often referred to as alternative), in combination with other alternative therapies, or in addition to conventional therapies (sometimes referred to as complementary)" (http://nccam.nih.gov/fcp/faq/index.html#what-is). As some of these strategies move into mainstream medicine, they may still continue to be described under the CAM label.

2002), but further research is necessary to demonstrate their efficacy in other symptoms such as fatigue, sedation, and nausea. The use of transcutaneous electrical nerve stimulation (TENs) units has received almost no formal research, yet based on anecdotal reports from patients and clinicians, such units may have a significant role to play in symptom control.

Research Directions: Perinatal Death

More children die in the neonatal period or immediately prior to birth than in any other period in childhood. Recent advances in prenatal diagnosis, prenatal treatment, and neonatal care have led to changes in the timing and nature of decisions that families make when confronted with a fetus or newborn infant with a lethal or potentially lethal condition. Little systematic descriptive information is available concerning the long-term impact on families of these decisions, the perceptions of parents of the benefits and harms of different life-sustaining and palliative interventions, or the best methods for communicating with families faced with these decisions. Likewise, little research has investigated the emotional impact of prenatal diagnosis on mothers and fathers, the effect of perinatal death on surviving or future siblings, and differences in effects on family members related to gender, culture, and socio-economic characteristics. More research in this area (Box 10.3) should help improve the care provided to a large group of bereaved families and should also contribute to a better understanding of decisionmaking about treatment choices (i.e., ending the pregnancy or trying to carry the fetus to term) and the consequences of different choices.

Despite the frequency of perinatal loss, population-based studies of the long-term impact of perinatal loss on parents are not available. Descriptive

---

BOX 10.3
Directions for Research on Perinatal Death and Bereavement

- Describe quality-of-life outcomes and self-perceptions of parenting skills in a population-based cohort of mothers and fathers up to five years after the perinatal loss.
- Describe gender differences and changes over time in coping mechanisms and parental perceptions of the benefits and harms of life-sustaining and palliative interventions for fetuses or infants with specific, prenatally or postnatally determined lethal diagnoses.
- Assess the long-term as well as the short-term effects on parent outcomes of interventions for parents who have sustained perinatal loss.
- Determine the effect of perinatal death on surviving or future siblings.
- Determine the impact of antenatal ultrasound on parental perceptions of pregnancy and of the prognosis for their baby.

research to assess parents' quality of life and perceptions of their role and skills as parents should follow them for at least five years after a perinatal death.

Because of the differing physical and emotional impact of pregnancy on women compared to men, fathers and mothers may respond differently to information concerning fetal or infant diagnosis and prognosis. They may also differ in the rates at which they comprehend or assimilate information. Such differences may amplify already significant emotional stress or pre-existing psychological disorders and may lead to confusion about the wishes of parents for interventions. Obstetricians, pediatricians, nurses, social workers, psychologists, and bereavement specialists would benefit from prospective studies that (1) investigate the coping mechanisms of parents who are confronted by an antenatal or postnatal fetal diagnosis that is potentially lethal and (2) explore parental perceptions of the benefits and burdens of different interventions (including palliative care) stratified by fetal or neonatal diagnosis and by timing of diagnosis.

Several perinatal interventions undertaken in the 1970s and 1980s were reported to benefit mothers during the first six months after a perinatal loss (Giles, 1970; Kennell et al., 1970; Parkes, 1980; Forrest et al., 1981, 1982). No data are, however, available on the long-term impact of these interventions, and no randomized trials have assessed the benefits of specific interventions (Chambers and Chan, 2000). Long-term (one to five years), prospective studies of parents who have received different interventions are needed. They should be stratified by fetal or neonatal diagnosis, reproductive history, and socioeconomic status and cultural characteristics. (See also the discussion below of directions for bereavement research.)

In addition to understanding parental experience with lethal or potentially lethal perinatal diagnosis or death, research attention also should extend to siblings subjected to the stress of perinatal loss and to the grief and parental chaos prompted by such loss. The committee located no longitudinal studies of parental perceptions of surviving siblings, self-perceptions of surviving siblings, or interactions between parents and surviving or later-born siblings.

Although the sensitivity and specificity of antenatal ultrasound diagnosis have been carefully defined (see, e.g., Sabbagha et al., 1985; Brocks and Bang, 1991; Chitty et al., 1991; Ewigman et al., 1993), little research (e.g., Cox et al., 1987; Michelacci et al., 1988; Cromie, 2001) documents the short-term and long-term emotional stress on parents of antenatal ultrasound, including when the procedure leads to a diagnosis of a lethal or potentially lethal condition. More research has focused on prenatal genetic testing and choices about pregnancy termination (see, e.g., Vintzileos and Egan, 1995; Bergsjo and Villar, 1997; Malone et al., 2000; Rillstone and Hutchison, 2001). Given the ubiquitous use of ultrasound and the known impact of emotional stress on pregnancy outcome, prospective studies should evaluate the emotional cost of antenatal ultrasound and the emotional care provided by obstetricians following ultrasound diagnosis of a lethal condition.

Research Directions: Sudden and Unexpected Death

In addition to infant death, the other large contributor to death in childhood is injury, both unintentional and intentional. Despite the development of sophisticated emergency medical services capacities that each year benefit thousands of seriously ill or injured children and their families, little is known about key aspects of the care provided to children who die and their survivors or about the consequences for emergency care providers of their involvement in child deaths. Box 10.4 summarizes several directions for research on sudden and unexpected death, and Appendix F also discusses research needs.

Resuscitation

When resuscitation should be terminated in children who have experienced cardiopulmonary arrest (CPA) is a continual subject of research and debate in emergency medicine. Continued efforts to establish predictors of resuscitation outcomes for out-of-hospital pediatric CPA are warranted to guide prehospital and emergency department care. One particular controversy involves the use of high-dose epinephrine (HDE) following cardiopulmonary arrest in children. The value of this intervention is not supported by

---

BOX 10.4
Directions for Research on Sudden and Unexpected Death

• Identify predictors of mortality in children during resuscitation in prehospital and emergency department settings.
• Continue to evaluate the benefits and harms of resuscitation measures for children who have experienced prolonged hypoxic–ischemic injury.
• Continue to assess the short- and long-term effects on bereaved parents of being present during attempted resuscitation of a child.
• Investigate the association between acute, sudden, or unexpected death of a child and the development by parents or siblings of more severe grief responses. Consider factors (e.g., nature of the death itself, family characteristics, support offered by emergency personnel) that may affect responses.
• Evaluate the short- and long-term effects of Critical Incident Stress Management or other interventions to lessen stress and emotional trauma for emergency care providers in the short and long term.

clinical research, yet HDE remains a pharmacologic option (Callaham et al., 1992; Dieckmann and Vardis, 1995; Patterson, 1999; Young and Seidel, 1999; AHA, 2000a).

Transient return of spontaneous circulation following prolonged resuscitation can trigger a tumultuous series of events, including admission to the pediatric intensive care unit (PICU) and subsequent decisions about withdrawal of life support, declaration of brain death, and organ donation. Although these events add stress to an already overwhelmingly stressful situation, it is possible that the time spent in intensive care benefits some families, for example, by helping them believe everything possible has been done to save their child. The consequences for families and for clinicians of predictably unsuccessful resuscitation efforts deserve systematic attention.

Several institutional studies have investigated issues related to family presence during attempted resuscitation (see, e.g., Meyer et al., 1998; Guzzetta et al., 2000; Clark et al., 2001). They suggest that families generally favor having the choice and that they tend to report afterwards that being present was helpful. These studies were, however, small, often retrospective, and limited in scope. Nonetheless, emergency medicine professionals are increasingly accepting and even encouraging parental presence, not only during resuscitation in the emergency department but also during other critical care procedures (AHA, 2000a). Given the vulnerability of parents during these high-intensity, often unsuccessful interventions, it seems prudent to undertake additional systematic research on the bereavement outcomes and other consequences of parental presence policies and their implementation. Prospective studies could follow families from the discussion of presence during resuscitation through their decisions, the procedures, and the aftermath, with follow-up during bereavement. The committee did not investigate differences in institutional protocols for family presence (among institutions that allowed or encouraged it), but if different approaches characterize different phases of family experience (e.g., discussion, presence, immediate and later bereavement support), it would be helpful to compare the effects on families and on health care personnel involved.

Sudden Death, Care Outside the Hospital, and Family Support

Each year, before or after a child's sudden and expected death, thousands of families encounter emergency medical personnel, police, staff of medical examiners' offices, and others who may positively support families in time of shock and grief—or whose behavior may unintentionally add to their pain and suffering. The committee identified little research on the aftermath of these encounters (see, e.g., Schmidt and Harrahill, 1995). Although it found examples of educational materials and policies intended to prepare these personnel to support survivors and avoid harm, the actual use and effectiveness of such materials and policies appears little investigated (Jaslow et al., 1997).

The committee recognizes that even retrospective, descriptive studies of the short-term and long-term effects on survivors of prehospital care may be costly and pose other practical and ethical challenges. Nonetheless, it encourages consideration of research on bereaved parents' and siblings' experiences and perceptions as a step toward identifying deficiencies in support and directions for improvement for personnel outside as well as inside the hospital. (Other questions about family experience following a child's sudden death are discussed in the section on bereavement research.)

Critical Incident Stress Management

Professionals who care for children who die suddenly and unexpectedly may also experience serious emotional distress. Critical Incident Stress Management (CISM) is a widely used strategy for providing acute psychological support for emergency medical services (EMS) and other public safety personnel involved in traumatic incidents such as child deaths, multiple deaths, and other especially difficult situations (Everly and Boyle, 1999; Everly, 2000; Lipton and Everly, 2002). Recent reviews of the literature on this strategy concluded that research tends to support the short-term effectiveness of certain critical incident debriefing approaches with emergency and other personnel involved in stressful incidents (Everly and Boyle, 1999; Everly and Mitchell, 2000). Research on long-term effects is limited. More research would be useful in assessing or clarifying the timing of interventions, the criteria for selecting personnel and situations for intervention, the consequences of different levels or types of training for those conducting the debriefings, and the interactions among complementary interventions.

Research Directions: Bereavement Care

As in other areas of bereavement research, the scientific basis for current practices with parents, siblings, or others following a child's death is limited (Stroebe et al., 1993, 2001b). Most studies are retrospective and relatively short term and suffer from the familiar limitations of late recall and abbreviated follow up. Research designs are also often inadequate in other ways (e.g., lack of control groups, small sample sizes), thus raising questions about the validity of the findings (Schut et al., 2001). One complication in intervention research is the relative (and fortunate) infrequency of child deaths in any single community. Possibly, Internet-based strategies can be explored as a means of involving larger numbers of family members.

> ## BOX 10.5
> ### Directions for Research on Bereavement Care
>
> - Develop appropriate, relevant, and culturally sensitive measures of grief and bereavement outcomes for parents, siblings, and the family as a unit.
> - Initiate prospective, long-term follow-up studies of bereaved families that begin before a child's death (when it can be anticipated) or immediately thereafter to help better understand common patterns and variations in bereavement and emotional reconstitution and to identify factors that put parents, siblings, and other family members at higher risk of complicated grief.
> - Clarify the criteria for diagnosing uncomplicated and complicated bereavement in parents and siblings (taking developmental stage into account).
> - Clarify the relationship between bereavement and posttraumatic stress disorder following a child's sudden and unexpected death and the implications for bereavement interventions.
> - Identify consequences for bereavement (parent, sibling, other) and the implications for bereavement interventions of (1) site of death; (2) cause of death (e.g., trauma, prematurity, chronic condition); (3) age, developmental status, and birth order of the child who dies; (4) age of parents and age, developmental status, and birth order of siblings; (5) family presence at the time of death and immediately after; (6) parental decisions about curative efforts, life-support interventions, and hospice or other end-of-life care; and (7) behavior of the child's care teams before, at the time of, and after death.
> - Evaluate different bereavement interventions, especially immediate interventions, to mitigate the trauma experienced by families and others following a child's sudden, violent death.
> - Examine the impact on bereavement of parents' and siblings' attributions of the cause of death (e.g., random fate, God's will, one's own or somebody else's fault).
> - Investigate the role of spirituality (as defined by individuals) in bereavement.

The discussions above of perinatal and sudden death have already suggested directions for bereavement research in these areas. Box 10.5 lists additional areas for investigation, including continued refinement of tools for measuring grief and bereavement.

The committee sees a pressing need to develop prospective research that studies over many years the experiences of parents, siblings, and other family members during a child's life-threatening illness and after a child's death (whether sudden or anticipated). Such research should help increase understanding of variations in grief and bereavement experiences, including patterns of complicated bereavement and associated risk and protective factors. Prospective research likewise may increase understanding of parents' willingness or reluctance to participate in bereavement support groups and seek other mental health services for themselves or for their surviving children.

Research also should consider the impact of a child's death as it affects not only parents and siblings individually but also as it affects the parents as a couple, the family as a unit, the extended family, and the family's larger network of support. Measures applicable to individuals (e.g., psychological symptoms) will not necessarily apply to the family unit, and measures of functioning will appropriately vary for parents, young siblings, adolescents, grandparents, and other family members.

As part of a research strategy, the concept of complicated grief or bereavement needs further attention, as do criteria for identifying complicated grief in bereaved parents and siblings. Complicated bereavement has been proposed as a specific mental disorder but is not yet accepted as a diagnostic category (Prigerson and Jacobs, 2001).

The sudden, unexpected death of a child may create symptoms similar to posttraumatic stress disorder in perhaps one-third of surviving family members (Peebles-Kleiger, 2000).[4] The experience of posttraumatic stress after a child's death requires continued investigation, as does the relationship of this stress to complicated bereavement. A better understanding is necessary of the characteristics of individuals (e.g., gender) and situations (e.g., death by homicide, family dysfunction) that are associated with more severe distress or differences in responses. This will help in identifying high-

---

[4]As set forth in the guide for diagnosing mental disorders (*Diagnostic and Statistical Manual of Mental Disorders*, Fourth Edition [DSM-IV], American Psychological Association, 1994), the criteria for diagnosing PTSD include

1. Exposure to a traumatic event with both of the following elements: experiencing, witnessing, or being confronted with an event involving actual or threatened death or serious injury or a threat to the physical integrity of oneself or another *and* responding with intense fear, helplessness, or horror;

2. Persistent reexperience of the event, for example, in recurrent, intrusive, and upsetting recollections or dreams, in the sense that the event is happening again, or in intense reactions to cues that symbolize or are similar to the event;

3. Persistent avoidance of reminders of the traumatic event as demonstrated by three or more of the following: efforts to avoid thoughts, feelings, or conversations associated with the trauma; efforts to avoid activities, places, or people that arouse recollections of the trauma; inability to remember key aspects of the event; feelings of detachment or estrangement; significantly reduced interest or participation in activities; restricted range of emotions (e.g., to feel love); or sense of a limited future (e.g., loss of expectations related to job, family, life span); and

4. Persistent, new symptoms of increased arousal including at least two of the following: trouble sleeping; irritability or anger, difficulties concentrating; hypervigilance and exaggerated startle responses; duration of symptoms for more than one month; or clinically significant distress or impairment in social, occupational, or other important functioning.

risk individuals in advance for special attention and support and in tailoring strategies to individuals.

More generally, the development of effective interventions depends on better knowledge of the range of reactions to the sudden death of a child and of the factors related to similarities and differences in bereavement experiences and outcomes in parents, siblings, and other family members. Do the same risk and protective factors pertain to adults and children? Some commonly identified or hypothesized risk factors include deaths that are violent, self-inflicted, publicized, or linked to a broader catastrophic event. Hypothesized protective factors include stronger immediate and extended family relationships, relative economic security, religious faith, and absence of past traumatic losses. Research suggests men and women grieve differently. Do they differ otherwise in risk and protective factors?

When death is anticipated, are there factors that predict different outcomes, for example, continuity in relationships with the child's physician or other caregivers, timely and accurate information, or access to psychosocial support services? The research by Wolfe and colleagues (2000a,b, 2001) discussed in Chapter 3 suggests some lines of inquiry. Ideally, these could be pursued using methods that do not depend entirely on after-death interviews with parents. In practice, as discussed elsewhere in this chapter, concurrent collection of information about end-of-life care for children is difficult because the timing of death is often uncertain and because interviews with children or parents during the child's last days or weeks may be unacceptable or infeasible.

Research Directions: Models of Care Delivery

The committee identified a critical need for more systematic information on the organization, delivery, and outcomes of care for children with life-threatening conditions and their families (Box 10.6). After considering written statements from advocacy groups, discussions with parents, research and other literature, and professional experience, the committee identified several consistent themes: confusion about available resources and their quality, fragmentation of services with consequent lack of coordination and continuity of care, uneven and limited access to valued services, and deficits in communication, symptom management, and bereavement care in organizations that care for children with fatal or potentially fatal conditions. The very availability of key services is not well documented. For example, despite the increasing availability of useful information on the Internet, families cannot easily and reliably discover whether a children's hospital has palliative care or pain management teams or which hospices have well-established pediatric programs—much less how that program performs in meeting child and family needs.

BOX 10.6
Directions for Research on Models of Care Delivery

• Identify and describe existing organizations or programs that offer pediatric palliative, end-of-life, and bereavement care, and delineate models of such care, including hospice/hospital partnerships, hospice/home health agency partnerships, inpatient consulting, and direct care programs.

• Conduct community-based case studies of the coordination and continuity of care experienced by children and families and the institutional and other factors associated with more and less positive experiences.

• Describe and assess current processes of care and outcomes (e.g., symptom control, satisfaction with care, preparation for death) in inpatient and home settings.

• Study and compare different modes of communicating with children and families about the diagnosis of a life-threatening illness, prognosis, treatment options (including palliative and end-of-life care), and related issues.

• Define and test strategies for improving coordination and continuity of care including interdisciplinary team care for children with advanced illness.

• Investigate innovative methods to support children, families, and providers in smaller communities and rural areas and promote continuity of local and regional specialty care including palliative, and end-of-life care.

Developing the research base for organizational and system improvement is perhaps the most difficult research challenge identified by the committee. Such research tends to be practically and methodologically difficult, expensive, and not a priority for clinicians, health care managers, or research funders. Recognizing these obstacles, the committee proposes an incremental research strategy that includes both the identification and description of innovative programs and the evaluation of these strategies within and across institutions and settings.

Collecting data on the availability and characteristics of pediatric palliative and hospice care programs is one important step. Another is community-based case studies that describe child and family experiences with care coordination and continuity. Such case studies should help researchers to develop and refine hypotheses about factors that support or discourage coordination and continuity for families receiving services from multiple professionals and providers. Interviews with parents, patients, social workers, and others can generate useful information, but case studies will provide a fuller picture and help refine questions for further investigation.

Concurrently with descriptive research must come the most important step: the definition and testing of discrete, innovative care processes and broader models of palliative, end-of-life, and bereavement care. (For purposes of this discussion, processes of care include activities focused on specific tasks or goals such as symptom assessment and documentation of discussions with parents; models of care include more comprehensive arrangements such as inpatient palliative care consultation services or inpatient hospice units.) Such evaluative research would, ideally, consider outcomes for children (e.g., levels of pain or anxiety, quality of life, continuity of care), families (e.g., satisfaction with care, understanding of diagnosis, prognosis, and treatment options), and providers (e.g., rates of specific problems such as unassessed symptoms).

Given the complexity and expense of organizing multi-site studies, especially in newer areas of investigation, evaluations will often focus on processes and models of care at single sites. Although generalization from single-site studies must be undertaken cautiously, controlled trials and other comparative studies within single institutions can help in the identification of more and less effective ways of providing care. One creative example is the small, randomized controlled trial, mentioned in Chapter 6, of a program providing parents of hospitalized premature infants with an interactive link with the neonatal intensive care unit and also Internet access to other resources.

Notwithstanding the challenges, multi-site, comparative studies are important to replicate and test the robustness of care models in different environments. If, as recommended earlier in this chapter, the NIH promoted research on palliative and end-of-life care based in pediatric cancer centers, neonatal network participants, and similar networks, this could facilitate comparative organizational as well as clinical studies.

Even multi-site studies that are not formally comparative may be a useful step in the development of systematic research initiatives. For example, although not comparative in design, the federally supported Medicaid demonstration projects described earlier in this report should provide individual evaluations of several home care and hospice models and suggest ideas for further investigation. Similarly, although focused primarily on adult care, the quality improvement initiative reported by Lynn and colleagues (2000) suggests opportunities for formal research to improve palliative and end-of-life care for children as well as adults (see Chapter 6).[5] For

---

[5]The quality improvement strategies described usually involved the testing of specific, focused organizational changes with small groups of patients during a relatively short period using existing information systems insofar as possible. Based on the results, a change might be abandoned or expanded or considered for more formal comparative research. An important practical difference between quality improvement projects and formal research is that the latter must meet requirements for the protection of human subjects—including special requirements for children—and obtain approval from Institutional Review Boards as described later in this chapter. When CQI projects should be considered research and be reviewed by IRBs is a topic of debate (see, e.g., Casarett et al., 2000, and comments and discussion by Cretin et al., 2000, and Hayley, 2000).

example, studies might compare the outcomes of different processes and structures for assessing, documenting, and managing pain and other symptoms, or they might test different procedures to improve the discussion, documentation, and implementation of care plans for children.

More generally, the research reviewed in Chapter 3 and the ideas and programs described in Chapters 4, 5, and 6 can suggest topics for organizational research into processes and models of care. For example, it would be useful to have additional research comparing outcomes for children and families associated with early versus late discussion of hospice or other options for care at the end-of-life.

Outcome and Performance Measures

One critical issue in organizational research is how to measure performance. For example, to what degree should investigators rely on assessments of patient or family satisfaction with care as indicators of the quality of care? Given the literature it reviewed and members' own experiences, the committee is concerned that families may greatly appreciate the care provided to their children without realizing that more could have been done, for example, to treat a child's pain effectively.

Thus, although it is appropriate to inquire about parents' satisfaction with the care provided to their child and their family and about the help they had making decisions, it is also important to inquire about what the child and family experienced and to continue efforts to develop and use other measures. These measures include valid, reliable, and feasible instruments for assessing physical and psychological symptoms and quality of life. (See also Appendix C and Box 10.1.)

Information and Communication

This report, consistent with other discussions of care for patients with life-threatening medical conditions, stresses the importance of timely and accurate information and communication geared to child and family needs and circumstances. Most studies of communication in this area have focused on adult patients and their families, but many of the findings about barriers to effective communication have broad relevance for child patients and their families.

This committee has stressed the importance of involving children in discussions and decisions about their care, consistent with their development stage and preferences and with sensitivity to family culture and values.

To further such involvement, strategies for communicating with seriously ill children need further systematic investigation. As discussed in Chapter 4, most of what has been written about children's understanding of death involves well children. Because children with advanced illness may have awareness and knowledge beyond their years, findings from studies of communication strategies involving well children need to be used with some caution. Rigorous research on communication with children made vulnerable by serious illness may raise ethical and practical challenges, but if carefully planned, reviewed, and conducted, it has the potential to help the research participants as well as children who follow them.

One persistent theme in statements of parents who have faced a child's life-threatening illness is that shock, fear, and grief interfere with their ability to absorb and process information during initial and subsequent conversations with clinicians. Little or no systematic research is available to guide the timing, pace, or style of communication with these parents. One example of research underway in this area is the PAICC project mentioned earlier. It asks parents about the value and timeliness of information provided through a written manual for parents and other means. The plan is to have 20 parents evaluate the material, revise the manual with that feedback, and proceed again with another cohort of 20 parents.

The usefulness of specific modes of communication with children and parents may vary depending on the purpose of the communication (e.g., giving bad news, developing care objectives and plans), the type of information to be communicated (e.g., medical, administrative), the recipient (e.g., young versus older child), the opportunity for repeated reference to the information, and other factors. Structured, face-to-face communication appears essential for some purposes, but other strategies including written materials, graphics, videos, and Internet-based tools may reinforce such communication and, for some purposes, substitute for it. These expectations are reasonable but should be further investigated.

Interdisciplinary Care Teams

Despite their seeming ubiquity and this committee's judgment of their importance, little rigorous research appears to have focused on the prevalence or functioning of different kinds of pediatric or adult palliative care teams or to have identified factors associated with more or less effective team performance in different contexts. Such systematic research as was identified by the committee focused primarily on primary care and chronic illness care (often as an element of primary care) (see e.g., Campbell et al.,

2001; Barrett et al., 2001; Roy-Byrne et al., 2001; Rost et al., 2000; but see also Shortell et al., 1994 on intensive care teams).[6] Team care is, however, often a part of a multi-element intervention in which the individual structural elements or processes are not separately evaluated.[7]

Although problems in coordination and continuity often arise when multiple providers (e.g., hospitals, home care agencies) are involved in a child's care, problems also arise within single organizations (e.g., as shifts change or clinicians from different disciplines interact with parents). As a starting point, it would be helpful to have more systematic information on the structure, composition, environment, and functioning of the lead care teams for children with life-threatening medical conditions and the characteristics of teams associated with better coordination and continuity for the dimensions of care identified in Chapters 4 and 5. In addition, an important question for pediatric palliative and end-of-life care is how care teams relate to each other during transitions in care (e.g., from inpatient to home hospice care) or when additional expertise (e.g., palliative care consultations) is needed.

Regional Programs

As discussed in Chapter 6, access to expertise in pediatric palliative care is limited by geography. Some children who die will be cared for through the end of life at specialized regional centers, but families will take other children home to be cared for by family members and local pediatricians and community hospitals that have limited preparation for and experience in providing palliative and end-of-life care. In Chapter 6, the committee

---

[6]Some relevant research may be categorized under related concepts or objectives such as care coordination or quality improvement. For example, team care is often associated with the use of formal clinical practice guidelines and quality improvement initiatives, and some studies suggest problems in the team care component of such initiatives, for example, staff turnover, physical separation, and responsibilities outside the team (Weissman et al., 1997; Hayward et al, 2000; see also Campbell E. et al., 1998).

[7]Some research has focused on the contributions or acceptance of specific categories of professionals (e.g., nurse practitioners, social workers, or genetic counselors) in different environments (see, e.g., Burl et al., 1994; Aquilino et al., 1999; Inati et al., 1994). Research not specifically focused on the effectiveness of multidisciplinary teams has pointed to potential problems for team functioning arising from differences in the views of physicians and nurses about what constitutes clinically or ethically appropriate care at the end of life (see Chapter 3). In its call for grant applications on quality of life for individuals at the end of life, the National Institute of Nursing Research mentioned "multidisciplinary interventions" and noted that research is need to support care systems that include multidisciplinary teams (NIH, 2000).

recommended strategies for supporting these professionals and organizations, including written protocols, family guides, and various forms of telemedicine. The federal government has supported research to investigate the potential of telemedicine to improve care for rural populations, including people receiving care at home for serious chronic illness. (See, e.g., Office for the Advancement of Telehealth at http://telehealth. hrsa.gov.) Although limited, this research can provide a foundation for studies related to pediatric palliative and end-of-life care specifically.

Research Directions: Financing Pediatric Palliative and End-of-Life Care

Chapter 7 has made clear that few systematic data are available to describe the financing of palliative and end-of-life care for children, much less evaluate systematically the effects of different financing policies or practices on that care. Thus, the committee's conclusions and recommendations about financing are based primarily on logic, experience, value judgments, and cautious generalization from studies involving adults. Although the committee believes it is appropriate to move to implement the recommendations, it also recognizes that further research and analysis are important to guide certain changes in financing policies and practices (Box 10.7).

Descriptive Research

More complete descriptive research on financing practices would help providers, managers, and policymakers better understand how care for children who die and their families is financed and how the situation for children differs from that for adults. The first steps should include a state-by-state inventory of variations in Medicaid coverage and reimbursement policies related to the elements of pediatric palliative and end-of-life care discussed in Chapter 7. Although a complete inventory is not feasible for private health plans given their large number, coverage and payment policies should be surveyed for a subset of representative plans or communities.

Next steps should also include some assessment of the extent to which written policies (including early periodic screening, detection, and treatment [EPSDT] policies) match implementation (e.g., whether claims administrators often deny claims for hospice and palliative services covered for children but not adult Medicaid beneficiaries). To be manageable, such an assessment might cover only a subset of states using a survey or case studies or both. Once the descriptive foundation is in place, the next step is to assess the impact of different coverage policies and reimbursement methods on cost, access, and quality of care for children who die and their families.

BOX 10.7
Directions for Research on Financing of Palliative, End-of-Life, and Bereavement Care

• Document variation in state Medicaid and private insurance coverage and reimbursement policies regarding pediatric palliative, end-of-life, and bereavement care:
—Survey and inventory all state Medicaid programs.
—Survey a representative sample of private insurance plans.
—Assess the extent to which written policies match their implementation (e.g., determinations about actual claims for physician, hospice, or home health services).
• Examine the effects of different Medicaid and private insurance coverage and reimbursement policies on access, cost and quality of care.
• Conduct studies to assess the appropriateness for pediatric populations of payment and coding systems created for adult populations (e.g., diagnosis-related groups, resource-based relative value scales)
• Develop diagnosis and severity-of-illness criteria for establishing eligibility for expanded pediatric hospice and palliative care benefits.
• Conduct prospective studies of palliative and end-of-life care to identify and compare costs associated with different care settings and specific interventions.
• Assess hospice access pathways (i.e., hospice referral patterns, characteristics of populations denied access, comparisons of costs and outcomes) and factors influencing those pathways.
• Assess the extent of diffusion of Medicare prospective payment methods for home health care to Medicaid and private insurance plans and the effects on quality of care and family burden.
• Develop a Medicaid hospice cost-reporting system to use in creating a hospice payment outlier system and for research on utilization and costs of hospice care.
• Develop simulation models as research tools that will assist in the estimation of cost and utilization effects of implementing changes in palliative care, end-of-life care, and bereavement benefits. (Note: This research development is dependent on recommendation to create a national data resource on palliative and end-of-life care.)

Payment, Coding, and Severity of Illness Systems or Measures

A number of Medicaid and private health plans have adopted or adapted payment and coding systems originally devised for Medicare (i.e., diagnosis-related groups [DRGs] for hospital care and the resource-based relative value scale [RBRVS] for physician care). Researchers and child health advocates have raised several concerns about the application of these schemes to children, as described in Chapter 7. Further studies are needed to examine whether state and private reimbursement systems based on

DRGs or the RBRVS properly categorize and weigh palliative and end-of-life services for children. Such research could also identify possible adjustments in these systems to correct any problems identified.

Chapter 7 made general suggestions about establishing children's eligibility for certain types of palliative services using diagnosis and severity-of-illness criteria. Analytic work is needed to identify reliable and valid approaches for establishing such criteria for payment purposes and to assess their feasibility, cost implications, and likely consequences for child and family access to palliative care.

Hospice

As discussed in Chapter 7, studies of hospice care for adults have identified serious limitations in Medicare's per diem payments for that care. For example, studies have documented hospice access problems for adult patients with particularly high-cost needs (e.g., those requiring expensive pain medications or other palliative therapies). Research is needed to document the extent of hospice access problems for pediatric patients, examine hospice referral patterns, and identify characteristics of patients who are denied access. To explore these issues, prospective studies using existing clinical networks (e.g., the Children's Oncology Group) for patient identification should be conducted.

In order to implement a payment outlier system for hospices (recommended by the committee in Chapter 7) and to facilitate research on utilization and costs of hospice care for adult and pediatric patients, a Medicaid hospice cost-reporting system should be created. Since many hospices do not currently maintain detailed data on number of hours or types of services provided by staff, Medicaid could begin by creating a cost-reporting system based on high-cost items that hospices are more likely to track (e.g., expensive medications, durable medical equipment).

Prospective Payment for Home Health Care

Because Medicare policies often influence state and private policies, studies are needed to examine how new Medicare prospective payments systems for home health care and other services have diffused to state Medicaid programs and private health plans and how these systems are affecting care for children with life-threatening medical conditions. A first phase of research would involve surveying Medicaid and private plans to assess their adoption of Medicare reimbursement methods. A second phase would investigate the impact of these payment approaches on family burden and quality of care for Medicaid-covered children.

Cost Implications of Family Choices

For reasons discussed earlier in this report, families should have choices about the site of death for children with fatal medical problems. To assess the cost implications of these choices, prospective studies are needed to identify and compare the costs of different home and inpatient care options for children expected to die from congenital anomalies, cancers, progressive neurological disorders, and other serious conditions. Existing studies based on Medicare beneficiaries' use of hospice care cannot be generalized to children and are, in any case, flawed by retrospective research designs that cannot control for selection bias (i.e., differences in preferences and other characteristics of those who choose hospice care).

Although the committee expects that the financing changes recommended in Chapter 7 will involve limited additional costs for the benefits expected, a simulation model would assist in estimating the cost and utilization effects of implementing different options. For example, the cost of eliminating the six-month prognosis requirement could be estimated.

Finally, as noted elsewhere in this chapter, long-term prospective research is needed to evaluate the effectiveness of bereavement interventions for parents and siblings. The estimated costs and long-term cost-effectiveness of alternative interventions should also be investigated if such studies are undertaken.

Research Directions: Educating Health Professionals

Despite several decades of research on methods for educating health care professionals, much uncertainty remains about methods that can be consistently applied to produce changes in knowledge and practice, especially changes that endure beyond the classroom or the continuing education program. One challenge for educators is that the knowledge, values, and actions they teach are not uniformly rewarded or reinforced in day-to-day practice.

Educational research is not always valued within academic departments or by research funders. Long-term follow-up of educational outcomes, in particular, tends to be expensive and logistically complicated. Nonetheless, given the huge investments in preparing health professionals for practice, research is essential to identify the effectiveness of different educational techniques and emphases in creating desired changes in knowledge, skills, attitudes, and especially, behaviors.

The committee expects that much research involving education in pediatric care, adult palliative care, and generally relevant attitudes or skills (e.g., empathy, interviewing patients) would be generalizable to education in pediatric palliative care. Nonetheless, in developing curricula or interventions for pediatric specialists in training or for established pediatric specialists, revisions or adjustments will have to be considered and evaluated to take into account the special emotional and other dimensions of caring for dying children and their families. For example, as discussed in Chapter 8, the use of standardized patients is now a common educational tool, but using child actors or volunteers to depict dying children might encounter practical and ethical obstacles. Standardized families can be used, and systematic research into the effectiveness of this strategy—and of different variants—would be helpful. The projects by Williams and colleagues (2001b, 2002) and Greenberg and colleagues (1993) discussed in Chapter 9 offer examples of how such standardized families might be used to improve skills in communicating bad news and informing family decisionmaking.

Box 10.8 lists several directions for educational research. The involvement of bereaved parents in educational programs should be investigated, both for its impact on trainees and for the consequences for the parents. Conversations with bereaved parents suggest that some have found consolation and strength in presenting their experiences and perspectives, answering questions, and otherwise helping to educate both clinicians-in-training and established clinicians. Self-selection of the most confident or educated parents is, however, a potential concern and should be taken into account in any research about the role of parents as educators.

Because it will take years for newly educated health professionals to dominate health care systems by numbers or other influence, it is important

---

BOX 10.8
Directions for Research on Educating Health Care Professionals

- Investigate the participation of bereaved parents in educational programs at all levels.
- Identify characteristics of pediatric care systems (e.g., inpatient hospice programs, links to hospice agencies) that promote and reinforce lessons learned about palliative and end-of-life care in all educational contexts, including continuing education.
- Establish priorities and strategies for research on the short-term and long-term effects of education to prepare health care professionals to work in interdisciplinary teams.
- Assess strategies to improve symptom management and increase professionals' awareness of how well their assessments and performance match the experiences and expectations of patients and family members.
- Assess educational strategies to improve physician comfort and skill in compassionately providing patients and families with accurate and complete information about diagnosis, prognosis, and treatment options (including palliative care).

to examine continuing education in pediatric palliative care for established clinicians. Further, research is needed to identify characteristics of pediatric care systems that promote and reinforce lessons learned about palliative and end-of-life care in all educational contexts. As noted above, without reinforcement, educational interventions may manage to create desired short-term results but fail to produce durable changes. Research questions include whether education programs are more effective when institutions have formal relationships with hospices, formal pediatric palliative care consultation programs, formal adult inpatient palliative care services (for institutions serving adults and children), or identified palliative care role models and educators.

This report has stressed the importance of team care to bring multiple clinical perspectives and skills to bear on the complex physical, emotional, spiritual, and practical needs of seriously ill or injured children and families. In addition to research on the performance of pediatric teams in different environments and contexts (including providing palliative, end-of-life, and bereavement care in hospitals or at home), research also should assess methods for successfully educating physicians, nurses, social workers, and others to function as effective members of health care teams.

Also stressed in this report is the importance of adequate and timely information for patients and families. As reviewed in Chapters 3 and 4, studies have suggested that clinicians may be reluctant to provide such information when the diagnosis and prognosis are grim. One study (Lamont and Christakis, 2001) suggested that clinicians may provide patients and families with misleadingly optimistic assessments and that younger adult patients were more likely to receive such misleading assessments than older adults. Another study involving physicians caring for adults found that they dreaded explicit discussion of patient prognosis, usually were not specific, and often waited until parents or families raised the issue (Christakis and Iwashyna, 1998). Other studies of adult and pediatric palliative care have identified discrepancies between physician assessments of care and the assessments of patients or family members (see, e.g., Wolfe et al., 2000b).

A variety of educational interventions—for example, role playing, standardized patients who provide feedback, and parents as teachers—could potentially promote greater clinician self-awareness and more explicit concern for the actual experiences and expectations of patients and family members. Studies of efforts to teach empathy that were conducted in the 1970s suggest strategies to assess and compare such educational interventions (Fine and Therrien, 1977; see also Spiro, 1992; Reiser, 1996; Halpern, 2001).

Finally, the development and evaluation of educational techniques to improve the use of proven symptom management strategies are important if their benefits are to reach children in need. In particular, although cognitive and behavioral strategies have demonstrated effectiveness in reducing pain and improving coping, teaching of these techniques to clinicians generally appears to lack the rigor and uniformity that characterize other clinical domains.

CHALLENGES OF RESEARCH ON PALLIATIVE AND END-OF-LIFE CARE FOR CHILDREN AND THEIR FAMILES

The paucity of information about palliative and end-of-life care for children and their families has several explanations. Although over 50,000 children die each year, many of these deaths result from severe injuries or sudden infant death syndrome (SIDS). The medical care actually provided to or consciously experienced by these children is limited compared to that of children with chronic medical conditions. For surviving family members, interactions with emergency medical personnel (particularly first responders) or ICU personnel are often relatively brief and poorly documented, which makes it difficult for researchers to use medical records retrospectively to assess the extent and quality of the information and emotional support provided to survivors.

Particularly for deaths involving infants and very young children, a considerable fraction of deaths result from an array of relatively or very uncommon congenital conditions. Even over several years and across multiple medical centers, it may be difficult to identify enough cases for each condition to allow productive prospective or retrospective analyses of the patterns and quality of palliative and end-of-life care for these children and their families. Combining information about children with different conditions may sometimes be a plausible strategy if the symptoms and other characteristics of each condition and the consequences for the children and families are similar. Nonetheless, accumulating enough cases for analysis may still take years.

Even when numbers are sufficient for study, however, retrospective analyses of medical records may be constrained by failures to document relevant aspects of care, for example, whether or not pain and other symptoms were explicitly assessed. Such lack of documentation, in itself, is an important finding with implications for day-to-day clinical practice and quality improvement efforts.

Another constraint is that although Medicare-related databases offer much comprehensive information about the types and costs of care provided to elderly adults, no comparable information is available for younger individuals covered by the 50-plus state Medicaid programs and thousands of private insurance plans. Other information sources, such as government surveys of home health and hospice agencies, may not include enough children to allow meaningful analyses.

Despite many differences, researchers studying end-of-life care and researchers studying children share a common challenge: their subjects are often unable to report directly on the care they have received or on their physical or emotional distress or well-being. Even for children old enough to report reliably, the effects of a life-threatening medical problem or its treatment may render them unconscious, confused, drowsy, fatigued, or otherwise not able to answer questions. As a result, researchers frequently rely on surrogates—usually the parents—to describe their perceptions of the patient's experience and quality of life (see Appendix C). Also, because the time of death is often unpredictable, researchers may be unable to assess patients' status at comparable points before death and may have to rely on the recollections of surrogates about a patient's status during the days, weeks, or months prior to death (see, e.g., Wolfe et al., 2000a,b). Nonetheless, surrogate reports and retrospective reports raise serious questions of validity and reliability, and researchers and research funders should consider alternatives whenever possible.

Another challenge is that research funders, who are accustomed to more stable research situations, measurement tools, clinical end points (e.g., remission, five-year survival), and already-conducted pilot testing, may be reluctant to support research that does not fit these patterns. In the committee's experience, they are also reluctant to fund the kinds of pilot studies that provide an essential base for more rigorous research. This puts researchers in this new and difficult arena in a classic "Catch-22" situation.

In addition, the conduct of medical or health services research involving children faces more stringent ethical and legal constraints than apply to research involving most adults. These are discussed below.

ETHICAL AND LEGAL ISSUES IN
RESEARCH INVOLVING CHILDREN

Policymakers, researchers, and ethicists have been working for decades to develop protections for people participating in research, especially "vulnerable" populations including children, prisoners, and those with serious cognitive or emotional problems. The first widely recognized principles for ethical research were the Nuremberg Code's directives for human experimentation, which were developed in 1947 by judges presiding over the trials of Nazi physicians accused of research atrocities (Shuster, 1997). These judges developed 10 principles for research, the first of which stated that it is absolutely essential that human subjects voluntarily consent to participation. The statement did not consider the involvement of children in research.

The 1964 Declaration of Helsinki from the World Medical Association called for parents of child participants in research to give their consent and for children's "assent" to be obtained when possible (WMA, 1964). In the United States, a national commission on protection of human subjects in research likewise proposed in 1977 that parental permission be required as well as assent in some form from children age 7 and over (USDHEW, 1977). Subsequent books, articles, and conferences have continued to explore ethical issues involved in research on children, the boundaries of permissible research, and strategies for protecting child research subjects (see, e.g., Stanley and Sieber, 1992; Grodin and Glantz, 1994; AAP, 1995a; Levine, 1995; Rosato, 2000).

If conducting research presents ethical questions, so does the *failure* to conduct research. As noted by the American Academy of Pediatrics in a statement on drug research, the "lack of studies in children presents the treating physician with an ethical dilemma. The physician must frequently either not treat children with potentially beneficial medications or treat them with medications based on adult studies or anecdotal empirical experience in children" (AAP, 1995a, p. 286).

Federally Funded Research

As set forth in Box 10.9, federal regulations adopted in 1983 and revised in 1991 set forth requirements related to children's participation as subjects of federally funded research (45 CFR 46; USDHSS, 1993). The regulations also provided for institutional review boards (IRBs) to be established by each research institution to review federally funded research that involves human subjects and determine whether proposed research meets federal standards.

Although the regulations and accompanying federal guidance encourage respect for a child's views about participating in research, they make clear that a research project may be approved without requiring that each child provide assent before enrollment (45 CFR 46.408[a]). The IRB must conclude in such cases that the research has the potential to produce an important direct benefit to the child, that such benefit is possible only in the research context, and that provisions are adequate for obtaining informed permission from the child's parents for the research.

The regulations also require that research conform to state laws and judicial decisions including those related to the age of consent for medical treatment. If an adolescent is considered legally competent under state law to consent to treatment, he or she can usually consent to research presenting equivalent risk.

In some situations (e.g., for research on children who have been abused), researchers and the IRB may seek alternatives to or reviews of parental permission for a child's participation in research. If a child is a ward of the state, additional limitations are imposed on his or her participation in

**BOX 10.9
Categories of Research Involving Children That May Be
Approved for Federal Funding**

Research Involving No Greater Than Minimal Risk (46.404)

"The Institutional Review Board (IRB) must find that the research involves no greater than minimal risk to children and that adequate provisions are made for soliciting the assent of the children and the permission of their parents or guardians."

**Research Involving Greater Than Minimal Risk That Has Potential to
Benefit the Research Subjects Directly (46.405)**

"The IRB must find that more than minimal risk to children is presented by an
intervention and then must also find that (a) the research may directly benefit the
individual research subjects, (b) the anticipated benefit is sufficient to justify the
risk, (c) the relation of the benefit to the risk is equally or more favorable as that
presented by available nonresearch alternatives, and (d) adequate provisions are
made for soliciting the assent of the children and the permission of their parents or
guardians."

**Research Involving Greater Than Minimal Risk That Has No Prospect
of Direct Benefit to Individual Subjects but Is Likely to Yield
Generalizable Knowledge (46.406)**

"The IRB must find that more than minimal risk to children is presented by an
intervention that is not expected to benefit the individual subject directly but that (a)
the increased risk is minor, (b) the experiences associated with the intervention
are reasonably similar to those inherent in the subject's actual or expected medical
situation, (c) the intervention is likely to yield generalizable knowledge about the
subject's condition that is vitally important to understand or ameliorate the condition, and (d) adequate provisions are made for soliciting assent of the children and
the permission of their parents or guardians."

Research That Is Not Otherwise Approvable (46.407)

"The IRB must conclude that the research does not meet the above requirements
but does present a reasonable opportunity to further the understanding, prevention, or alleviation of a serious problem affecting the health or welfare of children.
The research must then be judged by the Secretary of the Department of Health
and Human Services (after consultation with appropriate experts and opportunity
for public review and comment) to fit one of the categories described above *or* to
meet the following conditions of (a) presenting a reasonable opportunity for better
understanding, preventing, or alleviating a serious problem affecting the health or
welfare of children, (b) following sound ethical principles for research, and (c) including adequate provisions for soliciting the assent of children and the permission
of their parents or guardians."

SOURCE: 45 CFR 46 Protection of Human Subjects, Additional Protections for Children Involved as Subjects in Research, Subpart D, Sections 401–409. 56 FR 28032, June 18, 1991
(http://www.med.umich.edu/irbmed/FederalDocuments/hhs/HHS45CFR46.html).

research when the research involves more than minimal risk with no prospect of direct benefit to the child. The research must either be related to children's status as wards or be conducted in settings such as hospitals or schools where the majority of child research participants are not wards of the state (45 CFR 46.409). Also, a special advocate (other than the guardian) must be appointed for a child participating in such research. The committee understands that some states refuse to permit wards of the state to participate in research, even if no alternative treatment exists for the child's life-threatening illness.

Explanations of the proposed research are to be appropriate for the specific child's age, maturity, experience, and medical condition. The National Cancer Institute provides guidance for parents and guardians, including advice that parents not withhold information about the discomforts or risks involved in research and that they monitor whether the child really seems to understand the explanations being provided (NCI, 2001c).

Based on members' experiences and their conversations with other researchers, the committee believes that many IRBs, as presently constituted, may lack the expertise and background to evaluate proposals for research on pediatric palliative and end-of-life care. They may have unwarranted concerns about the potential of such research to cause harm to children and families. As described below, Congress has asked for a study that will investigate the competence of IRBs to assess research involving children.

Some research should soon be available to document positive responses by families to studies investigating their experiences and perspectives (Wolfe, 2001). As noted in a recent report on family perspectives on the quality of pediatric palliative care, "The families who participated in our assessment unanimously expressed gratitude for the opportunity to 'tell their stories' " (Contro et al., 2002, p. 18). Researchers in that study reported, however, that 20 of 63 families they reached declined to participate because it would be too painful.

Privately Funded Research

The regulations described in the preceding section apply to federally funded research involving children. Pediatric drug research promoted by the Food and Drug Administration is generally funded by pharmaceutical companies. As directed by Congress in the Children's Health Act of 2000, the FDA must apply Department of Health and Human Services requirements for federally funded research that involves children to privately funded studies of products regulated by the FDA. (The agency had long required IRB review of drug research submitted to it by private companies [Levine, 1988].)

In April 1, 2001, the FDA issued an interim rule to change its regulations accordingly (21 CFR 50 and 56; FDA, 2001a). The agency invited comment on several issues including children's participation in placebo-controlled trials, the definition of what constitutes a "minor increase over minimal risk" (and ways of measuring minor risk and determining when a minimal risk becomes a major risk), and ways to provide age-appropriate explanations of research to children.

The interim rule differs from the regulations governing federally funded research in certain respects. For research in the "not otherwise approvable" category (see Box 10.8) that is referred to the commissioner of the FDA for consideration, the agency may not be able to offer public review and comment if the research sponsor is unwilling to make public necessary information that is privileged under other FDA requirements.

Research that is neither federally funded nor conducted under the FDA provisions described earlier may be covered by state regulations and institutional policies requiring review of all research undertaken by its employees or students. In general, IRBs apply the same criteria to research proposals without reference to the source of funding.

Continuing Concerns about Children's Participation in Research

Policies about children's participation in research continue to prompt debate. The major issues involve

- the appropriateness of current regulations for children of different ages or intellectual and emotional maturity,
- the ethics of including children and other vulnerable subjects in research that is not expected to benefit these subjects directly,
- the definition of minimal risk,
- the extent of children's and adolescents' comprehension of information about the risks and benefits of treatments and participation in research,
- the potential for conflict between parent and child and the meaningfulness of "assent" or discussions about assent with a child when parents can override the child's wishes, and
- the performance of IRBs in evaluating research involving children.

The legislation reauthorizing the incentives for pediatric drug testing provided for an Institute of Medicine study to examine such issues and review federal regulations relating to research involving children. The results of this report are to be given to Congress by the close of 2003.

CONCLUSION

This chapter has proposed a range of research efforts to strengthen the very limited base of knowledge now available to guide those providing, organizing, financing, and monitoring palliative, end-of-life, and bereavement care for children and families. It has recommended strategies to promote relevant research in federally funded pediatric centers, networks, and similar structures. The intent is to increase the numbers of children and families involved in studies, encourage the development and use of common research methods, and increase the credibility and acceptance of the research findings.

The research directions proposed here focus on children who have conditions that are certain or likely to prove fatal, but investigation of some of the suggested research questions may involve participation by children who survive and their families. In some cases, such participation will reflect the unpredictability of certain life-threatening conditions and the requirements of prospective research designs. In other cases, it will reflect a focus on questions that affect the well being of children and families facing a life-threatening problem, whether or not that problem actually ends in death. In either case, when it is appropriate, including a larger group of children usually has methodological advantages.

Much of the research proposed here thus should provide knowledge that will inform and improve the care of children who survive as well as those who do not—and likewise will help every family that suffers with a seriously ill or injured child. Indeed, all of the recommendations in this report, if implemented, should help create a care system that all children and families can trust to provide capable, compassionate, and reliable care when they are in need.

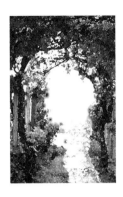

REFERENCES

AACCN (American Association of Critical-Care Nurses). 2001 (September 8). Written statement to the IOM committee on improving palliative and end-of-life care for children and their families, Washington, DC.

AACN (American Association of Colleges of Nursing). 1998. Peaceful Death: Recommended Competencies and Curricular Guidelines for End-of-Life Nursing Care. [Online]. Available: http://www.aacn.nche.edu/Publications/deathfin.htm [accessed March 31, 2002].

AACN. 2001 (September 24). Statement written by Geraldine Bednash to the IOM committee on improving palliative and end-of-life care for children and their families, Washington, DC.

AACN. 2002. End of Life Nursing Education Consortium. [Online]. Available: http://www.aacn.nche.edu/elnec [accessed March 31, 2002].

AAHPM (American Academy of Hospice and Palliative Medicine). 2000. UNIPACs. [Online]. Available: http://www.aahpm.org/unipac's.htm [accessed April 18, 2001].

AAHPM. 2001 (September 21). Statement written by Bruce P. Himelstein, Sarah Freiebert, Jeanne Lewandowski, Suzanne Toce, Kate Eastman, Dennis Johnson, and Javier Kane to the IOM committee on improving palliative and end-of-life care for children and their families, Washington, DC.

AAP (American Academy of Pediatrics). 1984. Guidelines for infant bioethics committees. *Pediatrics* 74(2):306–310.

AAP. 1987. Qualifications and utilization of nursing personnel delivering health services in schools. *Pediatrics* 79(4):647–648.

AAP. 1991. Guidelines for pediatric cardiology diagnostic and treatment centers. *Pediatrics* 87(4):576–580. [Online]. Available: http://www.aap.org/policy/03836.html [accessed March 31, 2002].

AAP. 1992. The medical home. *Pediatrics* 90(5):774.

AAP. 1994a. Death of a child in the emergency department. *Pediatrics* 93(5):861–862. [Online]. Available: http://www.aap.org/policy/00206.html [accessed December 12, 2001].

AAP. 1994b. Guidelines on forgoing life-sustaining medical treatment. *Pediatrics* 93(3):532–536. [Online]. Available: http://www.aap.org/policy/00118.html [accessed December 12, 2001].

392

AAP. 1995a. Informed consent, parental permission, and assent in pediatric practice. *Pediatrics* 95(2):314–331. [Online]. Available: http://www.aap.org/policy/00662.html [accessed December 12, 2001].

AAP. 1995b. *The Medical Home and Early Intervention: Linking Services for Children With Special Needs*. Elk Grove Village, IL: AAP Publications.

AAP. 1995c. Perinatal care at the threshold of viability. *Pediatrics* 96(5):974–976.

AAP. 1996. Ethics and the care of critically ill infants and children. *Pediatrics* 98(1):149–152.

AAP. 1997a. Alternative routes of drug administration—advantages and disadvantages (subject review). *Pediatrics* 100(1):143–152. [Online]. Available: http://www.aap.org/policy/970701.html [accessed October 4, 2001].

AAP. 1997b. Guidelines for the Pediatric Cancer Center and Role of Such Centers in Diagnosis and Treatment. *Pediatrics* 99(1):139–141.

AAP. 1997c. Noise: A hazard for the fetus and newborn. *Pediatrics* 100(4):724–727. [Online]. Available: http://www.aap.org/policy/re9728.html [accessed October 4, 2001].

AAP. 1997d. Religious objections to medical care. *Pediatrics* 99(2):279–281. [Online]. Available: http://www.aap.org/policy/re9707.html [accessed December 12, 2001].

AAP. 1998a. Issues in the Application of the Resource-Based Relative Value Scale System to Pediatrics: A Subject Review. [Online]. Available: http://www.aap.org/policy/re9818.html [accessed August 13, 2001].

AAP. 1998b. Pediatric workforce statement 1998 (August). *Pediatrics* 102(2):418–427. [Online]. Available: http://www.aap.org/policy/re9750.html [accessed December 12, 2001].

AAP. 1999a. Disclosure of illness status to children and adolescents with HIV infection. *Pediatrics* 103(1):164–166. [Online]. Available: http://www.aap.org/policy/re9827.html [accessed December 12, 2001].

AAP. 1999b. Care coordination: Integrating health and related systems of care for children with special health care needs. *Pediatrics* 104(4):978–981.

AAP. 1999c. Investigation and review of unexpected infant and child deaths. *Pediatrics* 104(5):1158–1160.

AAP. 1999d. Medicaid Reimbursement Survey. [Online]. Available: http://www.aap.org/research/medreim.htm [accessed April 19, 2002].

AAP. 2000a. Prevention and management of pain and stress in the neonate. *Pediatrics* 105(2): 454–461. [Online]. Available: http://www.aap.org/policy/re9945.html [accessed October 4, 2001].

AAP. 2000b. Changing concepts of sudden infant death syndrome: Implications for infant sleeping environment and sleep position. *Pediatrics* 105(3):650–656. [Online]. Available: http://www.aap.org/policy/re9946.html [accessed December 12, 2001].

AAP. 2000c. Child life services. *Pediatrics* 106(5):1156–1159. [Online]. Available: http://www.aap.org/policy/re9922.html [accessed December 12, 2001].

AAP. 2000d. Do not resuscitate orders in schools. *Pediatrics* 105(4):878–879. [Online]. Available: http://www.aap.org/policy/re9842.html [accessed December 12, 2001].

AAP. 2000e. Foregoing life-sustaining medical treatment in abused children. *Pediatrics* 106(5): 1151–1153. [Online]. Available: http://www.aap.org/policy/re0015.html [accessed December 12, 2001].

AAP. 2000f. Improving Access to Children's Health Insurance in the United States. [Online]. Available: http://www.aap.org/advocacy/chi2/us.pdf [accessed July 12, 2001].

AAP. 2000g. Palliative care for children. *Pediatrics* 106(2):351–357. [Online]. Available: http://www.aap.org/policy/re0007.html [accessed December 12, 2001].

AAP. 2000h. Race/ethnicity, gender, socioeconomic status—research exploring their effects on child health: A subject review. *Pediatrics* 105(6):1349–1351.

AAP. 2001a. The assessment and management of acute pain in infants, children, and adolescents. *Pediatrics* 108(3):793–797. [Online]. Available: http://www.aap.org/policy/ 9933.html [accessed October 4, 2001].

AAP. 2001b. Care of children in the emergency department: Guidelines for preparedness. *Pediatrics* 107(4):771–781.

AAP. 2001c. Distinguishing sudden infant death syndrome from child abuse fatalities. *Pediatrics* 107(2):437–441. [Online]. Available: http://www.aap.org/policy/re0036.html [accessed December 12, 2001].

AAP. 2001d. Institutional ethics committees. *Pediatrics* 107(1):205–209. [Online]. Available: http://www.aap.org/policy/re0017.html [accessed December 12, 2001].

AAP. 2001e. *RVRBS: What Is It and How Does It Affect Pediatrics?* Elk Grove Village, IL: AAP. [Online]. Available: http://www.aap.org/visit/pedrbrvs.htm [accessed August 2, 2001].

AAP. 2001f (September 8). Statement presented by G. Kevin Donovan to the IOM committee on improving palliative and end-of-life care for children and their families, Open Meeting. Washington, DC.

AAP, Critical Care Section. 2001a (September 8). Letter written by Deborah Mulligan-Smith to the IOM committee on improving palliative and end-of-life care for children and their families, Washington, DC.

AAP, Critical Care Section. 2001b (September 8). Statement presented by M. Michele Moss to the IOM committee on improving palliative and end-of-life care for children and their families, Open Meeting. Washington, DC.

Abbott KH, Sago JG, Breen CM, Abernathy AP, Tulsky JA. 2001. Families looking back: One year after discussion of withdrawal or withholding of life sustaining support. *Critical Care Medicine* 29(1):197–201.

Abele Meekin S, Klein JE, Fleischman AR, Fins JJ. 2000. Development of a palliative education assessment tool for medical student education. *Academic Medicine* 75:986–992.

ABIM (American Board of Internal Medicine). 1996a. *Caring for the Dying: Identification and Promotion of Physician Competency: Educational Research Documents.* Philadelphia: ABIM.

ABIM. 1996b. *Caring for the Dying: Identification and Promotion of Physician Competency: Personal Narratives.* Philadelphia: ABIM.

ABP (American Board of Pediatrics). 2001 (September 8). Statement presented by Ernest Krug III to the IOM (Institute of Medicine) committee on Children Who Die and Their Families, Open Meeting. Washington, DC.

ABP. 2002. [Online]. Available: http://www.abp.org/ABPINFO/abp.htm [accessed March 31, 2002].

ABP, Program Directors Committee. 2001 (September 26). Written statement from Edwin Forman, M.D. to the IOM committee on Children Who Die and Their Families, Washington, DC.

Abt Associates, 1991. *Reexamination of the Adequacy of Physician Supply Made in 1980 by the Graduate Medical Education National Advisory Committee (GMENAC) for Selected Specialties.* Cambridge, MA: Abt Associates, Inc.

ACEP (American College of Emergency Physicians). 2001 (September 19). Statement written by Marianne Gausche-Hill and Robert W. Schafermeyer to the IOM committee on improving palliative and end-of-life care for children and their families, Washington, DC.

ACGME (Accreditation Council on Graduate Medical Education). 2000 (September 26). [Online]. Available: http://www.acgme.org [accessed March 31, 2002].

ACP (American College of Physicians). 1997a. *Home Care Guide for Advanced Cancer*. PS Houts, ed. Philadelphia: ACP. [Online]. Available: http://www.acponline.org/public/ h_care/index.html [accessed August 11, 2001].

ACP (American College of Physicians). 1997b. *Home Care Guide for HIV and Aids*. PS Houts, ed. Philadelphia: ACP. [Online]. Available: http://www.acponline.org/public/hiv/ index.html [accessed August 11, 2001].

ACT (Association for Children with Life-Threatening and Terminal Conditions and Their Families) and the RCPCH (Royal College of Paediatrics and Child Health). 1997. A Guide to the Development of Children's Palliative Care Services. London: RCPCH.

Adams-Greenly, M. 1984. Helping children communicate about serious illness and death. *Journal of Psychosocial Oncology* 2(2):61–72.

Addington-Hall JM, Walker L, Jones C, Karlsen S, McCarthy M. 1998. A randomised controlled trial of postal versus interviewer administration of a questionnaire measuring satisfaction with and use of services received in the year before death. *Journal of Epidemiology and Community Health* 52(12):802–807.

Aetna Insurance. 2001. Important Consumer Disclosure Information: Texas. [Online]. Available: http://www.aetna.com/data/disclosures/tx_open_access.pdf [accessed March 31, 2002].

AHA (American Heart Association) in Collaboration with the International Liaison Committee on Resuscitation. 2000a. Guidelines 2000 for cardiopulmonary resuscitation and emergency cardiovascular care. *Circulation* 102(8 Suppl):1–374.

AHA. 2000b. Pediatric advanced life support. *Circulation* 102(Suppl):I-291–I-342.

AHCPR (Agency for Health Care Policy and Research [now Agency for Healthcare Research and Quality], U.S. Department of Health and Human Services). 1994 (March). *Management of Cancer Pain*. Clinical Practice Guideline No. 9. Publication No. 94–0592. Rockville, MD: AHCPR.

Ahmann E. 1998. Review of commentary: Two studies regarding giving "bad news." *Pediatric Nursing* 24(6):554–556.

Ahrens WR, Hart RG. 1997. Emergency physicians' experience with pediatric death. *American Journal of Emergency Medicine* 15(7):642–643.

Ahrens W, Hart R, Maruyama N. 1997. Pediatric death: Managing the aftermath in the emergency department. *Journal of Emergency Medicine* 15(5):601–603.

AHRQ (Agency for Healthcare Research and Quality). 2001a. Child Health Toolbox: Measuring Performance in Child Health Programs: Measuring Services for Children with Special Health Care Needs. [Online]. Available: http://www.ahrq.gov/chtoolbx/cshcn.htm [accessed August 17, 2001].

AHRQ, Center for Cost and Financing Studies. 2001b. *2000 Medical Expenditure Panel Survey: Compendium of Tables*. Rockville, MD. [Online]. Available: http://www.meps. ahrq.gov/Data_Pub/CompendiumTables/Table1_A2000PIT.PDF [accessed January 31, 2002].

AHRQ. 2001c. Telemedicine for the Medicare population: Pediatric, obstetric, and clinician-indirect home interventions. *Evidence Report/Technology Assessment (Summary)* No. 24, Supplement:1–32.

AHSRHP (Academy for Health Services Research and Health Policy). 2001. States extend coverage in programs in 2000. *State of the States Report* (Prepared for the Robert Wood Johnson Foundation's State Coverage Initiatives). Washington, DC: AHSRHP. Pp. 4–19.

Alderson P. 1993. *Children's Consent to Surgery*. Buckingham, UK: Buckingham Open University Press.

All Saints Healthcare System. 1998. *A New Employee's Handout: The Ethical Implications of Providing Religious and Sacramental Services in a Healthcare Environment.* Racine, WI. [Online]. Available: http://www.episcopalchurch.org/aehc/resource/ethics/handout.htm [accessed October 1, 2001].

Alpers A, Lo B. 1999. Avoiding family feuds: Responding to surrogate demands for life-sustaining interventions. *Journal of Law, Medicine, and Ethics* 27(1):74–80.

Altarescu G, Hill S, Wiggs E, Jeffries N, Kreps C, Parker CC, Brady RO, Barton NW, Schiffmann R. 2001. The efficacy of enzyme replacement therapy in patients with chronic neuronopathic Gaucher's disease. *Journal of Pediatrics* 138(4):539–547.

AMA (American Medical Association), Council on Ethics and Judicial Affairs. 1992. Treatment Decisions for Seriously Ill Newborns: Opinion 2.215. [Online]. Available: http://www.ama-assn.org/ama1/upload/mm/369/43b.pdf [accessed October 22, 2001].

AMA, Council on Ethics and Judicial Affairs. 1994a. Withholding or Withdrawing Life-Sustaining Medical Treatment E-2.20. [Online]. Available: http://www.ama-assn.org/apps/pf_online/pf_online?f_n=browse&doc=policyfiles/CEJA/E-2.20.HTM&&s_t=&st_p =&nth=1&prev_pol=policyfiles/CEJA/E-1.02.HTM&nxt_pol=policyfiles/CEJA/E-2.01.HTM& [accessed March 31, 2002].

AMA, Council on Ethics and Judicial Affairs. 1994b. *Ethics Committees in Health Care Institutions E-9.11.* Chicago: AMA.

AMA, Council on Ethics and Judicial Affairs. 1997. Medical fertility in end-of-life care E-2.037. *Code of Medical Ethics.* [Online]. Available: http://www.ama-assn.org/ama/pub/category/2503.html [accessed March 31, 2002].

AMA, Council on Ethics and Judicial Affairs. 2001. *Principles of Medical Ethics.* Chicago: AMA.

Amark K, Sunnegardh J. 1999. The effect of changing attitudes to Down's syndrome in the management of complete atrioventricular septal defects. *Archives of Diseases in Childhood* 81:151–154.

Ambuel B, Mazzone MF. 2001. Breaking bad news and discussing death. *Primary Care* 28(2):249–267.

American Heritage Dictionary. 1992. 3rd ed. Boston: Houghton Mifflin Company.

American Hospital Association. 2000. *Annual Survey Database—Fiscal Year 1998. (CD-ROM).* Chicago: AHA Health Forum.

Anand KJ, Barton BA, McIntosh N, Lagercrantz H, Pelausa E, Young TE, Vasa R. 1999. Analgesia and sedation in preterm neonates who require ventilatory support: Results from the NOPAIN trial. Neonatal outcome and prolonged analgesia in neonates. *Archives of Pediatric Adolescent Medicine* 153(4):331–338.

Andrews JS, Anderson GF, Han C, Neff JM. 1997. Pediatric carve outs. The use of disease-specific conditions as risk adjusters in capitated payment systems. *Archives of Pediatric and Adolescent Medicine* 151(3):236–242.

Aney C. 2001. Written, unpublished responses to survey of bereaved parents developed and distributed by J. Hilden and H. Janes-Hodder for Children's Oncology Group Parent Advocates Group. Used with permission.

Angell M. 1985. Cost containment and the physician. *Journal of the American Medical Association* 254(9):1203–1207.

APA (American Psychological Association). 1995. State Medicaid Reimbursement Standards for Psychologists. [Online]. Available: http://www.apa.org/practice/statemedicaid.html [accessed August 17, 2001].

APA. 2001a (February). Resolution on End-of-Life Issues and Care. [Online]. Available: http://www.apa.org/ppo/issues/eolresolu.html [accessed March 31, 2002].

APA and Society of Pediatric Psychology. 2001 (September 8). Statement presented by Daniel Armstrong to the IOM committee on improving palliative and end-of-life care for children and their families, Open Meeting. Washington, DC.

APHA (American Public Health Association). 2001. Criteria for assessing the quality of health information on the Internet. *American Journal of Public Health* 91(3):513–514.

APS (American Pain Society). 1995. Pediatric Chronic Pain: A Position Statement from the American Pain Society. *American Pain Society Bulletin, The Society.* [Online]. Available: http://www.ampainsoc.org/advocacy/pediatric.htm [accessed March 31, 2002].

APS. 1997. Treatment of pain at the end of life: A position statement from the American Pain Society. *APS Bulletin* 7(1). [Online]. Available: http://www.ampainsoc.org/pub/bulletin/jan97/treatment.htm.

Aquilino ML, Damiano PC, Willard JC, Momany ET, Levy BT. 1999. Primary care physician perceptions of the nurse practitioner in the 1990s. *Archives of Family Medicine* 8(3):224–227.

Armstrong-Dailey A, Goltzer SZ, eds. 1993. *Hospice Care for Children.* New York: Oxford University Press.

Armstong-Dailey A, Zarbock S, eds. 2001. *Hospice Care for Children.* New York: Oxford University Press.

Arnold W, Alexander S. 1997. Cost, work, reimbursement, and the pediatric nephrologist in the United States Medicare/End-Stage Renal Disease Program. *Pediatric Nephrology* 11(2):250–257.

Asch DA, Hansen-Flaschen J, Lanken PN. 1995. Decisions to limit or continue life-sustaining treatment by critical care physicians in the United States: Conflicts between physicians' practices and patients' wishes. *American Journal of Respiratory Critical Care Medicine* 151(2 Pt 1):288–292.

Asch DA, Faber-Langendoen K, Shea JA, Christakis NA. 1999. The sequence of withdrawing life-sustaining treatment from patients. *American Journal of Medicine* 107(2):153–156.

ASCO (American Society for Clinical Oncology). 2002. *ASCO Curriculum: Organizing Cancer Care—The Importance of Symptom Management.* Alexandria, VA: ASCO.

ASIM (American Society for Internal Medicine). 1981 (January). *Reimbursement for Physicians' Cognitive and Procedural Services: A White Paper.* Washington, DC: ASIM.

ASPH/O (American Society of Pediatric Hematology/Oncology). 2001 (September 18). Statement written by Beverly Lange to the IOM committee on improving palliative and end-of-life care for children and their families, Washington, DC.

Aston G. 2001. Mental health parity law nears expiration. *American Medical News.* 44(27):14.

Atkins D, DiGuiseppi CG. 1998. Broadening the evidence base for evidence-based guidelines. A research agenda based on the work of the U.S. Preventive Services Task Force. *American Journal of Preventive Medicine* 14(4):335–344.

Aurora P, Whitehead B, Wade A, Bowyer J, Whitmore P, Rees PG, Tsang VT, Elliott MJ, de Leval M. 1999. Lung transplantation and life extension in children with cystic fibrosis. *Lancet* 354(9190):1591–1593.

Averill RF, Muldoon JH, Ventress JC, Goldfield NI, Mullin RL, Fineran EC, Zhang MZ, Steinbeck B, Grant T. 1998. The evolution of case mix measurement using diagnosis related groups (DRGs). 3M HIS Working Paper. Study performed by 3M Health Information Systems and the National Association of Children's Hospitals and Related Institutions. [Online]. Available: http://www.3m.com/market/healthcare/his/us/documents/reports/evolcasemix5-98.pdf [accessed August 15, 2001].

Avery GB. 1998. Futility considerations in the neonatal intensive care unit. *Seminars in Perinatology* 22:216–222.

Avila R. 2001 (September 9). Statement and discussion with the IOM committee on improving palliative and end-of-life care for children and their families, Open Meeting. Washington, DC.

Avila S. 2001 (September 9). Statement and discussion with the IOM committee on improving palliative and end-of-life care for children and their families, Open Meeting. Washington, DC.

Baile WF, Kudelka AP, Beale EA, Glober GA, Myers EG, Greisinger AJ, Bast RC Jr., Goldstein MG, Novack D, Lenzi R. 1999. Communication skills training in oncology: Description and preliminary outcomes of workshops on breaking bad news and managing patient reactions to illness. *Cancer* 86(5):887–897.

Baile WF, Buckman R, Lenzi R, Glober G, Beale EA, Kudelka AP. 2000. SPIKES—a six-step protocol for delivering bad news: Application to the patient with cancer. *Oncologist* 5(4):302–311.

Balfour-Lynn IM, Martin I, Whitehead BF, Rees PG, Elliott MJ, deVal MR. 1997. Heart–lung transplantation for patients under 10 with cystic fibrosis. *Archives for Disabled Children* 76(1):38–40.

Ballantyne M, Stevens B, McAllister M, Dionne K, Jack A. 1999. Validation of the premature infant pain profile in the clinical setting. *Clinical Journal of Pain* 15(4):297–303.

Barnard D, Quill T, Hafferty FW, Arnold R, Plumb J, Bulger R, Field M. 1999. Preparing the ground: Contributions for care near the end of life. Working Group on the Pre-clinical Years of the National Consensus Conference on Medical Education for Care Near the End of Life. *Academic Medicine* 74(5):499–505.

Barr RG. 1994. Pain experience in children: Developmental and clinical characteristics. In: Wall PD, Melzack R, eds. *Textbook of Pain*, 3rd ed. London: Churchill Livingstone. Pp. 739–765.

Barrett J, Gifford C, Morey J, Risser D, Salisbury M. 2001. Enhancing patient safety through teamwork training. *Journal of Healthcare Risk Management* 21(4):57–65.

Bartel DA, Engler AJ, Natale JE, Misra V, Lewin AB, Joseph JG. 2000. Working with families of suddenly and critically ill children: Physician experiences. *Archives of Pediatric and Adolescent Medicine* 154(11):1127–1133.

Bartholome WG. 1995. (letter) Informed consent, parental permission, and assent in pediatric practice. *Pediatrics* 96:981–982.

Barzansky B, Veloski JJ, Miller R, Jonas HS. 1999. Education in end-of-life care during medical school and residency training. *Academic Medicine* 74(10):s102–s104.

Bauchner H, Waring C, Vinci R. 1991. Parental presence during procedures in an emergency room: Results from 50 observations. *Pediatrics* 87(4):544–548.

Bayer Institute for Health Care Communication. 2001. PREPARE to be Partners in Your Health Care: Six Steps to Help You Get More Out of Your Doctor's Visit. [Online]. Available: http://www.bayerinstitute.com/patient/index.htm [accessed May 28, 2002].

Bazelon (Bazelon Center for Mental Health Law). 1999. *Medicaid Formulary Policies: Access to High-Cost Mental Health Medications*. [Online]. Available: http://www.bazelon.org/formulary.html [accessed July 12, 2001].

BCBSRA (Blue Cross Blue Shield of the Rochester Area). 2002. CompassionateNet: A program for families with children facing a potentially life limiting condition, Rochester, NY. [Online]. Available: http://www.bcbsra.com/members/members_home.htm [accessed April 17, 2002].

Beauchamp TL, Childress JF. 1983. *Principles of Biomedical Ethics*, 2nd ed. New York: Oxford University Press.

Beauchamp TL, Childress JF. 1994. *Principles of Biomedical Ethics*, 4th ed. Oxford: Oxford University Press.

Behrman RE, Kliegman RM, Jenson HB. 2000. *Nelson Textbook of Pediatrics*, 16th ed. Philadelphia: WB Saunders.

Bergsjo P, Villar J. 1997. Scientific basis for the content of routine antenatal care. II. Power to eliminate or alleviate adverse newborn outcomes; some special conditions and examinations. *Acta Obstetricia et Gynecologica Scandinavica* 76(1):15–25.

Berland GK, Elliott MN, Morales LS, Algazy JI, Kravitz RL, Broder MS, Kanouse DE, Munoz JA, Puyol JA, Lara M, Watkins KE, Yang H, McGlynn EA. 2001. Health information on the Internet: Accessibility, quality, and readability in English and Spanish. *Journal of the American Medical Association* 285(20):2612–2621.

Bernstein D. 2000. Epidemiology of congenital heart disease. In: Behrman RE, Kliegman RM, Jenson HB, eds. *Nelson Textbook of Pediatrics*, 16th ed. Philadelphia: WB Saunders. Pp. 1362–1363.

Berwick D. 1989. Continuous quality improvement as an ideal in health care. *New England Journal of Medicine* 320:53–56.

Berwick D, Godfrey AB and Roessner J. 1990. *Curing Health Care: New Strategies for Quality Improvement*. San Francisco: Jossey-Bass Publishers.

Bidari PM. 1996. An incompetent child's right to have medical treatment terminated when there is uncontroverted evidence that medical assistance is futile. *Journal of Juvenile Law* 17:1.

Billings JA. 1998. What is palliative care? *Journal of Palliative Medicine* 1:73–83.

Billings JA, Block S. 1997. Palliative care in undergraduate medical education: Status report and future directions. *Journal of the American Medical Association* 278(9):733–738.

Blackhall LJ, Murphy ST, Frank G, Michel V, Azen S. 1995. Ethnicity and attitudes toward patient autonomy. *Journal of the American Medical Association* 274(10):820–825.

Blackhall LJ, Murphy ST, Frank G, Michel V, Azen S. 1999. Ethnicity and attitudes towards life sustaining technology. *Social Science and Medicine* 48(12):1779–1789.

Blackhall LJ, Murphy ST, Frank G, Michel V. 2001. Bioethics in a different tongue: The case of truth-telling. *Journal of Urban Health* 78(1):59–71.

Bleyer AW, Tejeda H, Murphy SB, Robison LL, Ross JA, Pollock BH, Severson RK, Brawley OW, Smith MA, Ungerleider RS. 1997. National cancer clinical trials: Children have equal access; adolescents do not. *Journal of Adolescent Health* 21:366–373.

Block S, Billings JA. 1998. Nurturing humanism through teaching palliative care. *Academic Medicine* 73(7):763–765.

BLS (Bureau of Labor Statistics, Department of Labor). 1999. Employee Benefits in Medium and Large Private Establishments, 1997. Bulletin 2517. Washington, DC: BLS.

BLS. 2000. Employee Benefits in State and Local Governments, 1998. Bulletin 2531.

Blue Cross Blue Shield Association. 2002. 2002 Blue Cross and Blue Shield Service Benefit Plan, p. 63. [Online]. Available: http://www.fepblue.org/pdf/2002sbp.pdf [accessed February 13, 2002].

Bluebond-Langner M. 1978. *The Private Worlds of Dying Children*. Princeton, NJ: Princeton University Press.

Bodenheimer T. 1997. The Oregon Health Plan—lessons for the nation: Second of two parts. *New England Journal of Medicine* 337(10):720–723.

Bookbinder M. 2001. Improving the quality of care across settings. In: Ferrell B, Coyle N, eds. *Textbook of Palliative Nursing*. Oxford: Oxford University Press. Pp. 503–530.

Bookbinder M, Coyle N, Kiss M, Layman Goldstein M, Holritz, Thaler H, Gianella A, Derby S, Brown M, Racolin M, Nah Ho M, Portenoy RK. 1996. Implementing national standards for cancer pain management: Program model and evaluation. *Journal of Pain & Symptom Management.* 12(6):334–347.

Bookbinder, M., Kiss, M., Coyle, N., Brown, M., Gianella, A., Thaler, H. 1995. Improving pain management practices. In: McGuire D, Yarbro C, Ferrell B, eds. *Cancer Pain Management*, 2nd ed. Boston: Jones and Bartlett. Pp. 321–362.

Bowen K, Marshall WN. 1998. Pediatric death certification. *Pediatric Adolescent Medicine* 152:852–854.

Bowman DH. 2001, December 5. Efforts link sick children to classes. *The Washington Post.* [Online]. Available: http://www.washingtonpost.com/ac2/wp-dyn?pagename=article& node=&contentId=A57677-2001Dec4 [accessed March 16, 2002].

Boyd R. 2000. Witnessed resuscitation by relatives. *Resuscitation* 43(3):171–176.

Breen CM, Abernathy AP, Abbott KH, Tulsky JA. 2001. Conflict associated with decisions to limit life-sustaining treatment in intensive care units. *Journal of General Internal Medicine* 16(5):283–289.

Brennan TA. 1991. Practice guidelines and malpractice litigation: Collision or cohesion? *Journal of Health Politics, Policy and Law* 16(1):67–85.

Briery BG, Rabian B. 1999. Psychosocial changes associated with participation in a pediatric summer camp. *Journal of Pediatric Psychology* 24(2):183–190.

Britton A, Russell R. 2002. Multidisciplinary team interventions for delirium in patients with chronic cognitive impairment (Cochrane Review). In: The Cochrane Library. Oxford: Update Software. [Online]. Available: http://www.cochrane.org/cochrane/revabstr/ ab000395.htm [accessed June 5, 2001].

Broaddus M, Ku L. 2000. Nearly 95 Percent of Low-Income Uninsured Children Now Are Eligible for Medicaid or SCHIP. Washington, DC: Center on Budget and Policy Priorities. [Online]. Available: http://www.cbpp.org/12-6-00schip.htm [accessed March 31, 2002].

Brock DW. 1989. Children's competence for health care decision-making. In: Kopelman LM, Moskop JC, eds. *Children and Health Care: Moral and Social Issues.* Dordrecht, The Netherlands: Kluwer Academic Publishers. Pp. 181–212.

Brocks V, Bang J. 1991. Routine examination by ultrasound for the detection of fetal malformations in a low risk population. *Fetal Diagnostic Therapies* 6:37–45.

Brodeur, D. 1998. Health care institutional ethics: Broader than clinical ethics. In: Monagle J, Thomasma, DC, eds. *Health Care Ethics: Critical issues for the 21st Century.* Gaithersburg, MD: Aspen. Pp. 497–504.

Brody H. 2000. Evidence-based medicine, nutritional support and terminal suffering. *American Journal of Medicine* 109:740–741.

Bromley BE, Blacher J. 1991. Parental reasons for out-of-home placement of children with severe handicaps. *Mental Retardation* 29(5):275–280.

Brosco JP. 1999. The early history of the infant mortality rate in America: A reflection upon the past and a prophecy of the future. *Pediatrics* 103(2):478–485.

Browman GP. 2001. Development and aftercare of clinical guidelines. The balance between rigor and pragmatism. *Journal of the American Medical Association* 286(12):1509–1511.

Brown KT. 1996. In the Matter of Baby K: The Fourth Circuit stretches EMTALA even further. *Mercer Law Review* 47:1173–1179.

Browning D. In press. Fragments of love: Exploration in the ethnography of suffering and professional caregiving. In: Berzoff J, Silverman P, eds. *End-of-Life Care for Social Workers.* New York: Columbia University Press.

Bruen BK. 2000. *Medicaid and Prescription Drugs: An Overview.* Prepared for the Kaiser Commission on Medicaid and the Uninsured. Washington, DC: The Urban Institute.

Bruen BK. 2002. *States Strive to Limit Medicaid Expenditures for Prescribed Drugs.* Prepared for the Kaiser Commission on Medicaid and the Uninsured. Washington, DC: The Urban Institute.

Bruera E, Neumann CM, Mazzocato C, Stiefel F, Sala R. 2000. Attitudes and beliefs of palliative care physicians regarding communication with terminally ill cancer patients. *Palliative Medicine* 14(4):287–298.

Bryant C. 1993. Role clarification: A quality improvement survey of hospital customers. *Journal of Healthcare Quality* 15(4):18–20.

Budetti PP, Kletke PR, Connelly JP. 1982. Current distribution and trends in the location pattern of pediatricians, family physicians and general practitioners between 1976 and 1979. *Pediatrics* 70:780–789.

Bukowski R. 1999. Cytoprotection in the treatment of pediatric cancer: Review of current strategies in adults and their application to children. *Medical and Pediatric Oncology* 32(2):124–34.

Bula K, Bula J. 2001. Written, unpublished responses to survey of bereaved parent developed and distributed by J. Hilden and H. Janes-Hodder for Children's Oncology Group Parent Advocates Group. Used with permission.

Bull MJ, Jervis LL. 1997. Strategies used by chronically ill older women and their caregiving daughters in managing posthospital care. *Journal of Advanced Nursing* 25(3):541–547.

Buntin MB, Newhouse JP. 1998. *Employer Purchasing Coalitions and Medicaid Experience with Risk Adjustment.* New York: The Commonwealth Fund.

Burck R. 1996. Feeding, withdrawing, and withholding: Ethical perspectives. *Nutritional Clinical Practices* 11(6):243–253.

Burl JB, Bonner A, Rao M. 1994. Demonstration of the cost-effectiveness of a nurse practitioner/physician team in long-term care facilities. *HMO Practices* 8(4):157–161.

Burns JP, Truog RD. 1997. Ethical controversies in pediatric critical care. *New Horizons* 5(1):72–84.

Burns JP, Mitchell C, Outwater KM, Geller M, Griffith JL, Todres ID, Truog RD. 2000. End-of-life care in the pediatric intensive care unit after the forgoing of life-sustaining treatment. *Critical Care Medicine* 28(8):3060–3066.

Burns JP, Mitchell C, Griffith JL, Truog RD. 2001. End-of-life care in the pediatric intensive care unit: Attitudes and practices of pediatric critical care physicians and nurses. *Critical Care Medicine* 29(3):658–664.

Bush JP, Harkins SW, eds. 1991. *Children in Pain: Clinical and Research Issues from a Development Perspective.* New York: Springer-Verlag.

Butler P. 2000. ERISA Complicates State Efforts to Improve Access to Individual Insurance for the Medically High Risk: Issue Brief. [Online]. Available: http://www.academyhealth. org/publications.htm [accessed July 12, 2001].

Butler S, Twohig JS. 2001. *New End-of-Life Benefits Models in Blue Cross and Blue Shield Plans.* Vienna, VA: Barksdale Ballard and Company.

Byock I. 1997. *Dying Well: The Prospect for Growth at the End of Life.* New York: Riverhead Books.

Cacciatore-Garard assisted by Kubler-Ross E. 2001. The power of compassion. Statement submitted to IOM committee on improving palliative and end-of-life care for children and their families, Open Meeting. Washington, DC.

Calhoun B, Hoeldke N. 2000. The perinatal hospice: Plowing the field of natal sorrow. *Supportive Voices.* [Online]. Available: http://www.careofdying.org/Home.html [accessed March 31, 2002].

Callaham M, Madsen CD, Barton CW, Saunders CE, Pointer J. 1992. A randomized trial of high-dose epinephrine and norepinephrine vs standard-dose epinephrine in prehospital cardiac arrest. *Journal of the American Medical Association* 268:2667–2672.

Campbell E, Sanson-Fisher RW. 1998. Breaking bad news. 3: Encouraging the adoption of best practices. *Behavioral Medicine* 24(2):73–80.

Campbell H, Hotchkiss R, Bradshaw N, Porteous M. 1998. Integrated care pathways. *British Medical Journal* 316:133–137.

Campbell SM, Hann M, Hacker J, Burns C, Oliver D, Thapar A, Mead N, Safran DG, Roland MO. 2001. Identifying predictors of high quality care in English general practice: Observational study. *British Medical Journal* 323(7316):784–787.

Candlelighters: Childhood Cancer Foundation. 2001 (September 8). Statement presented by Ruth Hoffman to the IOM committee on improving palliative and end-of-life care for children and their families, Open Meeting. Washington, DC.

CAPC (Center to Advance Palliative Care, Mt. Sinai Medical Center [New York City]). No date. Writing a Business Plan. [Online]. Available: http://www.capcmssm.org/topic/4/ [accessed July 20, 2001].

CAPC. No date. [Online]. Available: http://www.capcmssm.org [accessed November 12, 2000].

Caplan AL. 1992. Hard cases make bad law: The legacy of the Baby Doe controversy. In: Caplan AL, Blank RH, Merrick JC, eds. *Compelled Compassion: Government Intervention in the Treatment of Critically Ill Newborns*. Totowa, NJ: Humana Press. Pp. 105–122.

Capron AM. 2001. Brain death—well settled yet still unresolved. *New England Journal of Medicine* 344(16):1244–1246.

Carrese, JA, Rhodes LA. 2000. Bridging cultural differences in medical practice. The case of discussing negative information with Navajo patients. *Journal of General Internal Medicine* 15(2):92–96.

Carron AT, Lynn J, Keaney P. 1999. End-of-life care in medical textbooks. *Annals of Internal Medicine* 130(1):82–86.

Casarett, DJ, Daskal F, Lantos J. 1998. Experts in ethics? The authority of the clinical ethicist. *Hastings Center Report* 28(6):6–11.

Casarett D, Karlawish JH, Sugarman J. 2000. Should patients in quality-improvement activities have the same protections as participants in research studies? *Journal of the American Medical Association* 284(14):1786–1788.

Cassel CK, Ludden JM, Moon GM. 2000. Perceptions of barriers to high-quality palliative care in hospitals. *Health Affairs* 19(5):166–172.

CDC (Centers for Disease Control and Prevention). 1997. Rates of homicide, suicide and firearm death among children—26 industrialized countries. *Morbidity and Mortality Weekly Report* 46(5):101–105. [Online]. Available: http://www.cdc.gov/mmwr/PDF/wk/ mm4605.pdf [accessed December 13, 2001].

CDC. 1999a. Achievements in public health, 1900–1999: Control of infectious diseases. *Morbidity and Mortality Weekly Report*. July 30, 1999 / 48(29);621–629. (Also appeared in *Journal of the American Medical Association* 282(11):1029–1032, 1999.) [Online]. Available: http://www.cdc.gov/mmwr/preview/mmwrhtml/mm4829a1.htm [accessed March 22, 2001].

CDC. 1999b. Achievements in public health, 1900–1999: Healthier mothers and babies. *Morbidity and Mortality Weekly Report* 48(38)849–858. [Online]. Available: http:// www.cdc.gov/epo/mmwr/preview/mmwrhtml/mm4838a2.htm [accessed March 22, 2001].

Centerwall BS. 1995. Race, socioeconomic status, and domestic homicide. *Journal of the American Medical Association* 273(22):1755–1758.

Chaffee S. 2001. Pediatric palliative care. *Primary Care: Clinics in Office Practice* 28(2):365–390.

Chambers CT, Craig KD. 1999. Commentary—Parents as judges of their children's pain: Are they accurate? *Pediatric Pain Letter* 3(2):13–14. [Online]. Available: http:// www.pediatric-pain.ca/pplet/v3n2c.PDF [accessed April 15, 2002].

Chambers HM, Chan FY. 2000. Support for women/families after perinatal death. *Cochrane Database System Review* (2):CD000452. [Online]. Available: http://www.update-software.com/abstracts/ab000452.htm [accessed March 12, 2002].

Charon R. 2001. Narrative medicine: A model for empathy, reflection, profession, and trust. *Journal of the American Medical Association* 286(15):1897–1902.

Charon R, Banks JT, Connelly JE, Hawkins AH, Hunter KM, Jones AH, Montello M, Poirer S. 1995. Literature and medicine: Contributions to clinical practice. *Annals of Internal Medicine* 122:599–606.

Cherny NI, Portenoy RK. 1994. The management of cancer pain. *CA: A Cancer Journal for Clinicians* 44(5):263–303. [Online]. Available: http://pain.roxane.com/library/TMOCP/ [accessed December 13, 2001].

CHI (Children's Hospice International). 1991. *Home Care for Seriously Ill Children: A Manual for Parents*. Prepared by Moldow DG and Martinson IM. Alexandria, VA: CHI.

CHI. 2002. *Implementation Manual: Program for All-Inclusive Care for Children and Their Families (PACC)*. Alexandria, VA: CHI.

Child Life Council. 2001 (September 8). Statement presented by Christina Brown to the IOM committee on improving palliative and end-of-life care for children and their families, Open Meeting. Washington, DC.

ChIPPS (Children's International Project on Palliative/Hospice Services). 2001. *A Call for Change: Recommendations to Improve the Care of Children Living with Life-Threatening Conditions*. Alexandria, VA: National Hospice and Palliative Care Organization.

Chisholm CA, Pappas DJ, Sharp MC. 1997. Communicating bad news. *Obstetrics and Gynecology* 90(4.1):637–639.

Chitty LS, Hunt GH, Moore J, Lobb MO. 1991. Effectiveness of routine ultrasonography in detecting fetal structural abnormalities in a low risk population. *British Medical Journal* 303:1165–1169.

Chochinov HM, Breitbart W, eds. 2000. *Handbook of Psychiatry in Palliative Medicine*. New York: Oxford University Press.

Christakis DA, Wright JA, Koepsell TD, Emerson S, Connell FA. 1999. Is greater continuity of care associated with less emergency department utilization? *Pediatrics* 103(4):738–742.

Christakis DA, Mell L, Koepsell TD, Zimmerman FJ, Connell FA. 2001. Association of lower continuity of care with greater risk of emergency department use and hospitalization in children. *Pediatrics* 107(3):524–529.

Christakis DA, Wright JA, Zimmerman FJ, Bassett AL, Connell FA. 2002. Continuity of care is associated with high-quality care by parental report. *Pediatrics* 109(4):e54.

Christakis NA, Iwashyna TJ. 1998. Attitude and self-reported practice regarding prognostication in a national sample of internists. *Archives of Internal Medicine* 158(21):2389–2395.

CHSRP (Center for Health Services Research and Policy). 1999 (November). Part 1: Items and Services: Sample Purchasing Specifications. Washington, DC: George Washington University Medical Center. [Online]. Available: http://www.gwu.edu/~chsrp/sps/peds/nov99/part1.html [accessed July 23, 2001].

Clark AP, Calvin AO, Meyers TA, Eichhorn DJ, Guzzetta CE. 2001. Family presence during cardiopulmonary resuscitation and invasive procedures. A research-based intervention. *Critical Care Nursing Clinics of North America* 13(4):569–75.

Clatworthy S, Simon K, Tiedeman ME. 1999. Child drawing: Hospital—an instrument designed to measure the emotional status of hospitalized school-aged children. *Journal of Pediatric Nursing* 14(1):2–9.

Clay MC, Lane H, Willis SE, Peal M, Chakravarthi S, Poehlman G. 2000. Using a standard-ized family to teach clinical skills to medical students. *Teaching and Learning in Medicine* 12(3):145–149.

Clayton EW. 1995. What is really at stake in Baby K? A response to Ellen Flannery. *Journal of Law, Medicine, and Ethics* 23(1):13–14.

Clayton PJ, Halikas JA, Maurice WL. 1972. The depression of widowhood. *British Journal of Psychiatry* 120:71–77.

COG (Children's Oncology Group). [Online]. Available: http://www.childrensoncologygroup.org/ [accessed March 31, 2002].

COG End-of-Life Care Subcommittee. 2001 (September 8). Statement written by Joanne M. Hilden and Sarah Friebert to the IOM committee on improving palliative and end-of-life care for children and their families, Washington, DC.

Cohen, SR, Mount BM. 1992. Quality of life in terminal illness: Defining and measuring subjective well-being in the dying. *Journal of Palliative Care* 8(3):40–45.

Cohen SO, Walco GA. 1999. Dance/movement therapy for children and adolescents with cancer. *Cancer Practices* 7(1):34–42.

Coleman B. 2000. *Helping the Helpers: State Supported Services for Family Caregivers*. Washington, DC: AARP.

Coles R. 1990. *The Spiritual Life of Children*. Boston: Houghton Mifflin Company.

Collins J, Grier H, Kinney H, Berde CB. 1995. Control of severe pain in children with terminal malignancy. *Journal of Pediatrics* 126(4):653–657.

Conlon G. 2001 (September 9). Statement and discussion during open meeting with the IOM committee on improving palliative and end-of-life care for children and their families, Open Meeting. Washington, DC.

Conlon R. 2001. (September 9). Statement and discussion during open meeting with the IOM committee on improving palliative and end-of-life care for children and their families, Open Meeting. Washington, DC.

Connolly C. 2002 (March 19). FDA to suspend a rule on child drug testing agency. *Washington Post*, p. A10.

Cook A, Kornfield T, Gold M. 2000. *The Role of PBMs in Managing Drug Costs: Implications for a Medicare Drug Benefit*. Washington, DC: Mathematica Policy Research.

Cook LA, Watchko JF. 1996. Decision making for the critically ill neonate near the end of life. *Journal of Perinatology* 16(2 Pt 1):133–136.

Contro N, Larson J, Scofield S, Sourkes B, Cohen H. 2002. Family perspectives on the quality of pediatric palliative care. *Archives of Pediatric Adolescent Medicine* 156(1):14–19.

Corless IB. 2001. Bereavement. In: Ferrell B and Coyle N, eds. *Textbook of Palliative Nursing*. Oxford: Oxford University Press. Pp. 352–362.

Cornaglia C, Massimo L, Haupt R, Melodia, A., Sizemore, W., and Benedetti, C. 1984. Incidence of pain in children with neoplastic disease. *Pain* 2(suppl):S28.

Cotton P. 1992. "Basic benefits" have many variations, tend to become political issues. *Journal of the American Medical Association* 268(16):2139–2141.

Cox DN, Wittmann BK, Hess M, Ross AG, Lind J, Lindahl S. 1987. The psychological impact of diagnostic ultrasound. *Obstetrics & Gynecology* 70(5):673–676.

CPS (Canadian Paediatric Society). 2001. Guidelines for health care professionals supporting families experiencing a perinatal loss. *Paediatrics & Child Health* 6(71):469–477.

Crawley L, Payne R, Bolden J, Payne T, Washington P, Williams S. 2000. Palliative and end-of-life care in the African-American community. *Journal of the American Medical Association* 284:2518–2521.

Cretin S, Keeler EB, Lynn J, Batalden PB, Berwick DM, Bisognano M. 2000. Comment on: *JAMA* 283(17):2275–80 (Should patients in quality-improvement activities have the same protections as participants in research studies?). *Journal of the American Medical Association* 284(14):1786–1788.

Crimmins, TJ. Ethical issues in resuscitation. *Annals of Emergency Medicine* 22(2 pt 2):229–235.

Cromie WJ. 2001. Implications of antenatal ultrasound screening in the incidence of major genitourinary malformations. *Seminars in Pediatric Surgery.* 10(4):204–211.

CSHSC (Center for Studying Health System Change). 1999. Wall Street comes to Washington: Analysts' perspectives on the changing health care system. *Issue Brief* 21:1–4. Washington, DC: CSHCS.

Cubbin C, Pickle LW, Fingerhut L. 2000. Social context and geographic patterns of homicide among US black and white males. *American Journal of Public Health* 90(4):579–587.

Curtis JR, Patrick DL, Shannon SE, Treece PD, Engelberg RA, Rubenfeld GA. 2001. The family conference as a focus to improve communication about end of life care in the intensive care unit: Opportunities for improvement. *Critical Care Medicine* 29(2 Suppl): N26–33.

Cushing AM, Jones A. 1995. Evaluation of a breaking bad news course for medical students. *Medical Education* 29(6):430–435.

Daaleman TP, Frey B. 1998. Prevalence and patterns of physician referral to clergy and pastoral care providers. *Archives of Family Medicine* 7(6):548–553.

Daaleman TP, Nease DE Jr. 1994. Patient attitudes regarding physician inquiry into spiritual and religious issues. *Journal of Family Practice* 39(6):564–568.

Daaleman TP, VandeCreek L. 2000. Placing religion and spirituality in end-of-life care. *Journal of the American Medical Association* 284(19):2514–2517.

Dagi TF. 1995. Prayer, piety and professional propriety: Limits on religious expression in hospitals. *Journal of Clinical Ethics* 6(3):274–279.

Dana-Farber Cancer Institute. 2001. Inside the Institute. [Online]. Available: http://www.dana-farber.org/images/pdfs/abo_pub_inside091101.pdf [accessed March 31, 2002].

Danis M, Federman D, Fins JJ, Fox E, Kastenbaum B, Lanken PN, Long K, Lowenstein E, Lynn J, Rouse F, Tulsky J. 1999. Incorporating palliative care into critical care education: Principles, challenges, and opportunities. *Critical Care Medicine* 27(9):2068–2069.

Davies B. 1998. *Shadows in the Sun: The Experiences of Sibling Bereavement in Childhood.* Philadelphia: Brunner/Mazel.

Davies B. 2001. Supporting families in palliative care. In: Ferrell B and Coyle N, eds. *Textbook of Palliative Nursing.* Oxford: Oxford University Press. Pp. 363–373.

Davies B, Brennar P, Orloff S, Sumner L, Worden W. 2002. Addressing spirituality in pediatric hospice and palliative care. *Journal of Palliative Care* 18(1):59–67.

Dean RA. 1998. Occupational stress in hospice care: Causes and coping strategies. *American Journal of Hospital and Palliative Care* 15(3):151–154.

DeAngelis C, Feigin R, DeWitt T, First LR, Jewett EA, Kelch R. 2000. Final Report of the FOPE II Pediatric Workforce Workgroup. *Pediatrics* 106(5):1245–1255. [Online]. Available: http://www.aap.org/profed/WorkforceWorkgroupReportpdf.pdf [accessed March 31, 2002].

Dechairo-Marino AE, Jordan-Marsh M, Traiger G, Saulo M. 2001. Nurse/physician collaboration: Action research and the lessons learned. *Journal of Nursing Administration* 31(5):223–232.

Derish MT, Vanden Heuvel K. 2000. Mature minors should have the right to refuse life-sustaining medical care. *Journal of Law, Medicine & Ethics* 28:109–124.

Desnick RJ. 2001. Enzyme replacement and beyond. *Journal of Inherited Metabolic Disease* 24(2):251–265.

Dieckmann RA, Vardis R. 1995. High-dose epinephrine in pediatric out-of-hospital cardiopulmonary arrest. *Pediatrics* 95:901–913.

DoD (Department of Defense). 1999 (June 25). Hospital Reimbursement: TRICARE/ CHAMPUS DRG-Based Payment System. TRICARE/CHAMPUS Policy Manual 6010.47, Payments Policy. [Online] Available: http://www.tricare.osd.mil/POL/ C13S6_1B.PDF [accessed July 5, 2002].

Doka K, Morgan J, eds. 1993. *Death and Spirituality*. Amityville, NY: Baywood Publishing Company.

Dokken D. 2001 (September 9). Statement and discussion during open meeting with the IOM committee on improving palliative and end-of-life care for children and their families, Open Meeting. Washington, DC.

Donaldson MS. 2001. Continuity of care: A reconceptualization. *Medical Care Research and Review* 58(3):255–290.

Donaldson MS, Field MJ. 1998. Measuring quality of care at the end of life. *Archives of Internal Medicine* 158(2):121–128.

Dosanjh, S, Barnes J, Bhandari M. 2001. Barriers to breaking bad news around medical and surgical residents. *Medical Education* 35(3):197–205.

Dowdy MD, Robertson C, Bander JA. 1998. A study of proactive ethics consultation for critically and terminally ill patients with extended lengths of stay. *Critical Care Medicine* 26(2):252–259.

Downer K. 1996. Assessment of parental competence to consent to treatment for their child. *Nursing in Critical Care* 1(1):6–8 (review).

Doyle D, Hanks GWC, MacDonald N, eds. 1998. *Oxford Textbook of Palliative Medicine*, 2nd ed. Oxford: Oxford University Press.

Doyle D, Jeffrey D. 2000. *Palliative Care in the Home*. Oxford: Oxford Medical Publications.

Draper DA, Hurley RE, Lesser CS, Strunk BC. 2002. The Changing Face of Managed Care. *Health Affairs* 21(1):11–23.

Driscoll A. 2000. Managing post-discharge care at home: An analysis of patients' and their carers' perceptions of information received during their stay in hospital. *Journal of Advanced Nursing* 31(5):1165–1173.

Dubay L, Haley J, Kenney G. 2002a. Children's Eligibility for Medicaid and SCHIP: A View from 2000. [Online]. Available: http://www.urban.org/UploadedPDF/310435.pdf [accessed March 31, 2002].

Dubay L, Kenney G, Haley J. 2002b. Children's Participation in Medicaid and SCHIP: Early in the SCHIP Era. [Online]. Available: http://www.urban.org/UploadedPDF/310430.pdf [accessed March 31, 2002].

Duff RS, Campbell AGM. 1973. Moral and ethical dilemmas in the special-care nursery. *New England Journal of Medicine* 289:890–894.

Dugan D. 2001. Ethics committees in religious hospitals: A different landscape. *Park Ridge Center Bulletin*. [Online]. Available: http://www.parkridgecenter.org/cgibin/ShowPage. dll?MODE=2&ID=585 [accessed December 15, 2001].

Duke D. 1997. Infants may not receive adequate pain relief, caregivers believe. Washington University School of Medicine in St. Louis. [Online]. Available: http://wupa.wustl.edu/ nai/feature/1997/oct97-infantpain.html [accessed October 4, 2001].

Du Pen SL, Du Pen AR, Polissar N, Hansberry J, Kraybill BM, Stillman M, Panke J, Everly R, Syrjala K. 1999. Implementing guidelines for cancer pain management: Results of a randomized controlled clinical trial. *Journal of Clinical Oncology* 17(1):361–370.

Dyer KA. 2001. Ethical challenges of medicine and health on the Internet: A review. *Journal of Medical Internet Research* 3(2):e23.

Easson AM, Crosby JA, Librach SL. 2001. Discussion of death and dying in surgical textbooks. *American Journal of Surgery* 182(1):34–39.

Editorial. 2002 (July 1). Medicare physician payment: Time to act on E&M mess. *American Medical News*. [Online]. Available: http://www.ama-assn.org/sci-pubs/amnews/amn_02/edsa0701.htm [accessed July 5, 2002].

Eggly S, Afonso N, Rojas G, Baker M, Cardozo L, Robertson RS. 1997. An assessment of residents' competence in the delivery of bad news to patients. *Academic Medicine* 72(5): 397–399.

Ehman JW, Ott BB, Short TH, Ciampa RC, Hansen-Flaschen J. 1999. Do patients want physicians to inquire about their spiritual or religious beliefs if they become gravely ill? *Archives of Internal Medicine* 159(15):1803–1806.

Eichhorn DJ, Meyers TA, Mitchell TG, Guzzetta CE. 1996. Opening the doors: Family presence during resuscitation. *Journal of Cardiovascular Nursing* 10(4):59–70.

Eisenberg D. 1996. *Halachic issues regarding the futility of medical treatment: Applications to nutrition and hydration in the terminally ill patient*. San Francisco: The Institute for Jewish Medical Ethics of the Hebrew Academy of San Francisco.

Ellershaw J, Smith C, Overill S, Walker SE, Aldridge J. 2001. Care of the dying: Setting standards for symptom control in the last 48 hours of life. *Journal of Pain and Symptom Management* 21(1):12–17.

Emanuel LL, von Gunten CF, Ferris FD. 1999. *Education for Physicians on End of Life Care* (EPEC): *Participant's Handbook*. Princeton, NJ: EPEC Project, The Robert Wood Johnson Foundation and Chicago, IL: American Medical Association.

EMSCWS (Emergency Medical Services for Children, Washington State). 2000. Hospital Pediatric Capabilities in Washington State: Comparison of 1989 and 1999 Hospital Surveys. [Online]. Available: http://www.washingtonemsc.org/wahospi/wahospi.html [accessed March 16, 2002].

Epstein RM, Hundert EM. 2002. Defining and assessing professional competence. *Journal of the American Medical Association* 287(2):226–235.

Everly GS Jr. 2000. Crisis management briefings (CMB): Large group crisis intervention in response to terrorism, disasters and violence. *International Journal of Emergency Mental Health* 2:53–57.

Everly GS Jr, Boyle SH. 1999. Critical incident debriefing: A meta-analysis. *International Journal of Emergency Mental Health* 1(3):165–168.

Everly GS Jr., Mitchell, J.T. 2000. The debriefing "controversy" crisis intervention: A review of lexical and substantive issues. *International Journal of Emergency Mental Health* 2(4):211–225.

Ewigman BG, Crane JP, Frigoletto FD, LeFevre ML, Bain RP, McNellis D. 1993. Effect of prenatal ultrasound screening on perinatal outcome. *New England Journal of Medicine* 329(12):821–827.

Exner DV, Dries DL, Domanski MJ, Cohn JN. 2001. Lesser response to angiotensin-converting-enzyme inhibitor therapy in black as compared with white patients with left ventricular dysfunction. *New England Journal of Medicine* 344:1351–1357.

Eyman RK, Grossman HJ, Chaney RH, Call TL. 1993 (March). Survival of profoundly disabled people with severe mental retardation. *American Journal of Diseases of Children* 147(3):329–336.

Eysenbach G, Diepgen TL. 1999. Labeling and filtering of medical information on the Internet. *Methods of Information in Medicine*. 38(2):80–88.

Faber-Langendoen K. 1996. A multi-institutional study of care given to patients dying in hospitals: Ethical and practice implications. *Archives of Internal Medicine* 156(18):2130–2136.

Fadiman A. 1997. *The Spirit Catches You and You Fall Down*. New York: Farrar, Straus, and Giroux.

Farley DO, Zellman G, Ouslander JG, Reuben DB. 1999. Use of primary care teams by HMOs for care of long-stay nursing home residents. *Journal of American Geriatric Society* 47(2):139–144.

Farmer FL, Clarke LL, Miller MK. 1993. Consequences of differential residence designations for rural health policy research: The case of infant mortality. *Journal of Rural Health* 9(1):17–26.

Faw C, Ballentine R, Ballentine L, vanEys J. 1977. Unproved cancer remedies: A survey of use in pediatric outpatients. *Journal of the American Medical Association* 238:1536–1538.

FDA (Food and Drug Administration). 1998. Regulations requiring manufacturers to assess the safety and effectiveness of new drugs and biological products in pediatric patients. Final Rule. *Federal Register* 63(231):66631–66672, December 2, 1998. [Online]. Available: http://www.fda.gov/ohrms/dockets/98fr/120298c.txt[DOCID:fr02de98-24 [accessed December 14, 2001].

FDA. 2001a. Additional safeguards for children in clinical investigations of FDA-regulated products. Interim rule. *Federal Register* 66(79):20589–20600, April 24, 2001 [Online]. Available: http://www.fda.gov/OHRMS/DOCKETS/98fr/042401a.htm [accessed December 14, 2001].

FDA. 2001b. Docket No. 98N-0056: Update of List of Approved Drugs for Which Additional Pediatric Information May Produce Health Benefits in the Pediatric Population, May 20, 2001. [Online]. Available: http://www.fda.gov/cder/pediatric/peddrugsfinal.htm [accessed December 14, 2001].

FDA. 2001c. *The Pediatric Exclusivity Provision: January 2001.* Status Report to Congress. Washington, DC: U.S. Department of Health and Human Services. [Online]. Available: http://www.fda.gov/cder/pediatric/index.htm [accessed March 31, 2002].

Feder G, Eccles M, Grol R, Griffiths C, Grimshaw J. 1999. Clinical guidelines: Using clinical guidelines. *British Medical Journal* 318(7185):728–730.

Federal Interagency Forum on Child and Family Statistics. 2000. *America's Children: Key National Indicators of Children's Well-Being, 2000.* Washington, DC: U.S. Government Printing Office.

Feldstein BD. 2001. A piece of my mind: Toward meaning. *Journal of the American Medical Association* 286(11):1291–1292.

Fernandez CV, Rees EP. 1994. Pain management in Canadian level 3 neonatal intensive care units. *Canadian Medical Association Journal* 150(4):499–504.

Ferrell BR, Coyle N, eds. 2001. *Textbook of Palliative Nursing.* New York: Oxford.

Ferrell BR, Rhiner M, Shapiro B, Dierkes M. 1994. The experience of pediatric cancer pain Part I: Impact of pain on the family. *Journal of Pediatric Nursing* 9(6):368–379.

Ferrell BR, Virani R, Grant M, Borneman T. 2000. Analysis of pain content in nursing textbooks: Improving end-of-life care in nursing education. *Journal of Pain Symptom Management* 19:216–228.

Feudtner C. 2000. Dare we go gently: A piece of my mind. *Journal of the American Medical Association* 284(13):1621–1622.

Feudtner C, Christakis DA, Connell FA. 2000. Pediatric deaths attributable to complex chronic conditions: A population-based study of Washington State, 1980–1997. *Pediatrics* 106(1 Pt 2):205–209.

Feudtner C, Hays RM, Haynes G, Geyer JR, Neff JM, Koepsell TD. 2001. Deaths attributed to pediatric complex chronic conditions: National trends and implications for supportive care services. *Pediatrics* 107(6):e99.

Feudtner C, Silveira MJ, Christakis DA. 2002. Where do children with complex chronic conditions die? Patterns in Washington State, 1980–1998. *Pediatrics* 109(4):656–660.

Field M, Grigsby J. 2002. Telemedicine and remote patient monitoring. *Journal of the American Medical Association* [accepted for publication].

Fine DK. 2000. Government as god: An update on federal intervention in the treatment of critically ill newborns. *New England Law Review* 34:343.

Fine VK, Therrien ME. 1977. Empathy in the doctor–patient relationship: Skill training for medical students. *Journal of Medical Education* 52(9):752–757.

Finkbeiner AK. 1998. *Living With Loss Through the Years*. Baltimore, MD: Johns Hopkins University Press (paperback).

Finkelhor D, Ormrod RK. 2001. Child abuse reported to the police. *Juvenile Justice Bulletin* May 2001. [Online]. Available: http://www.ncjrs.org/html/ojjdp/jjbul2001_5_1/contents.html [accessed April 16, 2002].

Fins JJ. 1999. Commentary: From contract to covenant in advance care planning. *The Journal of Law, Medicine & Ethics* 27(1):46–51.

Finucane TE, Christmas C, Travis K. 1999. Tube feeding in patients with advanced dementia: A review of the evidence. *Journal of the American Medical Association* 282(14):1365–1370.

Fleischman A. 1998. Commentary: Ethical issues in pediatric pain management and terminal sedation. *Journal of Pain Symptom Management* 15(4):260–261.

Fleischman A, Nolan K, Dubler NN, Epstein MF, Gerben MA, Jellinek MS, Litt IF, Miles MS, Oppenheimer S, Shaw A, van Eys J, Vaughn VC. 1994. Caring for gravely ill children. *Pediatrics* 94(4):433–439.

Fleming M. 1999. A case study of child abuse and a parent's refusal to withdraw life sustaining treatment. *Human Rights* 26:12.

Fletcher JC. 1991. The bioethics movement and hospital ethics committees. *Maryland Law Review* 50:859–894.

Fletcher JC. 1997. Bioethics in a legal forum: Confessions of an "expert" witness. *Journal of Medicine and Philosophy* 22:297–324.

Fletcher RH, O'Malley MS, Fletcher SW, Earp JA, Alexander JP. 1984. Measuring the continuity and coordination of medical care in a system involving multiple providers. *Medical Care* 22(5):403–411.

Foley KM. 1994. The World Health Organization program in cancer pain relief and palliative care. In *Proceedings of the 7th World Congress on Pain: Progress in Pain Research and Management*. Vol 2, Gebhart GI, Hammond DL, Jensen TS, eds. Seattle, WA: IASP Press. Pp. 59–74.

Forrest GC, Claridge R, Baum JD. 1981. The practical management of perinatal death. *British Medical Journal* 282:31–32

Forrest GC, Standish E, Baum JD. 1982. Support after perinatal death: A study of support and counseling after perinatal bereavement. *British Medical Journal* 285:1475–1479.

Fost N. 1999. Decisions regarding treatment of seriously ill newborns. *Journal of the American Medical Association* 281:2041–2043.

Fowler EJ, Anderson GF. 1996. Capitation adjustment for pediatric populations. *Pediatrics* 98(1):10–17.

Fowler JW. 1981. *Stages of Faith*. San Francisco: Harper.

Fox HB, McManus MA. 1998. Improving state Medicaid contracts and plan practices for children with special needs. *Future Child* 8(2):105–118.

Fox HB, McManus MA, Limb SJ. 2000. *Access to Care for S-CHIP Children with Special Health Care Needs*. Washington, DC: HRSA (Health Resources and Services Administration), Maternal and Child Health Bureau.

Fox P. 1999. *End-of-Life Care in Managed Care Organizations*. Washington, DC: American Association of Retired Persons.

Fox S, Rainie L. 2002. *Vital Decisions: How Internet Users Decide What Information to Trust When They or Their Loved Ones Are Sick.* Washington, DC: Pew Internet and American Life Project. [Online]. Available: http://www.pewinternet.org/reports/pdfs/PIP_Vital_Decisions_May2002.pdf [accessed June 19, 2002].

Freund DA, Rossiter LF, Fox PD, Meyer JA, Hurley RE, Carey TS, Paul JE. 1989. Evaluation of the Medicaid competition demonstrations. *Health Care Financing Review* 11(2):81–97.

Fried BJ, Rundall TG. 1996. Managing Groups and Teams. In: Shortell SM, Kaluzny AD, eds. *Essentials of Health Care Management.* Albany, NY: Delmar. Pp. 163–197.

FSMB (Federation of State Medical Boards). 2002 (May 31). USMLE Clinical Skills Examination: Fact Sheet. [Online]. Available: http://www.fsmb.org [accessed June 21, 2002].

Furth SL, Hwang W, Yang C, Neu AM, Fivush BA, Powe NR. 2001. Relation between pediatric experience and treatment recommendations for children and adolescents with kidney failure. *Journal of the American Medical Association* 285(8):1027–1033.

Gabel J, Hurst K, Hunt K. 1998. Health benefits for the terminally ill: Reality and perception. *Health Affairs* 17(6):120–127.

Gage B, Dao T. 2000 (March). Medicare's Hospice Benefit: Use and Expenditures, 1996 Cohort. Report prepared for U.S. Department of Health and Human Services. [Online]. Available: http://aspe.hhs.gov/daltcp/reports/96useexp.htm [accessed July 5, 2002].

Galloway KS, Yaster M. 2000. Pain and symptom control in terminally ill children. *Pediatric Clinics of North America* 47(3):711–746.

Garg A, Buckman R, Kason Y. 1997. Teaching medical students how to break bad news. *Canadian Medical Association Journal* 156(8):1159–1164.

Garrett JM, Harris RP, Norburn JK, Patrick DL, Danis M. 1993. Life-sustaining treatments during terminal illness: Who wants what? *Journal of General Internal Medicine* 8(7):361–368.

Gerson AC, Joyner M, Fosarelli P, Butz A, Wissow L, Lee S, Marks P, N Hutton. 2001. Disclosure of HIV diagnosis to children: When, where, why and how. *Journal of Pediatric Health Care* 15(4):161–167.

Gerteis M, Edgman-Levitan S, Daley J, Delbanco TL (eds). 1993. *Through the Patient's Eyes: Understanding and Promoting Patient-centered Care.* San Francisco: Jossey-Bass.

Gibson B. 2001. Long-term ventilation for patients with Duchenne muscular dystrophy: Physicians' beliefs and practices. *Chest* 119(3):940–946.

Gifford E, Weech-Maldonado R, Short PF. 2001 (June 12). Encouraging Preventive Health Services for Young Children: The Effect of Expanding Coverage to Parents. Presentation at the Academy for Health Services Research and Health Policy Conference, Atlanta.

Giles P. 1970. Reactions of women to perinatal death. *Australia New Zealand Journal of Obstetrics and Gynecology* 10:207–210

Gill JM, Mainous AG III. 1998. The role of provider continuity in preventing hospitalizations. *Archives of Family Medicine* 7(4):352–357.

Gill JM, Mainous AG III, Nsereko M. 2000. The effect of continuity of care on emergency department use. *Archives of Family Medicine* 9(4):333–338.

Gillick MR. 2001. Artificial nutrition and hydration in the patient with advanced dementia: Is withholding treatment compatible with traditional Judaism? *Medical Ethics* 27:12–15.

Gilligan T, Raffin TA. 1996. How to withdraw mechanical ventilation: More studies are needed. *American Journal of Critical Care* 5(5):323–325.

Gillon R. 1997. Clinical ethics committees—pros and cons. *Journal of Medical Ethics* 23(4):203–204.

Girgis AM, Sanson-Fisher RW. 1995. Breaking bad news: Consensus guidelines for medical practitioners. *Journal of Clinical Oncology* 13(9):2449–2456.

Gittler J. 1998. Title V of the Social Security Act and state programs for children with special health care needs. In: *Implementing Title V CSHCN Programs: A Resource Manual for State Programs*. Maternal and Child Health Bureau, U.S. Department of Health and Human Services, Rockville, MD. [Online]. Available: http://cshcnleaders.ichp.edu/ CSHCNProgramManual/02%20TITLE%20V%20Legislative%20History.pdf [accessed July 12, 2001].

Glaser BG, Strauss AL. 1965. *Awareness of Dying*. Chicago: Aldine Publishing.

Glover JJ, Rushton CH. 1995. Introduction: From Baby Doe to Baby K: Evolving challenges in pediatric ethics. *Journal of Law, Medicine, and Ethics* 23:5–6.

Goh AY, Mok Q. 2001. Identifying futility in a pediatric critical care setting: A prospective observational study. *Archives for Disabled Children* 84(3):265–268.

Gold M, Franks P, Erickson P. 1996. Assessing the health of the nation: The predictive validity of a preference-based measure and self-rated health. *Medical Care* 34(2):163–177.

Goldman A. 1996. Home care of the dying child. *Journal of Palliative Care* 12(3):16–19.

Goldman A. 1998. Life-threatening illnesses and symptom control in children. In: Doyle D, Hanks GWC, MacDonald N, eds. 1998. *Oxford Textbook of Palliative Medicine*, 2nd ed. Oxford: Oxford University Press. Pp.1033–1043.

Goldman A, ed. 1999. *Care of the Dying Child*. Oxford: Oxford University Press (paperback).

Goldman A. 2000. Integrating palliative and curative approaches in the care of children with life-threatening illnesses: Interview with Ann Goldman. *Innovations in End-of-Life Care* 2(2). [Online]. Available: http://www2.edc.org/lastacts/archives/archivesMarch00/ featureinn.asp [accessed November 26, 2001].

Goldman A, Christie D. 1993. Children with cancer talk about their own death with their families. *Pediatric Hematology and Oncology* 10(3):223–231.

Goldstein B, Merkens M. 2000. End-of-life in the pediatric intensive care unit: Seeking the family's decision of when and how, not if. *Critical Care Medicine* 28(8):3122–3123.

Gomez CF. 1996. Hospice and home care: Opportunities for training. In: *Care for the Dying: Identification and Promotion of Physician Competency: Educational Resource Document*. Philadelphia: American Board of Internal Medicine.

Gramelspacher GP, Zhou XH, Hanna MP, Tierney WM. 1997. Preferences of physicians and their patients for end of life care. *Journal of General Internal Medicine* 12(6):346–351.

Gray JE, Safran C, Davis RB, Pompilio-Weitzner G, Stewart JE, Zaccagnini L, Pursley D. 2000. Baby CareLink: Using the Internet and telemedicine to improve care for high-risk infants. *Pediatrics* 106(6):1318–1324.

Greenberg LW, Ochsenschlager D, Cohen GJ, Einhorn AH, O'Donnell R. 1993. Counseling parents of a child dead on arrival: A survey of emergency departments. *American Journal of Emergency Medicine* 11(3):225–229.

Greenberg LW, Ochsenschlager D, O'Donnell R, Mastruserio J, Cohen GJ. 1999. Communicating bad news: A pediatric department's evaluation of a simulated intervention. *Pediatrics* 103(6):1210–1217.

Grimaldo DA, Wiener-Kronish JP, Jurson T, Shaughnessy TE, Curtis JR, Liu LL. 2001 (July). A randomized, controlled trial of advanced care planning discussions during preoperative evaluations. *Anesthesiology* 95(1):43–50, discussion 5A.

Grimshaw JM, Shirran L, Thomas R, Mowatt G, Fraser C, Bero L, Grilli R, Harvey E, Oxman A, O'Brien MA. 2001. Changing provider behavior: An overview of systematic reviews and interventions. *Medical Care* 39(8 Suppl 2):II2–45.

Grodin MA, Glantz LH, eds. 1994. *Children as Research Subjects: Ethics and Law*. New York: Oxford University Press.

Gruskin A, Williams RG, McCabe ER, Stein F, Strickler J, Chesney RW, Mulvey HJ, Simon JL, Alden ER. 2000. Final report of the FOPE II Pediatric Subspecialists of the Future Workgroup. *Pediatrics* 106(5):1224–1244.

Gruttadaro DE, Ross EC, Honberg R. 2001. Legal Protections and Advocacy Strategies for People with Severe Mental Illnesses in Managed Care Systems. NAMI (National Alliance for the Mentally Ill). [Online]. Available: http://www.nami.org/legal/ManagedCare.pdf [accessed April 15, 2002].

Guyer B, Freedman MA, Strobino DM, Sondik EJ. 2000. Annual summary of vital statistics: Trends in the health of Americans during the 20th century. *Pediatrics* 106(6):1307–1317.

Guzzetta CE, Taliaferro E, Proehl JA. 2000. Family presence during invasive procedures and resuscitation. *Journal of Trauma* 49(6):1157–1159.

Haight BK, Burnside I. 1993. Reminiscence and life review: Explaining the differences. *Archive of Psychiatric Nursing* 7(2):91–98.

Halamka J. 2001. Inside a virtual nursery. *Health Management Technology* 22(6):37–38. [Online]. Available: http://www.healthmgttech.com/archives/h0601nursery.htm [accessed March 31, 2002].

Halpern J. 2001. *From Detached Concern to Empathy: Humanizing Medical Practice*. New York: Oxford University Press.

Hansen HE, Biros MH, Delaney NM, Schug VL. 1999. Research utilization and interdisciplinary collaboration in emergency care. *Academic Emergency Medicine* 6(4):271–279.

Hansen P, Cornish P, Kayser K. 1998. Family conferences as forums for decision making in hospital settings. *Social Work in Health Care* 27(3):57–74.

Hanson RM, Phythian MA, Jarvis JB, Stewart C. 1998. The true cost of treating children. *Medical Journal of Australia* 169:S39–S41. [Online]. Available: http://www.mja.com.au/public/issues/oct19/casemix/hanson/hanson.html [accessed August 16, 2001].

Hardart K, Heller KS, Solomon MZ for the Initiative for Pediatric Palliative Care (IPPC). 2002. Clinicians' perspectives on pediatric palliative care: What hinders, what helps. Unpublished manuscript. Newton, MA: Education Development Center, Inc.

Harper BC. 1977. *Death: The Coping Mechanism of the Health Professional*. Greenville, SC: Southeastern University Press.

Harper BC. 1993. Staff support. In: Armstrong-Dailey A, Goltzer SZ, eds. *Hospice Care for Children*. New York: Oxford University Press. Pp. 184–197.

Harris RP, Helfand M, Woolf SH, Lohr KN, Mulrow CD, Teutsch SM, Atkins D. 2001. Current methods of the U.S. Preventive Services Task Force: A review of the process. *American Journal of Preventive Medicine* 20(3 Suppl):21–35.

Harrison AM, Botkin J. 1999. Can pediatricians define and apply the concept of brain death? *Pediatrics* 103(6):e82.

Harrison H. 1993. The principles for family-centered neonatal care. *Pediatrics* 92(5):643–650.

Hart RG, Ahrens WR. 1998. Coping with pediatric death in the emergency department by learning from parental experience. *American Journal of Emergency Medicine* 16(1):67–68.

Hartman RG. 2000. Adolescent autonomy: Clarifying an ageless conundrum. *Hastings Law Journal* 51:1265.

Harvard Medical School. 2002. Program in Palliative Care and Education. [Online]. Available: http://www.hms.harvard.edu/cdi/pallcare/program.html [accessed March 15, 2002].

Haslam RHA. 2000. Congenital Anomalies of the Central Nervous System. In: Behrman RE, Kliegman RM, Jenson HB, eds. *Nelson Textbook of Pediatrics*, 16th ed. Philadelphia: WB Saunders. Pp. 1803–1813.

Hawkins LA. 1992. Living will statutes: A minor oversight. *Virginia Law Review* 78:1581–1615.

Hay MW. 1989. Principle in building spiritual assessment tools. *American Journal of Hospice Care* 6:25–31.

Hayley DC. 2000. Comment on: *JAMA* 2000 May 3; 283(17):2275–2280 (Should patients in quality-improvement activities have the same protections as participants in research studies?). *Journal of the American Medical Association* 284(14):1787–1788.

Hayward R, Forbes D, Lau F, Wilson D. 2000. *Strengthening Multidisciplinary Health Care Teams: Final Evaluation Report 2000.* Calgary, Alberta, Canada: Department of Health and Wellness. [Online]. Available: http://www.health.gov.ab.ca/key/phc/projects/independent/StrengtheningEvaluation.pdf [accessed January 11, 2002].

HCFA/CMS (Health Care Financing Administration, now Centers for Medicare and Medicaid Services, Department of Health and Human Services). 1994. 418.88(c) Standard: Spiritual Counseling State Operations Manual, Appendix M: Survey Procedures and Interpretive Guidelines for Hospices. p. M39. [Online]. Available: http://www.hcfa.gov/pubforms/07_som/somap_m.htm [accessed October 26, 2001].

HCFA/CMS). 1997 (September 22). Implementation of Section 1931 of the Social Security Act. Letter from Sally K. Richardson, Director, Center for Medicaid and State Operations to State Medicaid Director. [Online]. Available: http://www.hcfa.gov/medicaid/wrdl922.htm [accessed August 17, 2001].

HCFA/CMS. 1999 (December). Program Memorandum: Issues Related to Critical Care Policy. [Online]. Available: http://www.hcfa.gov/pubforms/transmit/b994360.htm [accessed August 17, 2002].

HCFA/CMS. 2000a. 1915(b) Freedom of Choice Waivers. [Online]. Available: http://www.hcfa.gov/medicaid/hpg3.htm [accessed August 17, 2001].

HCFA/CMS. 2000b. A Profile of Medicaid: Chartbook 2000. [Online]. Available: http://www.hcfa.gov/stats/2Tchartbk.pdf [accessed March 31, 2002].

HCFA/CMS. 2000c. Information Letters from Thomas Hamilton to Five State Medicaid Officials Clarifying a Children's Hospice Initiative Grant Opportunity. Baltimore, MD: June 8, 2000. [Online]. Available: http://www.hcfa.gov/medicaid/chi6800.htm [accessed March 31, 2002].

HCFA/CMS. 2000d. Medicare Coverage Policy, Clinical Trials: Final National Coverage Decision. [Online]. Available: http://www.hcfa.gov/coverage/8d2.htm [accessed August 17, 2001].

HCFA/CMS. 2000e. Medicare ESRD Dialysis Patients: Patient Profile: Table 1. [Online]. Available: http://www.hcfa.gov/medicare/esrdtab1.htm [accessed January 30, 2002].

HCFA/CMS. 2000f. Medicare program: Changes to the hospital inpatient prospective payment systems and fiscal year 2001 rates. *Federal Register* 65(148):47104–47153, August 1, 2000.

HCFA/CMS. 2000g. State Children's Health Insurance Program (SCHIP): Aggregate Enrollment Statistics for the 50 States and the District of Columbia for Federal Fiscal Year (FFY) 2000. [Online]. Available: http://www.hcfa.gov/init/children.htm [accessed July 22, 2001].

HCFA/CMS. 2001a. Disabled and Elderly Health Programs Group. [Online]. Available: http://www.hcfa.gov/medicaid/f2hrates.htm [accessed July 3, 2001].

HCFA/CMS. 2001b. Hospice services. [Online]. Available: http://www.hcfa.gov/medicaid/ltc2.htm [accessed August 13, 2001].

HCFA/CMS. 2001c. Medicaid and EPSDT. [Online]. Available: http://www.hcfa.gov/medicaid/epsdthm.htm [accessed July 3, 2001].

HCFA/CMS. 2001d. Medicaid: A Brief Summary. [Online]. Available: http://www.hcfa.gov/pubforms/actuary/ormedmed/default4.htm [accessed August 13, 2001].

HCFA/CMS. 2001e (June 8). Medicare program; five-year review of work relative value units under the physician fee schedule. Proposed Notice. *Federal Register* 66(11):31027–31084. [Online]. Available: http://www.hcfa.gov/regs/pfs/fr08jn01.htm [accessed August 2, 2001].

HCFA/CMS. 2001f (August 20). Protocols for External Quality Review of Medicaid Managed Care Organizations and Prepaid Health Plans. Notice of Proposed Rulemaking: Medicaid Managed Care; 42 CFR Part 400, et.al. [Online]. Available: http://www. hcfa.gov/medicaid/omchmpg.htm [accessed March 31, 2002].

HCFA/CMS. 2001g. Revision of Medicare Reimbursement for Telehealth Services. Program Memorandum Intermediaries and Carriers. Transmittal AB-01-69, May 1, 2001. [Online]. Available: http://www.hcfa.gov/pubforms/transmit/AB0169.pdf [accessed March 31, 2002].

Heim M, Martinowitz U, Horoszowski H, Springman P. 1986. Summer camps for haemophilic children and adolescents. *International Journal of Adolescent Medicine & Health* 2(4):281–284.

Henig NR, Faul JL, Raffin TA. 2001. Biomedical ethics and the withdrawal of advanced life support. *Annual Review in Medicine* 52:79–92.

Herlan ER. 1998. *The Legal Framework of Responding to DNR Orders on School Grounds*. Palm Beach Gardens, FL: LRP Publications.

Herndon C, Fike DS, Anderson AC, Dole EJ. 2001. Pharmacy student training in United States hospices. *American Journal of Hospice & Palliative Care* 18(3):181–186.

Hersh WR, Helfand M, Wallace J, Kraemer D, Patterson P, Shapiro S, Greenlick M. 2001. Clinical outcomes resulting from telemedicine interventions: A systematic review. BMC Medical Informatics and Decision Making 1(5). [Online]. Available: http://www. biomedcentral.com/1472-6947/1/5 [accessed February 5, 2002].

Heyl-Martineau T. 2001 (September 9). Statement and discussion with IOM committee on improving palliative and end-of-life care for children and their families, Open Meeting. Washington, DC.

Higginson I. 1993. *Clinical Audit in Palliative Care*. New York: Radcliffe Medical Press.

Higginson I, Hearn J, Webb D. 1996. Audit in palliative care: Does practice change? *European Journal of Cancer Care* 4:233–236.

Hilden JM, Tobin DR. 2002. *Children with Life-Threatening Illness: A Manual for Parents*. Albany, NY: The Life Institute Press.

Hilden JM, Emanuel EJ, Fairclough DL, Link MP, Foley KM, Clarridge BC, Schnipper LE, Mayer RJ. 2001a. Attitudes and practices among pediatric oncologists regarding end-of life care: Results of the 1998 American Society of Clinical Oncology survey. *Journal of Clinical Oncology* 19(1):205–212.

Hilden J, Himelstein BP, Freyer DR, Friebert S, Kane JR. 2001b. End-of-life care: Special issues in pediatric oncology. In: Foley KM, Gelband H, eds. *Improving Palliative Care for Cancer*. Washington, DC: National Academy Press. Pp. 161–198.

Hilden JM, Watterson J, Chrastek J. 2001c. Tell the children. *Journal of Clinical Oncology* 19(2):595–596.

Himelstein BP, Hilden J. 2001.When a child is dying: Smallest patients offer the biggest lesson. *Finding Our Way: Living with Dying in America*. [Online]. Available: http:// www.findingourway.net/Articles/article_child.html [accessed January 15, 2002].

Himelstein BP, Hilden JM, Kane J, Tobin DR, Larson DG. 2002. *Pediatric Advanced Illness Coordinated Care Program Training Manual*. Albany, NY: The Life Institute Press.

Hinds PS, Oakes L, Furman W. 2001. End-of-life decision making in pediatric oncology. In: Ferrell BR, Coyle N, eds. *Textbook of Palliative Nursing*. New York: Oxford University Press. Pp. 450–460.

Hoffman C, Pohl M. 2000. *Health Insurance Coverage in America: 1999 Data Update.* Washington, DC: Kaiser Commission on Medicaid and the Uninsured.

Hoffman W. 2001. Issues to consider when ending life support. *ACP-ASIM Observer* (American College of Physicians-American Society of Internal Medicine). [Online]. Available: http://www.acponline.org/journals/news/may01/lifesupport.htm [accessed March 31, 2002].

Hoffpauir SP. 2001. Do not resuscitate orders in schools. Alabama Association of School Boards, June 1, 2001. [Online]. Available: http://www.theaasb.org/education_ law.cfm? docID=687 [accessed October 18, 2001].

Holahan J, Rangarajan S, Schirmer M. 1999. Medicaid managed care payment rates in 1998. *Health Affairs* 18(3):217–227.

Holder AR. 1983. Parents, courts, and refusal of treatment. *Journal of Pediatrics* 103(4):515–521.

Holder AR. 1987. Minors' rights to consent to medical care. *Journal of the American Medical Association* 257:3400–3402.

Hopp FP, Duffy SA. June 2000. Racial variations in end-of-life care. *Journal of the American Geriatrics Society* 48(6):658–663.

Horn SD, Hopkins DP, eds. 1994. *Clinical Practice Improvement: A Technology for Delivering Cost-Effective Quality Health Care.* Washington, DC: Faulkner and Gray.

Horwitz ET. 1979. Of love and laetrile: Medical decision-making in a child's best interests. *American Journal of Law & Medicine* 5:271–294.

Hosenpud JD, Bennett LE, Keck BM, Edwards EB, Novick RJ. 1998. Effect of diagnosis on survival benefit of lung transplantation for end-stage lung disease. *Lancet* 351(9095):24–27.

Hospice to offer videoconferencing service. 2001. *Technology in Practice.* [Online]. Available: http://www.technologyinpractice.com/html/news/NewsStory.cfm?DID=7295 [accessed March 31, 2002].

Hostetler-Lelaulu S. 1999. On the Edge. You Just Don't Get It: Lissencephaly Network's Gripe page. [Online]. Available: http://www.lissencephaly.org/articles/gripe/gripe2.htm [accessed November 11, 2001].

Houts PS. 1997. *ACP Home Care Guide for Young Persons with Cancer.* PS Houts, ed. Philadelphia: Penn State University. [Online] Available: http://www.hmc.psu.edu/ pedsonco/Homeguide.html [accessed August 11, 2001].

Howe EG. 1999. Ethics consultants: could they do better? *Journal of Clinical Ethics* 10(1):13–25.

Hoyert D, Freedman MA, Strobino DM, Guyer B. 2001. Annual summary of vital statistics: 2000. *Pediatrics* 108(6):1241–1255.

HPNA (Hospice and Palliative Nurses Association). 2001 (September 19). Statement written by Molly A. Poleto to the IOM committee on improving palliative and end-of-life care for children and their families, Washington, DC.

Hunt AM. 1990. A survey of signs, symptoms, and symptom control in 30 terminally ill children. *Developmental Medicine and Child Neurology* 32(4):341–346.

Hunt AM, Burne R. 1995. Medical and nursing problems of children with neurodegenerative disease. *Palliative Medicine* 9(1):19–26.

Huskamp HA, Buntin MB, Wang V, Newhouse JP. 2001. Providing care at the end of life: Do Medicare rules impede good care? *Health Affairs* 20(3):204–211.

Hussey JM. 1997. The effects of race, socioeconomic status, and household structure on injury mortality in children and young adults. *Maternal and Child Health Journal* 1(4): 217–227.

Hwang HC, Stallones L, Keefe TJ. 1997. Childhood injury deaths: Rural and urban differences, Colorado 1980–1988. *Injury Prevention* 3(1):35–37.

Hygeia. 2001 (September 8). Statement presented by Michael R. Berman to the IOM committee on improving palliative and end-of-life care for children and their families, Open Meeting. Washington, DC.

Hynan, MT. 1996. Helping parents cope with a high-risk birth: Terror, grief, impotence and anger. Paper presented at November 10, 1996, meeting of the National Perinatal Association, Nashville, TN. [Online]. Available: http://www.uwm.edu/People/hynan/MINNAEP.html [accessed April 11, 2001].

Inati MN, Lazar EC, Haskin-Leahy L. 1994. The role of the genetic counselor in a perinatal unit. *Seminars in Perinatology* 18(3):133–139.

Inkelas M. 2001. *Incentives in a Specialty Care Carve-Out*. Santa Monica, CA: RAND.

IOM (Institute of Medicine). 1984. *Bereavement: Reactions, Consequences, and Care*. Osterweis M, Green M, eds. Washington, DC: National Academy Press.

IOM. 1990a. *Clinical Practice Guidelines: Directions for a New Program*. Lohr KN, Field M, eds. Washington, DC: National Academy Press.

IOM. 1990b. *Medicare: A Strategy for Quality Assurance*. Lohr KN, ed. Washington, DC: National Academy Press.

IOM. 1991. *The Computer-Based Patient Record: An Essential Technology for Health Care*. Dick RS, Steen EB, eds. Washington, DC: National Academy Press.

IOM. 1992. *Guidelines for Clinical Practice: From Development to Use*. Field M, Lohr KN, eds. Washington, DC: National Academy Press.

IOM. 1993. *Emergency Medical Services for Children*. Durch JS, KN Lohr, eds. Washington, DC: National Academy Press.

IOM. 1995. *Strategies for Assuring the Provision of Quality Services Through Managed Care Delivery Systems to Children with Special Health Care Needs: Workshop Highlights*. Harris-Wehling J, Ireys HT, Heagarty M, eds. Washington, DC: National Academy Press.

IOM. 1996a. *Paying Attention to Children in a Changing Health Care System*. Ein Lewin M, Altman S, eds. Washington, DC: National Academy Press.

IOM. 1996b. *Telemedicine: A Guide to Assessing Telecommunications in Health Care*. Field MJ, ed. Washington, DC: National Academy Press.

IOM. 1997. *Approaching Death: Improving Care at the End of Life*. Field MJ, Cassel CK, eds. Washington, DC: National Academy Press.

IOM. 1998. *America's Children: Health Insurance and Access to Care*. Edmunds M, Coye MJ, eds. Washington, DC: National Academy Press.

IOM. 2000a. *America's Health Care Safety Net: Intact but Endangered*. Ein Lewin M, Altman S, eds. Washington, DC: National Academy Press.

IOM. 2000c. *Enhancing Data Systems to Improve the Quality of Cancer Care*. Hewitt M, Simone JV, eds. Washington, DC: National Academy Press.

IOM. 2000d. *Extending Medicare Reimbursement in Clinical Trials*. Aaron HJ, Gelband H, eds. Washington, DC: National Academy Press.

IOM. 2001a. *Coverage Matters: Insurance and Health Care*. Washington, DC: National Academy Press.

IOM. 2001b. *Crossing the Quality Chasm*. Washington, DC: National Academy Press.

IOM 2001c. *Improving Palliative Care for Cancer*. Foley KM, Gelband H, eds. Washington, DC: National Academy Press.

IOM 2002. *Unequal Treatment: Confronting Racial and Ethnic Disparities in Health Care*. Smedley B, Stith AY, Nelson AR, eds. Washington, DC: National Academy Press.

Ireys HT. 1996. Children with special health care needs: Dimensions of the population. In: Ein Lewin M, Altman S, eds. *Paying Attention to Children in a Changing Health Care System*. Washington, DC: National Academy Press. Pp 64–73.

Irish DP, Lundquist KF, Nelson VJ, eds. 1993. *Ethnic Variations in Dying, Death, and Grief: Diversity in Universality.* Washington, DC: Taylor & Francis.

Iverson K. 1999. *Grave Words: Educational Models for Notifying Survivors After Sudden, Unexpected Deaths.* Tuscon, AZ: Galen Press.

Jackson B, Gibson T, Staeheli J. 2000. Hospice Benefits and Utilization in the Large Employer Market. The Medstat Group. Online. Available: http://aspe.hhs.gov/daltcp/reports/empmkt.htm [accessed July 12, 2001].

Jadad AR, Gagliardi A. 1998. Rating health information on the Internet: Navigating to knowledge or to Babel? *Journal of the American Medical Association* 279(8):611–614.

Jaslow D, Barbera JA, Johnson E, Moore W. 1997. Termination of nontraumatic cardiac arrest resuscitative efforts in field: A national survey. *Academic Emergency Medicine* 4(9):904–907.

JCAHO (Joint Commission on Accreditation of Healthcare Organizations). 1995, 1998. *Comprehensive Accreditation Manual for Hospitals.* Chicago.

JCAHO. 2001. Pain Standards for 2001. [Online]. Available: http://www.jcaho.org/standard/pm.html [accessed May 27, 2002].

Jecker NS, Carrese JA, Pearlman RA. 1995. Caring for patients in cross-cultural settings. *Hastings Center Report* 25(1):6–14.

Jeffrey T, Berger MD. 1998. Culture and ethnicity in clinical care. *Archives of Internal Medicine* 158:2085–2090.

Jenkins PC, Flanagan MF, Jenkins KJ, Sargent JD, Canter CE, Chinnock RE, Vincent RN, Tosteson AN, O'Connor GT. 2000. Survival analysis and risk factors for mortality in transplantation and staged surgery for hypoplastic left heart syndrome. *Journal of the American College of Cardiology* 36(4):1178–1185.

Johnson BH, Jeppson ES, Redburn L. 1992. *Caring for Children and Families. Guidelines for Hospitals.* Bethesda, MD: Association for the Care of Children's Health.

Joint Working Party of the Association for Children with Life-Threatening or Terminal Conditions and Their Families and the Royal College of Paediatrics and Child Health. 1997. *A Guide to the Development of Children's Palliative Care Services.* Bristol, England.

Jones NE, Pieper CF, Robertson LS. 1992. The effect of legal drinking age on fatal injuries of adolescents and young adults. *American Journal of Public Health* 82:112–115.

Jones NS. 1999. *Access to Home Health Services Under Medicare's Interim Payment System.* Washington, DC: National Health Policy Forum. Issue Brief No. 744, July 13. [Online]. Available: http://www.nhpf.org/pdfs/8-744+(web).pdf [accessed June 5, 2002].

Jonsen AR, Siegler M, Winslade W. 1998. *Clinical Ethics,* 4th ed. New York: McGraw-Hill.

Jonsen AR, Toulmin SE. 1988. *The Abuse of Casuistry: A History of Moral Reasonings.* Berkley, CA: University of California Press.

Jost TS. 1998. Public financing of pain management: Leaky umbrellas and ragged safety nets. *Journal of Law, Medicine & Ethics* 26(4):290–307.

Jurkovich GJ, Pierce B, Pananen L, Rivara FP. 2000. Giving bad news: The family perspective. *Journal of Trauma* 48(5):865–873.

Kaczorowski JM. 1989. Spiritual well-being and anxiety in adults diagnosed with cancer. *Hospice Journal* 5:105–116.

Kahn D, Richardson DK, Gray JE, Bednarek F, Rubin LP, Shah B, Frantz ID III, Pursley DM. 1998. Variation among neonatal intensive care units in narcotic administration. *Archives of Pediatrics and Adolescent Medicine* 152(9):844–851.

Kaiser Commission on Medicaid and the Uninsured. 2001. *Medicaid: A Primer.* Washington, DC: The Henry J. Kaiser Family Foundation. [Online]. Available: http://www.kff.org/content/2001/2248/2248.pdf [accessed August 8, 2001].

Kane B. 1979. Children's concepts of death. *Journal of Genetic Psychology* 11:497–515.

Kaluzny AD. 1985. Design and management of disciplinary and interdisciplinary groups in health services: Review and critique. *Medical Care Review* 42(1):77–112.

Karlawish JH, Quill T, Meier DE. 1999. A consensus-based approach to providing palliative care to patients who lack decision-making capacity. ACP-ASIM End-of-Life Care Consensus Panel. American College of Physicians-American Society of Internal Medicine. *Annals of Internal Medicine* 130(10):835–840.

Karpinski, M. 2000. *Quick Tips For Caregivers*. Medford, OR: Healing Arts Communications.

Katz A, Gardner M, Wright G, House P, Wellenstein G, Hwang C, Richards S. 2001 (February). State Primary Care Provider Study. Seattle, WA: Health Policy Analysis Program, University of Washington. [Online]. Available: http://depts.washington.edu/hpap/Publications/PCP_Study/pcp_study.html [accessed July 8, 2002].

Kaufman M, Connolly C. 2002 (April 20). U.S. backs pediatric tests in reversal on drug safety. *Washington Post*, p. A03.

Kaye N, Curtis D, Booth M. 2000. *Certain Children with Special Health Care Needs: An Assessment of State Activities and Their Relationship to HCFA's Interim Criteria*. Portland, ME: National Academy for State Health Policy.

Kazak AE, Penati B, Boyer BA, Himelstein B, Brophy P, Waibel MK, Blackall GF, Daller R, Johnson K. 1996. A randomized controlled prospective outcome study of a psychological and pharmacological intervention protocol for procedural distress in pediatric leukemia. *Journal of Pediatric Psychology* 21(5):615–631.

Kedziera P. 2001. Hydration, thirst, and nutrition. In: Ferrell BR, Coyle N, eds. *Textbook of Palliative Nursing*. New York: Oxford University Press. Pp. 156–163.

Keenan HT, Diekema DS, O'Rourke PP, Cummings P, Woodrum DE. 2000. Attitudes toward limitation of support in a pediatric intensive care unit. *Critical Care Medicine* 28(5):1590–1594.

Kellerman J, Katz E. 1977 The adolescent with cancer: Theoretical, clinical and research issues. *Journal of Pediatric Psychology* 2(3):127–131.

Kelly S, Marshall PA, Sanders LM, Raffin TA, Koenig BA. 1997. Understanding the practice of ethics consultation: Results of an ethnographic multi-site study. *Journal of Clinical Ethics* 8(2):136–149.

Kennell JH, Slyter H. Klaus MH. 1970. The mourning response of parents to the death of a newborn. *New England Journal of Medicine* 283:344–349.

Kenny G. 1999. Assessing children's spirituality: What is the way forward? *British Journal of Nursing* 8(1):28, 30–32.

Kenny NP, Frager G. 1996. Refractory symptoms and terminal sedation of children: Ethical issues and practical management. *Journal of Palliative Care* 12(3):40–45.

Kernberg PF, Chazan SE, Normandin L. 1998. The Children's Play Therapy Instrument (CPTI). Description, development, and reliability studies. *Journal of Psychotherapeutic Practice and Research* 7(3):196–207.

KFF (Kaiser Family Foundation). 2002 (May). Trends and Indicators in the Changing Health Care Marketplace: Chartbook. [Online]. Available: http://www.kff.org/content/2002/3161/3161.pdf [accessed May 20, 2002].

Khaneja S, Milrod B. 1998. Educational needs among pediatricians regarding caring for terminally ill children. *Archives of Pediatric and Adolescent Medicine* 152(9):909–914.

King WD, Nichols MH, Hardwick WE, Palmisano PA. 1994. Urban/rural differences in child passenger deaths. *Pediatric Emergency Care* 10(1):34–36.

Kingsbury RJ. 2001. Palliative Sedation: May We Sleep Before We Die? The Center for Bioethics and Human Dignity. [Online]. Available: http://www.bioethix.org/newsletter/012/012kingsbury.htm [accessed October 30, 2001].

Kirschbaum MS. 1996. Life Support Decisions for Children: What Do Parents Value? *Advances in Nursing Science* 19(1):51–71.

Kittiko WJ. 2001 (September 9). Statement and discussion with the IOM committee on improving palliative and end-of-life care for children and their families, Open Meeting. Washington, DC.

Klass D. 1988. *Parental Grief: Solace and Resolution*. New York: Springer Publishing.

Knebel, A., Solomon, M., Tilden, V, Rushton, C and Sabatier, K. 2001 (November). Challenges and opportunities when conducting interdisciplinary palliative and end-of-life care research. Panel Presentation. Sigma Theta Tau Annual Meeting. Indianapolis, IN.

Koenig HG, Idler E, Kasl S, Hays J, George LK, Musick M, Larson DB, Collins T, Benson H. 1999. Religion, spirituality, and medicine: A rebuttal to skeptics. *International Journal of Psychiatry in Medicine* 29:123–131.

Kohrman A, Wright CE, Frader JE, Grodin MA, Porter IH, Wagner, VM. 1995. Informed consent, parental permission, and assent in pediatric practice. *Pediatrics* 95:314–439.

Komiske BK. 1999. *Designing the World's Best: Children's Hospitals*. Victoria, Australia: Images Publishing.

Kopelman LM, Irons TG, Kopelman AE. 1988. Neonatologists judge the "Baby Doe" regulations. *New England Journal of Medicine* 318:677–683.

Kosecoff J, Kahn KL, Rogers WH, Reinisch EJ, Sherwood MJ, Rubenstein LV, Draper D, Roth CP, Chew C, Brook RH. 1990. Prospective Payment System and Impairment at Discharge. *Journal of the American Medical Association* 264(15):1980–1983.

Krahn GL, Hallum A, Kime C. 1993. Are there good ways to give "bad news"? *Pediatrics* 91(3):578–582.

Krakauer, EL. 2000. Cultural difference, trust, and optimum care for minority patients. In: *Forum: Ethics and Risk Management Concerns*. [Online]. Available: http://www.rmf. harvard.edu/publications/forum/v20n4/fv20n4-a4/body.html [accessed December 10, 2001].

Krakauer EL, Truog RD. 1997. Mistrust, racism, and end-of-life treatment. *Hastings Center Report* 27(3):23–25.

Kramer S, Meadows AT, Pastore G, Jarrett P, Bruce D. 1984. Influence of place of treatment on diagnosis, treatment and survival in three pediatric solid tumors. *Journal of Clinical Oncology* 2(8):917–923.

Kraus NA, Machlin S, Kass BL. 1999. Use of Healthcare Services, 1996. Rockville, MD: Agency for Health Care Policy and Research. MEPS, Research Findings No. 7. AHCPR Pub. No. 99-0018.

Krechel SW, Bildner J. 1995. CRIES: A new neonatal postoperative pain measurement score. Initial testing of validity and reliability. *Paediatric Anaesthesia* 5:53–61.

Kristina's Mom. No date. Labor and Delivery Wish List. [Online]. Available: http://www. asfhelp.com/ASF_files/support_group_files/abiding_heart_files/wish.htm [accessed January 27, 2001].

Ku L. 1990 (August). Who is paying the big bills? Very high cost pediatric hospitalizations in California, 1987. SysteMetrics/McGraw-Hill. Prepared for the U.S. Department of Health and Human Services. [Online]. Available: http://aspe.hhs.gov/daltcp/reports/bigblles.htm [accessed July 12, 2001].

Kubler-Ross E. 1983. *On Children and Death*. New York: MacMillan Publishing Company.

Kuhse H. 1987. *The Sanctity-of-Life Doctrine in Medicine*. Oxford: Oxford University Press.

Kurland G, Orenstein DM. 2001. Lung transplantation and cystic fibrosis: The psychosocial toll. *Pediatrics* 107(6):1419–1420. [Online]. Available: http://www.pediatrics.org/cgi/content/full/107/6/1419 [accessed March 31, 2002].

Lakin KC, Anderson L, Prouty R. 1998. Children and youth receiving residential services for persons with developmental disabilities outside their family home: Trends from 1977 to 1997. In: Prouty R, Lakin CK, eds. *Residential Services for Persons with Developmental Disabilities: Status and Trends Through 1997*. Minneapolis: University of Minnesota Research and Training Center on Community Living. [Online]. Available: http://ici2. coled.umn.edu/rtc/risp97/ [accessed November 8, 2001].

Lambrew JM. 2001. *Health Insurance: A Family Affair: A National Profile and State-by-State Analysis of Uninsured Parents and Their Children*. New York: The Commonwealth Fund.

Lamont EB, Christakis NA. 2001. Prognostic disclosure to patients with cancer near the end of life. *Annals of Internal Medicine* 134(12):1096–105.

Landa AS. 2002. Doctors backing bill to require pediatric tests for drugs. *American Medical News* 45(19):5, 8.

Landon BE, Epstein AM. 2001. For-profit and not-for-profit health plans participating in Medicaid. *Health Affairs* 20(3):162–171.

Lane JL, Ziv A, Boulet JR. 1999. A pediatric clinical skills assessment using children as standardized patients. *Archives of Pediatric Adolescent Medicine* 153(6):637–644.

Langston C, Cooper ER, Goldfarb J, Easley KA, Husak S, Sunkle S, Starc TJ, Colin AA. 2001. Human immunodeficiency virus-related mortality in infants and children: Data from the Pediatric Pulmonary and Cardiovascular Complications of Vertically Transmitted HIV (P^2C^2) Study. *Pediatrics* 107(2):328–338.

Lantos J. 1987. Baby Doe five years later: Implications for child health. *New England Journal of Medicine* 317:444–447.

Lantos JD, Singer PA, Walker RM, Gramelspacher GP, Shapiro GR, Sanchez-Gonzalez MA, Stocking CB, Miles SH, Siegler M. 1989. The illusion of futility in clinical practice. *American Journal of Medicine* 87:81–84.

Lantos JD, Berger AC, Zucker AR. 1993. Do-not-resuscitate orders in a children's hospital. *Critical Care Medicine* 21(1):52–55.

Lantos JD, Tyson JE, Allen A, Frader J, Hack M, Korones S, Merenstein G, Paneth N, Poland RL, Saigal S, Stevenson D, Truog RD, Van Marter LJ. 1994. Withholding and withdrawing life sustaining treatment in neonatal intensive care: Issues for the 1990s. *Archives of Disease in Childhood, Fetal and Neonatal Edition* 71(3):F218–223.

Laramie County (Wyoming) School District. 1996. Administrative Regulation for Do Not Resuscitate Orders. Board Policies: Chapter VIIIm Students (Section 25). Adopted 7/1/96. [Online]. Available: http://www.laramie1.k12.wy.us/policies/chapter8/policy8-25.htm [accessed April 16, 2002].

Larson DG, Tobin DR. 2000. End of life conversations. *Journal of the American Medical Association* 284(12):1573–1577.

Lee MA, Brummel-Smith K, Meyer J, Drew N, London MR. 2000. Physician orders for life-sustaining treatment (POLST): Outcomes in a PACE program. Program for All-Inclusive Care for the Elderly. *Journal of the American Geriatrics Society* 48:1219–1225.

Legislative Audit Council (South Carolina). 2000, 2001. A review of selected Medicaid issues: Fraud and Abuse, Prescription Drug Costs, Funding. [Online]. Available: http://www.state.sc.us/sclac/Reports/2001/Medicaid.pdf [accessed August 17, 2001].

Leibowitz A, Buchanan J, Mann J. 1992. A randomized trial to evaluate the effectiveness of a Medicaid HMO. *Journal of Health Economics* 11(3):235–257.

Lemeshow S, Klar J, Teres D. 1995. Outcome prediction for individual intensive care patients: Useful, misused, or abused? *Intensive Care Medicine* 21(9):770–776.

Lemons JA, Bauer CR, Oh W, Korones S, Papile L, Stoll BJ, Verter J, Temprosa M, Wright LL, Ehrenkranz RA, Fanaroff AA, Stark A, Carlo W, Tyson JE, Donovan EF, Shankaran S, Stevenson DK for the NICHD Neonatal Research Network. 2001. Very low birth weight outcomes of the National Institute of Child Health and Human Development Neonatal Research Network from January 1995 through December 1996. *Pediatrics* 107(1):e1. [Online]. Available: http://www.pediatrics.org/cgi/content/full/107/1/e1 [accessed September 27, 2001].

Leuthner SR, Pierucci R. 2001. Experience with neonatal palliative care consultation at the Medical College of Wisconsin-Children's Hospital of Wisconsin. *Journal of Palliative Medicine* 4(1):39–47.

Levetown M. 1998. Pediatric Supportive Care, The Butterfly Program: A Report to the Health Care Financing Administration. No city or publisher.

Levetown M. 2001. Pediatric care: The inpatient/ICU perspective. In: Ferrell BR, Coyle N, eds. *Textbook of Palliative Nursing*. New York: Oxford University Press. Pp. 570–581.

Levetown M, Carter MA. 1998. Child-centered care in terminal illness: An ethical framework. In: Doyle D, Hanks GWC, MacDonald N, eds. *Oxford Textbook of Palliative Medicine*, 2nd ed. Oxford: Oxford University Press. Pp. 1107–1117.

Levetown M, Pollack MM, Cuerdon TT, Ruttimann UE, Glover J. 1994. Limitations and withdrawals of medical intervention in pediatric critical care. *Journal of the American Medical Association* 272(16):1271–1275.

Levine C. 1998. *Rough Crossings: Family Caregivers' Odysseys Through the Health Care System*. New York: United Hospital Fund.

Levine RJ. 1995. Adolescents as research subjects without permission of their parents or guardians: Ethical considerations. *Journal of Adolescent Health* 17(5):287–297.

Levine RJ. 1988. *Ethics and Regulation of Clinical Research*, 2nd ed. New Haven, CT: Yale University Press.

Lewis, B. 1992. *Kids with Courage: True Stories About Young People Making a Difference*. Minneapolis: Free Spirit Publishing Co.

Lewis CC. 1981. How adolescents approach decisions: Changes over grades seven to twelve and policy implications. *Child Development* 52:538–544.

Lewis MA, Lewis CE. 1990. Consequences of empowering children to care for themselves. *Pediatrician* 17:63–67.

Li L, Irvin E, Guzman J, Bombardier C. 2001. Surfing for back pain patients: The nature and quality of back pain information on the Internet. *Spine* 26(5): 545–557.

Liben S, Goldman A. 1998. Home care for children with life-threatening illness. *Journal of Palliative Care* 14(3):33–38.

Linke D. 2002, April 12. Hospice taking long-term cases; agency now helps care for kids with "life-limiting" ills. *Chicago Tribune*, p. 7.

Lipton H, Coleman M. 2000a. Bereavement practice guidelines for health care. *International Journal of Emergency Mental Health* 2(1):1–13.

Lipton H, Coleman M. 2000b. Bereavement practice guidelines for health care professionals in the emergency department. *International Journal of Emergency Mental Health* 2(1):19–31.

Lipton H, Everly GS. 2002. Mental health needs for providers of emergency medical services for children: A report of a consensus panel. *Prehospital Emergency Care* 6:15–21.

Ljungman G, Gordh T, Sorensen S, Kreuger A. 1999. Pain in paediatric oncology: Interviews with children, adolescents and their parents. *Acta Paediatrica* 88(6):623–630.

Ljungman G, Gordh T, Sorensen S, Kreuger A. 2000. Pain variations during cancer treatment in children: A descriptive survey. *Pediatric Hematology and Oncology* 17(3):211–221.

Lo B, Ruston D, Kates LW, Arnold RM, Cohen CB, Faber-Langendoen K, Pantilat SZ, Puchalski CM, Quill TR, Rabow MW, Schreiber S; Sulmasy DP, Tulsky JA. 2002. Discussing religious and spiritual issues at the end of life: A practical guide for physicians. *Journal of the American Medical Association* 287:749–754.

Loder PA. 2001 (September 8). Statement on behalf of The Compassionate Friends to the IOM committee on improving palliative and end-of-life care for children and their families, Open Meeting. Washington, DC.

Lohiya GS, Tan-Figueroa L, Kohler H. 2002. End-of-life decisions in a developmental center: A retrospective study. *Western Journal of Medicine* 176(1):20–22.

Lohr KN, Eleazer K, Mauskopf J. 1998. Health policy issues and applications for evidence-based medicine and clinical practice guidelines. *Health Policy* 46(1):1–19.

Lonowski SC. 1995. Recognizing the right of terminally-ill minors to refuse life sustaining medical treatment: The need for legislative guidelines to give full effect to minors' expanded rights. *University of Louisville Journal of Family Law* 34:421–445.

Loza EL. 2000. Access to pharmaceuticals under Medicaid managed care: Federal law compiled and state contracts compared. *Food and Drug Law Journal* 55(3):449–476.

Lundin T.1984. Morbidity following sudden and unexpected bereavement. *British Journal of Psychiatry* 144:84–88.

Lyckholm LJ, Coyne P, Smith TJ. Palliative Care Program, Medical College of Virginia Campus of Virginia Commonwealth University. 2001. *Pioneer Programs in Palliative Care: Nine Case Studies*. New York: Milbank Memorial Fund and Robert Wood Johnson Foundation. [Online]. Available: http://www.milbank.org/pppc/0011pppc.html [accessed March 20, 2002].

Lynch J, Eldadah MK. 1992. Brain-death criteria currently used by pediatric intensivists. *Clinical Pediatrics* 31(8):457–460.

Lynn J, Harrell F Jr, Cohn F, Wagner D, Connors AF Jr. 1997. Prognoses of seriously ill hospitalized patients on the days before death: Implications for patient care and public policy. *New Horizons* 5(1):56–61.

Lynn J, O'Mara A. 2001. Reliable, high quality, efficient end-of-life care for cancer patients: Economic issues and barriers. In: Foley KM, Gelband H, eds. *Improving Palliative Care for Cancer*. Washington, DC: National Academy Press. Pp. 67–95.

Lynn J, Schuster JL, Kabcenell A. 2000. *Improving Care for the End of Life: A Sourcebook for Health Care Managers and Clinicians*. Oxford: Oxford University Press.

Lynn J, Teno JM, Harrell FE Jr. 1995. Accurate prognostications of death: Opportunities and challenges for clinicians. *The Western Journal of Medicine* 163(3):250–257.

Maddison DC, Viola A. 1968. The health of widows in the year following bereavement. *Journal of Psychosomatic Research* 12:297–330.

MacFarlane GD, Venkataramanan R, McDiarmid SV, Pirsch JD, Scheller DG, Ersfeld DL, Fitzsimmons WE. 2001. Therapeutic drug monitoring of tacrolimus in pediatric liver transplant patients. *Pediatric Transplantation* 5(2):119–124.

Make-a-Wish Foundation. [Online]. Available: http://www.wish.org/home/frame_aboutus.htm [accessed March 31, 2002].

Make-A-Wish Foundation. 2001 (September 8). Statement presented by Michele R. Atkins to the IOM committee on improving palliative and end-of-life care for children and their families, Open Meeting. Washington, DC.

Malone FD, Berkowitz RL, Canick JA, D'Alton ME. 2000. First-trimester screening for aneuploidy: Research or standard of care? *American Journal of Obstetrics & Gynecology* 182(3):490–496.

Maragakis EM. 1996. EMTALA rears its ugly head: The case of Baby K. *Utah Law Review* 47:1099–1130.

Margolis PA, Cook RL, Earp JA, Lannon CM, Keyes LL, Klein JD. 1992. Factors associated with pediatricians' participation in Medicaid in North Carolina. *Journal of the American Medical Association* 267(14):1942–1946.

Marquis MS, Long SH. 2000. Who helps employers design their health insurance benefits? *Health Affairs (Millwood)* 9(1):133–138.

Martin JA, Hoyert DL. 2001. The National Fetal Death File. Submitted for publication. Washington, DC: Division of Vital Statistics, National Center for Health Statistics, Centers for Disease Control and Prevention.

Martin JA, Parks MM. 1999. Trends in twin and triplet births. *NVSR* 47(24). [Online]. Available: http://www.cdc.gov/nchs/data/nvsr/nvsr47/nvs47_24.pdf [accessed September 3, 2001].

Martinson I. 1993. A home care program. In: Armstrong-Dailey A, Goltzer SZ, eds. *Hospice Care for Children*. New York: Oxford University Press. Pp. 231–247.

Martinson IM. 1993. Hospice care for children: Past, present, and future. *Journal of Pediatric Oncological Nursing* 10(3):93–98.

Martinson IM, Campos RG. 1991. Long-term responses to a sibling's death from cancer. *Journal of Adolescent Research* 6:54–69.

Maruyama N. 1997. (October 18). Your child is dead. *American College of Emergency Physicians News*.

Massie AM. 1993. Withdrawal of treatment for minors in a persistent vegetative state: Parents should decide. *Arizona Law Review* 35:173.

Mays GP, Hurley RE, Grossman JM. 2001. Consumers face higher costs as health plans seek to control drug spending. Center for Studying Health System Change Issue Brief #45. [Online]. Available: http://www.hschange.org/CONTENT/389/ [accessed March 22, 2002].

McCabe MA. 1996. Involving children and adolescents in medical decision making: Developmental and clinical considerations. *Journal of Pediatric Psychology* 21:505–516.

McCabe MA, Rushton CH, Glover J, Murray MG, Leikin S. 1996. Implications of the Patient Self-Determination Act: Guidelines for involving adolescents in medical decision making. *Journal of Adolescent Health* 19(5):319–324.

McCallum DE, Byrne P, Bruera E. 2000. How children die in hospital. *Journal of Pain Symptom Management* 20(6):417–423.

McCullough LB. 1988. An ethical model for improving the patient–physician relationship. *Inquiry* 25(4):454–468.

McGrath P. 1987. An assessment of children's pain: A review of behavioral, physiological and direct scaling techniques. *Pain* 31(2):47–176.

McGrath P. 1990. *Pain in Children: Nature, Assessment and Treatment*. New York: Guilford Publications.

McGrath P. 1998. Pain control. In: Doyle D, Hanks GWC, MacDonald N, eds. *Oxford Textbook of Palliative Medicine*, 2nd ed. Oxford: Oxford University Press. Pp.1013–1031.

McGrath PJ, Hsu E, Capelli M, Luke B, Goodmen JT, Dunn-Geier J. 1990. Pain from paediatric cancer: A survey of an outpatient oncology clinic. *Journal of Psychosocial Oncology* 8:109–124.

MCHB (Maternal and Child Health Bureau, U.S. Department of Health and Human Services). 1998. Implementing Title V CSHCN Programs: A Resource Manual for State Programs. [Online]. Available: http://cshcnleaders.ichp.edu/CSHCNProgramManual/default.htm [accessed July 12, 2001].

MCHB, Division of Services for Children with Special Healthcare Needs. 2000a. *Medical Home Development*. [Online]. Available: http://mchb.hrsa.gov/html/medicalhome.html [accessed October 10, 2001].

MCHB. 2000b. Guidance and forms for the Title V application/annual report: Part one. [Online]. Available: http://www.mchb.hrsa.gov/html/blockgrant.html [accessed August 13, 2001].

McLeod SD. 1998. The quality of medical information on the Internet: A new public health concern. *Journal of the American Medical Association* 116(12):1663–1665.

McManus M, Flint S, Kelly R. 1991. The adequacy of physician reimbursement for pediatric care under Medicaid. *Pediatrics* 87(6):909–920.

Mcpherson M, Arango P, Fox H, Lauver C, McManus M, Newacheck PW, Perrin JM, Shonkoff JP, Strickland B. 1998. A new definition of children with special health care needs. *Pediatrics* 102(1 Pt 1):117–123.

Meadow W, Frain L, Ren Y, Lee G, Soneji S, Lantos J. 2002. Serial assessment of mortality in the neonatal intensive care unit by algorithm and intuition: Certainty, uncertainty, and informed consent. *Pediatrics* 109(5):878–886.

Meadow W, Reimshisel T, Lantos J. 1996. Birth weight-specific mortality for extremely low birth weight infants vanishes by four days of life: Epidemiology and ethics in the neonatal intensive care unit. *Pediatrics* 97(5):636–643.

Meadows AT, Kramer S, Hopson R, Lustbader E, Jarrett P, Evans AE. 1983. Survival in childhood acute lymphocytic leukemia: Effect of protocol and place of treatment. *Cancer Investigation* 1(1):49–55.

Medical Board of California. 2000. *1999–2000 Annual Report.* [Online]. Available: http://www.medbd.ca.gov/99_00annualreport.pdf [accessed March 30, 2002].

MedPAC (Medicare Payment Advisory Commission). 1998a (March). *Report to the Congress: Medicare Payment Policy. Volume 1: Recommendations.* Washington, DC: MedPAC.

MedPAC. 1998b (June). *Report to the Congress: Selected Medicare Issues.* Washington, DC: MedPAC.

MedPAC. 1999 (June). *Report to the Congress: Selected Medicare Issues.* Washington, DC: MedPAC.

MedPAC. 2000a (November). *Report to the Congress: Improving Risk Adjustment in Medicare.* Washington, DC: MedPAC.

MedPAC. 2000b (June). *Report to the Congress: Selected Medicare Issues.* Washington, DC: MedPAC.

MedPAC. 2001 (March). *Report to the Congress: Medicare Payment Policy.* Washington, DC: MedPAC.

MedPAC. 2002 (May). *Report to the Congress: Medicare Beneficiaries' Access to Hospice.* Washington, DC: MedPAC.

Meier DE, Morris J, Morrison S. 2000. The Lilian and Benjamin Hertzberg Palliative Care Institute, Mount Sinai School of Medicine. In *Pioneer Programs in Palliative Care: Nine Case Studies.* New York: Milbank Memorial Fund and Robert Wood Johnson Foundation. Pp. 139-160. [Online]. Available: http://www.milbank.org/pppc/0011pppc.html [accessed March 20, 2002].

Meisel A, Snyder L, Quill T. 2000. Seven legal barriers to end-of-life care: Myths, realities, and grains of truth. *Journal of the American Medical Association* 284(19):2495–501.

Mejia RE, Pollack MM. 1995. Variability in brain death determination practices in children. *Journal of the American Medical Association* 274:550–553.

Mendeloff EN. 1998. Pediatric and adult lung transplantation for cystic fibrosis. *Journal of Thoracic and Cardiovascular Surgery* 115(2):404–414.

Merck Manual of Diagnosis and Therapy, Seventeenth Edition. 2001. Beers MH, Berkow R., eds. [Online]. Available: http://www.merck.com/pubs/mmanual.

Mermann AC, Gunn DB, Dickinson GE. 1991. Learning to care for the dying: A survey of medical school and a model course. *Academic Medicine* 66(1):35–38.

Meyer MH, Derr P, Hatfield, MO. 1998. *The Comfort of Home: An Illustrated Step-by-Step Guide for Caregivers.* Portland, OR: CareTrust Publications.

Michelacci L, Fava GA, Grandi S, Bovicelli L, Orlandi C, Trombini G. 1988. Psychological reactions to ultrasound examination during pregnancy. *Psychotherapy & Psychosomatics.* 50(1):1–4.

Mickan S, Rodger S. 2000. Characteristics of effective teams: A literature review. *Australian Health Review* 23(3):201–208.

Miller DK, Duckro PN, Videen SD, Chibnall JT. 2001. *Supportive–Affective Groups for Patients with Life-Threatening Medical Conditions: A Spiritual–Emotional–Relational Approach to Helping Patients "Live Until They Die."* St. Louis, MO: Saint Louis University School of Medicine.

Miller VL, Rice JC, De Voe M, Fos PJ. 1998. An analysis of program and family costs of case managed care for technology-dependent infants with bronchopulmonary dysplasia. *Journal of Pediatric Nursing* 13(4):244–251.

Miser AW, Dothage JA, Wesley RA, Miser JS. 1987. The prevalence of pain in a pediatric and young adult cancer population. *Pain* 29(1):73–83.

MISS (Mothers in Sympathy and Support). 2001 (September 8). Statement presented by Richard K. Olsen to the IOM committee on improving palliative and end-of-life care for children and their families, Open Meeting. Washington, DC.

Mitchell C, Truog RD. 2000. From the files of a pediatric ethics committee. *Journal of Clinical Ethics* 11:112–120.

Mitchell I, Nakielna E, Tullis E, Adair C. 2000. Cystic fibrosis: End-stage care in Canada. *Chest* 118(1):80–84.

Moore DL. 1995. Challenging parental decisions to overtreat children. *Health Matrix* 5:311.

Morrison RS, Meier DE. 1995. Managed care at the end of life. *Trends in Health Care Law Ethics* 10(1-2):91–96.

Morrow WR. 2000. Cardiomyopathy and heart transplantation in children. *Current Opinions in Cardiology* 15(4):216–223.

Motheral B, Fairman KA. 2001. Effect of a three-tier prescription copay on pharmaceutical and other medical utilization. *Medical Care* 39(12):1293–1304.

Motheral BR, Henderson R. 2000. The effect of a closed formulary on prescription drug use and costs. *Inquiry* 36(4):481–491.

Muelleman RL, Mueller K. 1996. Fatal motor vehicle crashes: Variations of crash characteristics within rural regions of different population densities. *Journal of Trauma* 41(2):315–320.

Muldoon JH. 1999. Structure and performance of different DRG classification systems for neonatal medicine. *Pediatrics* 103(1 Supl E):302–318.

NACHRI (National Association of Children's Hospitals and Related Institutions). [Online]. Available: http://www.childrenshospitals.net/nachri/.

NACHRI. 1998. *NACHRI Annual Survey: Part II.* Alexandria, VA: National Association of Children's Hospitals and Related Institutions.

NACHRI. 1999. *Serving the Nation's Children: 1999 Chart Book of Children's Hospitals.* Alexandria, VA: National Association of Children's Hospitals and Related Institutions.

NACHRI. 2001a (September 8). Statement presented by Susan Dull to the IOM committee on improving palliative and end-of-life care for children and their families, Open Meeting. Washington, DC.

NACHRI. 2001b. Report: All Children Need Children's Hospitals. [Online]. Available: http://www.childrenshospitals.net/nachri/abouth/ACReport.pdf [accessed March 31, 2002].

NAMI (National Alliance for the Mentally Ill). 2001. The Mental Health Equitable Treatment Act of 2001 (S. 543). [Online]. Available: http://www.nami.org/update/20010406.html [accessed August 17, 2001].

NAPHCC (National Association of Pediatric Home and Community Care). 2001 (September 8). Statement presented by Dorothy Page to the IOM committee on improving palliative and end-of-life care for children and their families, Open Meeting. Washington, DC.

NASEMSD (National Association of State Emergency Medical Services Directors). 2001 (September 5). Statement written by Dia Gainor to the IOM committee on improving palliative and end-of-life care for children and their families, Washington, DC.

NASHP (National Academy for State Health Policy). 2001. *Medicaid Managed Care: A Guide for States*, 5th ed. Portland, ME: National Academy for State Health Policy.

NASMD (National Association of State Medicaid Directors). 1999. State by State Impact of the OBRA 1989 EPSDT Provisions. [Online]. Available: http://medicaid.aphsa.org/research/epsdtissue.htm [accessed August 17, 2001].

NASN (National Association of School Nurses). 1996. Issue Brief: School Nurses and the Individuals with Disabilities Education Act (IDEA). [Online]. Available: http://www.nasn.org/briefs/idea.htm [accessed June 8, 2001].

NASN. 2000. Do Not Resuscitate. [Online]. Available: http://www.nasn.org/positions/resuscitate.htm [accessed March 31, 2002].

NASW (National Association of Social Workers). 2000. NASW Develops Bereavment Guidelines for Emergency Rooms. [Online]. Available: http://www.socialworkers.org/pressroom/2000/041000.htm [accessed March 31, 2002].

NASW. 2001 (September 8). Statement presented by Mirean Coleman to the IOM committee on improving palliative and end-of-life care for children and their families, Open Meeting. Washington, DC.

National Academy on Aging. 1997. Facts on Long-Term Care. Washington, DC.

National Tay-Sachs and Allied Diseases Association. 2001 (September 8). Statement presented by Carol and Eric Zimmerman to the IOM committee on improving palliative and end-of-life care for children and their families, Open Meeting. Washington, DC.

NCCD (Nordic Center for Classification of Disease). 2001. NordDRG — The Nordic DRG-System. WHO Collaborating Centre for the Classification of Diseases in the Nordic Countries, Uppsala University, Finland. [Online]. Available: http://www.pubcare.uu.se/nordwho/verksam/norddrge.htm [accessed July 26, 2001].

NCHS (National Center for Health Statistics, Centers for Disease Control and Prevention). 1997. *Revision: State Definitions and Reporting Requirements for Live Births, Fetal Deaths, and Induced Terminations of Pregnancy*. PHS 98-1119. Washington, DC: U.S. Department of Health and Human Services. [Online]. Available: http://www.cdc.gov/nchs/data/itop97.pdf.

NCHS, 1999. Vital Statistics of the United States—1995 Mortality, Technical Appendix. [Online]. Available: http://www.cdc.gov/nchs/about/major/dvs/mortdata.htm].

NCHS. 2000a. *Health United States 2000*. Washington, DC. [Online]. Available: http://www.cdc.gov/nchs/data/hus/hus00.pdf.

NCHS. 2000b. Infant mortality statistics from the 1998 period linked birth/infant death data set. *National Vital Statistics Report* 48(12):1–8. [Online]. Available: http://www.cdc.gov/nchs/data/nvsr/nvsr48/nvs48_12.pdf. [accessed March 31, 2002].

NCHS. 2001a. Deaths: Final Data for 1999. *National Vital Statistics Report* 49(8):1–15. [Online]. Available: http://www.cdc.gov/nchs/data/nvsr/nvsr49/nvsr49_08.pdf.

NCHS. 2001b. Deaths: Leading Causes for 1999. [Online]. Available: http://www.cdc.gov/nchs/data/nvsr/nvsr49/nvsr49_11.pdf.

NCHS. 2001c. *Health United States 2001*. [Online]. Available: http://www.cdc.gov/nchs/data/hus/hus01.pdf.

NCHS, 2001d. Vital Statistics System. Statistics Compiled by the Office of Statistics and Programming, National Center for Injury Prevention and Control. [Online]. Available: http://webapp.cdc.gov/sasweb/ncipc/leadcaus.html.

NCHS. 2001e. Vital Statistics System. Statistics Compiled by the Office of Statistics and Programming, National Center for Injury Prevention and Control. [Online]. Available: http://webapp.cdc.gov/sasweb/ncipc/mortrate.html [accessed October 15, 2001].

NCI (National Cancer Institute). 1999. Cancer Incidence and Survival Among Children and Adolescents: United States SEER Program 1975–1995. [Online]. Available: http://seer.cancer.gov/publications/childhood.

NCI. 2001a. Childhood Acute Lymphoblastic Leukemia: Treatment—Health Professionals. [Online]. Available: http://www.cancer.gov/cancer_information/cancer_type/leukemia/ [accessed October 1, 2001].

NCI. 2001b. Clinical Trials and Insurance Coverage: A Resource Guide. [Online]. Available: http://cancertrials.nci.nih.gov/understanding/indepth/insurance/ [accessed August 17, 2001].

NCI. 2001c. Understanding Trials: Children's Assent to Clinical Trial Participation: Special Considerations. [Online]. Available: http://cancertrials.nci.nih.gov/understanding/indepth/protections/assent/index.html [accessed December 17, 2001].

NCOD (National Commission on Orphan Diseases). 1989. Report of the National Commission on Orphan Diseases, Publication Number HRP-090-7248. Washington, DC: U.S. Government Printing Office.

NCSL (National Council of State Legislatures). 2001a (July 23). Fact Sheet: Prompt Payment. [Online] Available: http://www.hpts.org/info/info.nsf [accessed March 20, 2002].

NCSL. 2001b (August 1). News Release: Report Signals Reversal of Fortunes. Washington, DC: NCSL. [Online]. Available: http://www.ncsl.org/programs/press/2001/pr010801.htm [accessed August 10, 2001].

NEA (National Education Association). 1994. Policy on "Do Not Resuscitate Order." [Online]. Available: http://www.nea.org/esp/resource/safecare.htm [accessed October 10, 2001].

Nealy EA. 1995. Medical decision-making for children: A struggle for autonomy. SMU Law Review 49:133.

Needlman RD. 2000. Part II: Growth and Development. In: Behrman RE, Kliegman RM, Jenson HB, eds. Nelson Textbook of Pediatrics, 16th ed. Philadelphia: WB Saunders. Pp. 23–65.

Nelson EC, Batalden PB, Ryer JC, eds. 1998. Joint Commission Clinical Improvement Action Guide. Oakbrook Terrace, IL: Joint Commission on the Accreditation of Healthcare Organizations.

Nelson LJ, Rushton CH, Cranford RE, Nelson RM, Glover JJ, Truog RD. 1995. Forgoing medically provided nutrition and hydration in pediatric patients. Journal of Law, Medicine, and Ethics 23(1):33–46.

Nelson RM, Shapiro RS. 1995. The role of an ethics committee in resolving conflict in the neonatal intensive care unit. Journal of Law, Medicine, and Ethics 23(1):27–32.

Newacheck PW. 2000. Access to health care for children with special health care needs. Pediatrics 105(4):760–766.

Newacheck PW, Strickland B, Shonkoff JP, Perrin JM, McPherson M, McManus M, Lauver C, Fox H, Arango P. 1998. An epidemiologic profile of children with special health care needs. Pediatrics 102(1):117–123.

NHPCO (National Hospice and Palliative Care Organization), Children's International Project on Palliative/Hospice Services (ChIPPS). 2000. Compendium of Pediatric Palliative Care. Alexandria, VA: NHPCO.

NHPCO. 2001 (September 8). Statement presented by Stephen R. Connor to the IOM committee on improving palliative and end-of-life care for children and their families, Open Meeting. Washington, DC.

NHTSA (National Highway Traffic Safety Administration). 2000. Traffic Safety Facts 2000: Children. Washington, DC: U.S. Department of Transportation. [Online]. Available: http://www-nrd.nhtsa.dot.gov/departments/nrd-30/ncsa/factshet.html [accessed December 12, 2001].

NICCYD (National Information Center for Children and Youth with Disabilities). 1996 (October). The education of children and youth with special needs: What do the laws say? News Digest 15:1–16. (ND15). [Online]. Available: http://www.nichcy.org/pubs/newsdig/nd15txt.htm [accessed June 19, 2002].

NICHD (National Institute of Child Health and Human Development). 2000. Cooperative Multicenter Neonatal Research Network. [Online]. Available: http://grants.nih.gov/grants/guide/rfa-files/RFA-HD-00-010.html [accessed March 19, 2002].

NIDDK (National Institute of Diabetes and Digestive and Kidney Diseases). 2001. Research needs in pediatric kidney disease: 2000 and beyond. Research Updates in Kidney and Urologic Health. [Online]. Available: http://www.niddk.nih.gov/health/kidney/Research_Updates/win00-01/needs.htm [accessed March 19, 2002].

NIH (National Institutes of Health). 1998. Program Announcement: NIH Policy and Guidelines on the Inclusion of Children as Participants in Research Involving Human Subjects, March 6, 1998. [Online]. Available: http://grants.nih.gov/grants/guide/notice-files/not98-024.html [accessed December 14, 2001].

NIH. 2000. Program Announcement: Quality of Life for Individuals at the End of Life, August 2, 2000. [Online]. Available: http://grants.nih.gov/grants/guide/pa-files/PA-00-127.html [accessed January 10, 2002].

NIH. 2001a. Office on AIDS Research. [Online]. Available: http://www.nih.gov/od/oar/public/public.htm [accessed March 31, 2002].

NIH. 2001b. Program Announcement: Research on Emergency Medical Services for Children, January 25, 2001. [Online]. Available: http://grants.nih.gov/grants/guide/pa-files/PA-01-044.html [accessed March 11, 2002].

NIMH (National Institute of Mental Health). 1998. Parity in Financing Mental Health Services: Managed Care Effects on Cost, Access, and Quality: An Interim Report to Congress by the National Advisory Mental Health Council. NIH Publication No. 98-4322. [Online]. Available: http://www.nimh.nih.gov/research/prtyrpt/index.html [accessed March 20, 2002].

NINR (National Institute for Nursing Research), NCI, NIAID (National Institute for Allergy and Infectious Diseases), NIMH, OAM (Office of Alternative Medicine). 1997. Management of symptoms at the end of life. NIH Guide 26(40). [Online]. Available: http://grants1.nih.gov/grants/guide/pa-files/PA-98-019.html [accessed April 16, 2002].

Nitschke R, Humphrey GB, Sexauer CL, Catron B, Wunder S, Jay S. 1982. Therapeutic choices made by patients with end-stage cancer. Journal of Pediatrics 101(3):471–476.

Nitschke R, Meyer WH, Huszti HC. 2001. When the tumor is not the target, tell the children. Journal of Clinical Oncology 19(12):595–596.

NMHA (National Mental Health Association). 2001. NHMA Legislative Alert. [Online]. Available: http://www.nmha.org/newsroom/system/lal.vw.cfm?do=vw&rid=371 [accessed September 12, 2001].

NMRP (National Medicolegal Review Panel, National Institute of Justice). 1999 (November). Death Investigation: A Guide for the Scene Investigator: Research Report. Washington, DC: Department of Justice.

NOPMC (National Organization of Parents of Murdered Children). 2001 (September 8). Statement presented by Ruth Hoffman to the IOM committee on improving palliative and end-of-life care for children and their families, Open Meeting. Washington, DC.

NORD (National Organization for Rare Disorders). 2001 (September 8). Statement presented to the IOM committee on Care of Children Who Die and Their Families, Open Meeting. Washington, DC.

North Carolina Division of Medical Assistance, North Carolina Department of Health and Human Services. 1999. Hospital Services Manual. Chapter Eight: Reimbursement and Billing. [Online]. Available: http://www.dhhs.state.nc.us/dma/ [accessed July 25, 2001].

NPTR (National Pediatric Trauma Registry). 2001. Biannual Report. [Online]. Available: http://www.nptr.org/page3.htm [accessed December 13, 2001].

NRC (National Research Council). 1996. Children with special health care needs: Dimensions of the population. In: *Paying Attention to Children in a Changing Health Care System*. Washington, DC: National Academy Press. Pp. 64–73.

Nuland S. 1994. *How We Die*. New York: Knopf Publishing.

OAT (Office for the Advancement of Telehealth). 2001. *2001 Report to Congress on Telemedicine: Payment Issues*. Rockville, MD: U.S. Department of Health and Human Services. [Online]. Available: http://telehealth.hrsa.gov/pubs/report2001/pay.htm#tab1 [accessed April 17, 2002].

Oberman M. 1996. Minor rights and wrongs. *Journal of Law, Medicine & Ethics* 24(2):127–38.

O'Brien K, Hackler J, Telfair J. 2001 (June 11). Presentation to the IOM committee on improving palliative and end-of-life care for children and their families, Open Meeting. Washington, DC.

O'Connell M, Watson S. 2001. Medicaid and EPSDT. Presented at National Assistive Technology Conference, April 4–6, 2001, Austin, TX. [Online]. Available: http://www.nls.org/conf/epsdt.htm [accessed August 17, 2001].

Office of Technology Assessment (OTA). 1987. *Technology-Dependent Children: Hospital v. Home Care—A Technical Memorandum*. OTA-TM-H-38. Washington, DC: U.S. Government Printing Office.

OIG (Office of Inspector General). 2001 (December). The Physician's Role in Medicare Home Health. Washington, DC: U.S. Department of Health and Human Services. [Online]. Available: http://oig.hhs.gov/oei/summaries/oei-02-00-00620s.pdf [accessed April 17, 2002].

Oleske JM, Czarniecki L. 1999. Continuum of palliative care: Lessons from caring for children infected with HIV-1. *Lancet* 354(9186):1287–1291.

O'Neil EH and the Pew Health Professions Commission. 1998 (December). *Recreating Health Professional Practice for a New Century: The Fourth Report of the Pew Health Professions Commission*. San Francisco: Pew Health Professions Commission.

Opie A. 1997. Effective team work in health care: A review of issues discussed in recent research literature. *Health Care Annals* 5(1):62–70.

Orenstein JB. 2000. A farewell to arm. *Annals of Emergency Medicine* 36(5):536–537.

Organization of Neonatal–Perinatal Training Program Directors. 2001 (September 8). Written statement by William E. Truog to the IOM committee on improving palliative and end-of-life care for children and their families, Washington, DC.

Orloff S. 2001. Incorporating children in an adult hospice program. In: Armstrong-Daley A, Zarbock S, eds. *Hospice Care for Children*, 2nd ed. New York: Oxford University Press. Pp. 353–377.

Otten AL. 1998. Mental health parity: What can it accomplish in a market dominated by managed care? New York City: Milbank Memorial Fund. [Online]. Available: http://www.milbank.org/mrparity.html [accessed August 17, 2001].

Pan CX, Morrison RS, Meier DE, Natale DK, Goldhirsch SL, Kralovec P, Cassel CK. 2001. How prevalent are hospital-based palliative care programs? Status report and future directions. *Journal of Palliative Medicine* 4(3):315–324.

Papadatou D. 1997. Training health professionals in caring for dying children and grieving families. *Death Studies* 21(6):575–600.

Paris JJ, Crone RK, Reardon F. 1990. Physicians' refusal of requested treatment: The case of Baby L. *New England Journal of Medicine* 322:1012.

Parker D, Maddocks I, Stern L. 1999. The role of palliative care in advanced muscular dystrophy and spinal muscular atrophy. *Journal of Paediatrics & Child Health* 35(3): 245–250.

Parker PA, Baile WF, de Moor C, Lenzi R, Kudelka AP, Cohen L. 2001. Breaking bad news about cancer: Patients' preferences for communication. *Journal of Clinical Oncology* 19(7):2049–2056.

Parkes CM. 1975. Determinants of outcome following bereavement. *Omega* 6:303–323.

Parkes CM. 1980. Bereavement counseling—does it work? *British Medical Journal* 281:3–6.

Parkes CM. 1998. Bereavement. In: Doyle D, Hanks GWC, MacDonald N, eds. *Oxford Textbook of Palliative Medicine*. Oxford: Oxford University Press. Pp. 995–1010.

Parkes CM, Laungani P, Young B, eds. 1997. *Death and Bereavement Across Cultures*. London: Routledge.

Patrick DL, Erickson P. 1993. *Health Status and Health Policy*. New York: Oxford University Press.

Patrick DL, Engelberg RA, Curtis JR. 2001. Evaluating the quality of dying and death. *Journal of Pain Symptom Management* 22(3):717–726.

Patterson MD. 1999. Resuscitation update for the pediatrician. *Pediatric Clinics of North America* 46:1285–1303.

Paulson, MA. 2001. Ask Dr. Paulson: Questions and answers. *We Need Not Walk Alone* (magazine of the Compassionate Friends) Summer 2001:22.

Payne SM, Restuccia JD. 1987. Policy issues related to prospective payment for pediatric hospitalization. *Health Care Finance Review* 9(1):71–82.

PCN (Pediatric Chaplains Network). 1999a. Competencies and Code of Ethics. [Online]. Available: http://www.pediatricchaplains.org/007Documents.htm [accessed October 2, 2001].

PCN. 1999b. Demonstrated Competencies of a Pediatric Chaplain. [Online]. Available: http://www.pediatricchaplains.org [accessed October 2, 2001].

PCN. 2001 (September 8). Statement presented by Dane R. Sommer to the IOM committee on improving palliative and end-of-life care for children and their families, Open Meeting. Washington, DC.

PDIA (Project on Death in America). 2001a. [Online] Available: http://www.soros.org/death/newsletter8/socialnewsletter.html [accessed March 6, 2002].

PDIA. 2001b. Transforming the Culture of Dying. [Online]. Available: http://www.soros.org/death/prJuly3-01.html [accessed March 6, 2002].

Pearson HA, Johnson S, Simpson BJ, Gallagher M. 1997. A residential summer camp for children with vertically transmitted HIV/AIDS: A six-year experience at the Hole in the Wall Gang Camp. *Pediatrics* 100(4):709–713.

Peebles-Kleiger MJ. 2000. Pediatric and neonatal intensive care hospitalization as traumatic stressor: Implications for intervention. *Bulletin of the Menninger Clinic* 64(2):257–280.

Pellegrino ED. 2000. Decision to withdraw life-sustaining treatment: A moral algorithm. *Journal of the American Medical Association* 283(8):1065.

Pendergrass T, Davis S. 1981. Knowledge and use of "alternative" cancer therapies in children. *American Journal of Pediatric Hematology/Oncology* 3:339–345.

Penkower JA. 1996. The potential right of chronically ill adolescents to refuse life saving medical treatment: Fatal misuse of the mature minor doctrine. *DePaul Law Review* 45:1165–1216.

Perkins J. 1999. Fact Sheet: Early and Periodic Screening, Diagnosis and Treatment. Washington, DC: National Health Law Program. [Online]. Available: http://www.healthlaw.org/pubs/19990323epsdtfact.html [accessed July 19, 2001].

Perkins J, Kulkarni M. 2000. Addressing Home and Community-Based Waiver Waiting Lists Through the Medicaid Program. Washington, DC: National Health Law Program.

Perot R, Youdelman M. 2001. Racial, Ethnic, and Primary Language Data Collection in the Health Care System: An Assessment on Federal Policies and Practices. [Online]. Available: http://www.cmwf.org [accessed October 15, 2001].

Peroutka SJ. 2000. Analysis of Internet sites for migraine. Presented at 42nd annual scientific meeting of the American Headache Society. Montreal, Quebec, Canada.

Perrin JM, Kuhlthau K, Walker DK, Stein REK, Newacheck PW, Gortmaker SL. 1997. Monitoring health care for children with chronic conditions in a managed care environment. *Maternal and Child Health Journal* 1(1):15–23.

Peteet JR, Abrams HE, Ross DM, Stearns NM. 1991. Presenting a diagnosis of cancer: Patients' views. *Journal of Family Practice* 32(6):564–566.

Pierucci RL, RS Kirby, SR Leuthner. 2001. End-of-life care for neonates and infants: The experience and effects of a palliative care consultation service. *Pediatrics* 108(3): 653–660. [Online]. Available: http://www.pediatrics.org/cgi/content/full/108/3/653 [accessed October 4, 2001].

Pinkerton JV, Finnerty JJ, Lombardo PA, Rorty MV, Chapple H, Boyle RJ. 1997. Parental rights at the birth of a near-viable infant: Conflicting perspectives. *American Journal of Obstetrics and Gynecology* 177:283–288.

Pless JE.1983. The story of Baby Doe. *New England Journal of Medicine* 309:664.

Pollack MM, Cuerdon TT, Patel KM, Ruttimann UE, Getson PR, Levetown M. 1994. Impact of quality-of-care factors on pediatric intensive care unit mortality. *Journal of the American Medical Association* 272(12):941–946.

Post SG. 2001. Tube feeding and advanced progressive dementia. *Hastings Center Report* 31(1):36–42.

Post SG, Puchalski CM, Larson DB. 2000. Physicians and patient spirituality: professional boundaries, competency, and ethics. *Annals of Internal Medicine* 132:578–583.

Povar GJ. 1991. Evaluating ethics committees: What do we mean by success? *Maryland Law Review* 50:904.

PPRC (Physician Payment Review Commission). 1988 (March). *Annual Report to Congress 1988*. Washington, DC: Physician Payment Review Commission.

PPRC. 1993. *Annual Report to Congress 1993*. Washington, DC: Physician Payment Review Commission.

PPRC. 1994. *Annual Report to Congress 1994*. Washington, DC: Physician Payment Review Commission.

PPRC. 1995. *Annual Report to Congress 1995*. Washington, DC: Physician Payment Review Commission.

PPRC. 1997. *Annual Report to Congress 1997*. Washington, DC: Physician Payment Review Commission.

Presbyterian Health Plan. 2001. *Welcome to Your 2001/2002 Presbyterian Health Plan.* [Online]. Available: http://web1.phs.org/intel/exclusions.htm [accessed March 31, 2002].

President's Commission (President's Commission for the Study of Ethical Problems in Medicine and Biomedical and Behavioral Research). 1981. *Defining Death.* Washington, DC: U.S. Government Printing Office.

President's Commission. 1983. *Deciding to Forego Life-Sustaining Treatment.* Washington, DC: U.S. Government Printing Office.

Prestowitz M, Streett L. 2000. *A History of Medi-Cal Physician Payment Rates.* Oakland, CA: Medi-Cal Policy Institute.

Prigerson HG, Jacobs SC. 2001. Perspectives on care at the close of life. Caring for bereaved patients: "All the doctors just suddenly go." *Journal of the American Medical Association* 286(11):1369–1376.

Prigerson HG, Silverman GK, Jacobs SC, Maciejewski PK, Kasl SV, Rosenheck RA. 2001. Traumatic grief, disability and the underutilization of health services. *Primary Psychiatry* 8(5):61–66.

Promoting Excellence. 2001 (May). Promoting Excellence in End of Life Care: Interim Report. Missoula, MT: Robert Wood Johnson Foundation National Program Office/ [Online]. Available: http://www.promotingexcellence.org/navigate/frameset12.html. [accessed October 4, 2001].

ProPAC (Prospective Payment Assessment Commission). 1989 (June). *Medicare Prospective Payment and the American Health Care System: Report to the Congress*. Washington, DC: ProPAC.

ProPAC. 1996, March 1. *Report and Recommendations to the Congress*. Washington, DC: ProPAC.

Ptacek JT, Eberhardt TL. 1996. Breaking bad news: A review of the literature. *Journal of the American Medical Association* 276(6):496–502.

Ptacek JT, Fries EA, Eberhardt TL, Ptacek JJ. 1999. Breaking bad news to patients: Physicians' perceptions of the process. *Support and Care for Cancer* 7(3):113–120.

Puchalski CM, Romer AL. 2000. Taking a spiritual history allows clinicians to understand patients more fully. *Journal of Palliative Medicine* 3(1):129–137.

Puntillo KA, Benner P, Drought T, Drew B, Stotts N, Stannard D, Rushton C, Scanlon C, White C. 2001. End of life issues in intensive care units: A national random survey of nurses' knowledge and beliefs. *American Journal of Critical Care* 10(4):216–229.

Qualls SH, Czirr R. 1988. Geriatric health teams: Classifying models of professional and team functioning. *Gerontologist* 28(3):372–376.

Quill TE, Lo B, Brock DW. 1997. Palliative options of last resort. A comparison of voluntary stopping eating and drinking, terminal sedation, physician-assisted suicide, and voluntary active euthanasia. *Journal of the American Medical Association* 278:2099–2104.

Rabow MW, Hardie GE, Fair JM, McPhee SJ. 2000. End-of-life care content in 50 textbooks from multiple specialties. *Journal of the American Medical Association* 283(6):771–778.

Randall F, Downie RS. 1999. *Palliative Care Ethics: A Companion for All Specialties*, 2nd ed. Oxford: Oxford University Press.

Randolph AG, Zollo MB, Wigton RS, Yeh TS. 1997. Factors explaining variability among caregivers in the intent to restrict life-support interventions in a pediatric intensive care unit. *Critical Care Medicine* 25(3):435–439.

Randolph AG, Zollo MB, Egger MJ, Guyatt GH, Nelson RM, Stidham GL. 1999. Variability in physician opinion on limiting pediatric life support. *Pediatrics* 103(4):e46.

Randolph L, ed. 1997. *Physician Characteristics and Distribution in the US*. Chicago, IL: American Medical Association.

Rebagliato M, Cuttini M, Broggin L, Berbik I, de Vonderweid U, Hansen G, Kaminski M, Kollee LAA, Kucinskas A, Lenoir S, Levin A, Persson J, Reid M, Saracci R. 2000. Neonatal end-of-life decision making: Physicians' attitudes and relationship with self-reported practices in 10 European countries. *Journal of the American Medical Association* 284(19):2451–2459.

Reiser SJ. 1996. Science, pedagogy, and the transformation of empathy in medicine. In: *Empathy and the Practice of Medicine*, Spiro, HM, McCrea Curnen MG, Peschel E, St. James, D., eds. New Haven: Yale University Press. Pp. 121–132.

Reisinger AL, Colby DC, Schwartz A. 1994. Medicaid physician payment reform: Using the Medicare fee schedule for Medicaid payments. *American Journal of Public Health* 84(4):553–560.

Rhiner M, Ferrell BR, Shapiro B, Dierkes M. 1994. The experience of pediatric cancer pain. Part II: Management of pain. *Journal of Pediatric Nursing* 9(6):380–387.

Richardson DK. 2001. A woman with an extremely premature newborn. *Journal of the American Medical Association* 286(12):1498–1505.

Ricketts TC. 2000. The changing nature of rural health care. *Annual Review of Public Health* 21:639–657.

Ries LAG, Smith MA, Gurney JG, Linet M, Tamra T, Young JL, Bunin GR (eds). 1999. Cancer Incidence and Survival among Children and Adolescents: United States SEER Program 1975–1995, National Cancer Institute, SEER Program. NIH Pub. No. 99-4649. Bethesda, MD.

Ries LAG, Eisner MP, Kosary CL, Hankey BF, Miller BA, Clegg L, Edwards BK, eds. 2001. SEER Cancer Statistics Review, 1973–1998. Bethesda, MD: National Cancer Institute.

Rigoglioso RL. Family Caregivers in New York Report Lack of Essential Training and Support. *Last Acts Electronic Newsletter.* [Online]. Available: http://www.lastacts.org/statsite/3903la%5Feln%5Fnewsletter.html [accessed October 16, 2000].

Rillstone P, Hutchinson SA. 2001. Managing the reemergence of anguish: Pregnancy after a loss due to anomalies. *Journal of Obstetrical, Gynecological and Neonatal Nursing* 30(3):291–298.

Robinson SM, Mackenzie-Ross S, Campbell Hewson GL, Egleston CV, Prevost A. 1998. Psychological effect of witnessed resuscitation on bereaved relatives. *Lancet* 352(9128): 614–617.

Robinson WM, Ravilly S, Berde C, Wohl ME. 1997. End-of-life care in cystic fibrosis. *Pediatrics* 100(2):205–209.

Rojas-Burke J. 1999 (November 30). Oregon Health Plan faces cuts to relieve strain on its budget. *The Oregonian,* D01.

Romand JL. 1989. *Children Facing Grief: Letters from Bereaved Brothers and Sisters.* St. Meinrad, IN: Abbey Press.

Romer AL, Solomon MZ. 2000. Ready or Not Video and Study Guide for Medical School Faculty. Boston, MA: Education Development Center.

Romer AL, Heller KS, Solomon MZ, Weissman D. 2002. *Innovations in End-of-Life Care,* vol. 3. New York: Mary Ann Liebert Publishing Company.

Ronald McDonald House. 2002. [Online]. Available: http://www.rmhc.com/home/index.html [accessed March 31, 2002].

Rosato J. 1996. The ultimate test of autonomy: Should minors have the right to make decisions regarding life-sustaining treatments? *Rutgers Law Review* 49:1–103.

Rosato J. 2000. The ethics of clinical trials: A child's view. *Law and Medical Ethics* 28(4):362–378.

Rosauer J. 1999. *Experiencing Death at Home.* [Online]. Available: http://www.lissencephaly.org/articles/parent/death1.htm [accessed March 31, 2002].

Rosenau N. 2000. Do we really mean families for *all* children? Permanency planning for children with developmental disabilities. Vol. 11(2). Minneapolis: University of Minnesota, Research and Training Center on Community Living, Institute on Community Integration, College of Education and Human Development. [Online]. Available: http://ici.umn.edu/products/prb/112/ [accessed January 15, 2002].

Rosenbaum S, Markus A, Sonosky C, Repasch L. 2001 (May). *State Benefit Design Choices Under SCHIP — Implications for Pediatric Health Care. Policy brief #2.* SCHIP Policy Studies Project, George Washington University, Center for Health Services Research and Policy. [Online]. Available: http://www.gwhealthpolicy.org/downloads/SCHIP_brief2.pdf [accessed August 17, 2001].

Rost K, Nutting P, Smith J, Werner J, Duan N. 2000. Improving depression outcomes in community primary care practice: A randomized trial of the QUEST intervention: Quality enhancement by strategic teaming. *Journal of General Internal Medicine* 16(3):143–149.

Rousar-Thompson P. 2001. Written, unpublished responses to survey of bereaved parent developed and distributed by J. Hilden and H. Janes-Hodder for Children's Oncology Group Parent Advocates Group. Used with permission.

Roy-Byrne PP, Katon W, Cowley DS, Russo J. 2001. A randomized effectiveness trial of collaborative care for patients with panic disorder in primary care. *Archives of General Psychiatry* 58(6):869–876.

Rubenfeld G, Curtis R. 2000. *Managing Death in the ICU: The Transition From Cure to Comfort*. New York: Oxford University Press.

Rubenstein LB, Kahn KL, Reinisch EJ, Sherwood MJ, Rogers WH, Kamberg C, Draper D, Brook RH. 1990. Changes in quality of care for five diseases measured by implicit review, 1981–1986. *Journal of the American Medical Association* 264(15):1974–1979.

Rubin BK, Geiger DW. 1991. Pulmonary function, nutrition, and self-concept in cystic fibrosis summer campers. *Chest* 100(3):649–654.

Rubin SS, Malkinson R. 2001. Parental response to child loss across the life cycle: Clinical and research perspectives. In: Stroebe MS, Hansoon RO, Stroebe W, Schut H, eds. *Handbook of Bereavement Research: Consequences, Coping, and Care*. Washington, DC: American Psychological Association. Pp. 219–240.

Rushton CH. 2001. Pediatric palliative care: Coming of age. In: Solomon MZ, Romer AL, Heller KS, Weissman DE, eds. *Innovations in End-of-Life Care: Practical Strategies and International Perspectives*, vol. 2. Larchmont, NY: Mary Ann Liebert. Pp. 167–170.

Rushton CH. In press. The other side of caring: Caregiver suffering. In: Carter B, Levetown M, eds. *Palliative Care for Infants, Children and Adolescents: A Practical Handbook*. Baltimore: Johns Hopkins University Press.

Rushton CH, Hogue EE. 1993. When parents demand everything. *Pediatric Nursing* 19(2):180–183.

Rushton CH, Will J, Murray M. 1994. To honor and obey: DNR orders and the school. *Pediatric Nursing* 20(6):581–585.

Rushton CH, Terry P. 1995. Neuromuscular blockade and ventilator withdrawal: Ethical controversies. *American Journal of Critical Care* 4(2):112–115.

Rushton CH, Brooks-Brunn JA. 1997. Environments that support ethical practice. *New Horizon* 5(1):20–29.

Rushton CH, Lynch ME. 1992. Dealing with advance directives for critically ill adolescents. *Critical Care Nurse* 12:31–37.

RWJF. 2001 (February). Preparing future nurses and doctors to care for the dying. *State Initiatives in End-of Life Care*.

Sabatino CP. 1999. Survey of state EMS-DNR laws and protocols. *Journal of Law, Medicine, and Ethics* 27(4):297–315.

Sabbagha RE, Sheikh Z, Tamura RK, DalCompo S, Simpson JL, Depp R, Gerbie AB. 1985. Predictive value, sensitivity, and specificity of ultrasonic targeted imaging for fetal anomalies in gravid women at high risk for birth defects. *American Journal of Obstetrics & Gynecology* 152(7 Pt 1):822–827.

Sacchetti A, Lichenstein R, Carraccio CA, Harris RH. 1996. Family member presence during pediatric emergency department procedures. *Pediatric Emergency Care* 12(4):268–271.

Sachdeva RC, LS Jefferson, Coss-Bu J, Brody BA. 1996. Resource consumption and the extent of futile care among patients in a pediatric intensive care unit setting. *Journal of Pediatrics* 128(6):742–747.

Sackett D, Wennberg J. 1997. Choosing the best research design for each question. *British Medical Journal* 315:1636.

Salganicoff A, Keenan PS, Liska D. 1998. Kaiser Commission on Medicaid and the Uninsured, Child Health Facts: National and State Profiles of Coverage. [Online]. Available: http://www.kff.org/content/archive/2105/childfacts.pdf [accessed March 31, 2002].

SAM (Society for Adolescent Medicine). 1995. A position statement of the society for adolescent medicine. *Journal of Adolescent Health* 16:413.

Scala MC. 2001. I'm not contagious. *We Need Not Walk Alone* (newsletter of The Compassionate Friends) 24(2):4–6.

Schaefer C, Quesenberry CP Jr, Wi S. 1995. Mortality following conjugal bereavement and the effects of a shared environment. *American Journal of Epidemiology* 141:1142–1152.

Schechter NL, Berde CB, Yaster M, eds. 2002. *Pain in Infants, Children and Adolescents, 2nd ed.* Baltimore: Williams and Wilkins.

Schechter NL, Blankson V, Pachter LM, Sullivan CM, Costa L. 1997. The ouchless place: No pain, children's gain. *Pediatrics* 99(6):890–894.

Schmall VL, Cleland M, Sturdevant M. 2000. *The Caregiver Helpbook.* Portland: Legacy Caregiver Services.

Schmidt TA, Harrahill MA. 1995. Family response to out-of-hospital death. *Academic Emergency Medicine* 2(6):513–518.

Schniederman LJ, Gilmer T, Teetzel HD. 2000. Impact of ethics consultations in the intensive care setting: A randomized, controlled trial. *Critical Care Medicine* 28(12):3920–3924.

Schneiderman LJ, Jecker NS, Jonsen AR. 1990. Medical futility: Its meaning and ethical implications. *Annals of Internal Medicine* 112(12):949–954.

Schut H, Stroebe MS, von den Bout J, Terheggen M. 2001. The efficacy of bereavement interventions: Determining who benefits. In: Stroebe MS, Hansoon RO, Stroebe W, Schut H, eds. *Handbook of Bereavement Research: Consequences, Coping, and Care.* Washington, DC: American Psychological Association. Pp. 705–737.

Schwartz RM, Michelman T, Pezzullo J, Phibbs CS. 1991. Explaining resource consumption among non-normal neonates. *Health Care Financing Review* 13(2):19–28.

Schwartz RS. 2001. Racial profiling in medical research. *New England Journal of Medicine* 344(18):1392–1393.

Schweitzer SO, Mitchell B, Landsverk J, Laparan L. 1993. The costs of a pediatric hospice program. *Public Health Report* 108(1):37–44.

Scott ME. 1998. Play and therapeutic action. Multiple perspectives. *Psychoanalytic Study of Children* 53:94–101.

Seguin JH, Claflin KS, Topper WH. 1993. Impact of a resource-based relative value scale fee schedule on reimbursements to neonatologists. *Journal of Perinatology* 13(3):217–222.

Sell L, Devlin B, Bourke SJ, Munro NC, Corris PA, Gibson GJ. 1993. Communicating the diagnosis of lung cancer. *Respiratory Medicine* 87:61–63.

Sexton PR, Stephen SB. 1991. Postpartum mothers' perceptions of nursing interventions for perinatal grief. *Neonatal Network* 9(5):47–51.

Shapiro DL, Rosenberg JD. 1984. The effect of federal regulations regarding handicapped newborns: A case report. *Journal of the American Medical Association* 252:2031–2033.

Shapiro L. 2000. Molecular basis of genetic disorders. In: Behrman RE, Kliegman RM, Jenson HB, eds. *Nelson Textbook of Pediatrics,* 16th ed. Philadelphia: WB Saunders. Pp. 313–317.

Shelp EE. 2001. Pastoral care as a community endeavor: A sustaining presence through care team ministry. *Park Ridge Center Bulletin.* Pp. 7–8.

Shelton TL, Jeppson ES, Johnson BH. 1987. *Family-Centered Care for Children with Special Health Care Needs.* Bethesda, MD: Association for the Care of Children's Health.

Shelton TL, Stepanek JS. 1994. *Family-Centered Care for Children Needing Specialized Health and Developmental Services.* Bethesda, MD: Association for the Care of Children's Health.

Shepardson LB, Gordon HS, Ibrahim SA, Harper DL, Rosenthal GE. 1999 (January). Racial variation in the use of do-not-resuscitate orders. *Journal of General Internal Medicine* 14(1):15–20.

Sherck JP, Shatney CH. 1996. ICU scoring systems do not allow prediction of patient outcomes or comparison of ICU performance. *Critical Care Clinics* 12(3):515–523.

SHHV/SBC (Society for Health and Human Values/Society for Bioethics Consultation Task Force on Standards for Bioethics Consultation). 1998. Core Competencies for Health Care Ethics Consultation. Glenview, IL: American Society for Bioethics and Humanities.

Shortell SM, Zimmerman JE, Rousseau DM, Gillies RR, Wagner DP, Draper EA, Knaus WA, Duffy J. 1994. The performance of intensive care units: Does good management make a difference? *Medical Care* 32(5):508–525.

Shortell SM, Bennett CL, Byck GR. 1998. Assessing the impact of continuous quality improvement on clinical practice: What it will take to accelerate progress. *Milbank Quarterly* 76(4):593–624.

Shuster E. 1997. Fifty years later: The significance of the Nuremberg Code. *New England Journal of Medicine* 337(20):1436–1440.

Sibling Connection. 2000. Anniversary Reactions: Jonathan. [Online]. Available: http://www.counselingstlouis.net/page5.html [accessed March 31, 2002].

Sibling Corner. 2001. I still remember the day. [Online]. Available: http://www.portlandtcf.org/NL112001_4.html [accessed March 31, 2002].

SIDS Alliance. 2001 (September 8). Statement presented by Deborah Boyd to the IOM committee on improving palliative and end-of-life care for children and their families, Open Meeting. Washington, DC.

Silberberg M. 2001. Respite Care: State Policy Trends and Model Programs. [Online]. Available: http://www.caregiver.org/national_center/exec_sum_2001_04.html [accessed March 31, 2002].

Silverman PR. 2000. *Never Too Young To Know: Death in Children's Lives.* Oxford: Oxford University Press.

Silverman WA. 1982. A hospice setting for humane neonatal death. *Pediatrics* 69:239–240.

Sine D, Sumner L, Gracy D, von Gunten CF. 2001. Pediatric extubation: "Pulling the tube." *Journal of Palliative Medicine* 4(4):519–524.

Singh GK, Yu SM. 1995. Infant mortality in the United States: Trends, differentials, and projections, 1950 through 2010. *American Journal of Public Health* 85(7):957–964.

Skeels JF. 1990. The right of mature minors in Illinois to refuse life-saving medical treatment. *Loyola Chicago Law Journal* 21:1199.

Skelton JR, Macleod JAA, Thomas CP. 2001. Teaching literature and medicine to medical students, part II: Why literature and medicine? *Lancet* 356:2001–2003.

Smith DG, Wigton RS. 1987. Modeling decisions to use tube feeding in seriously ill patients. *Archive of Internal Medicine* 147(7):1242–1245.

Smith G, O'Keeffe J, Carpenter L, Doty P, Kennedy G, Burwell B, Mollica R, Williams L. 2000. Introduction. *Understanding Medicaid Home and Community Services: A Primer.* [Online]. Available: http://aspe.hhs.gov/daltcp/reports/primerpt.htm#Chap1 [accessed March 20, 2002].

Smith T, Rees H. Making Family Centered Care A Reality. [Online]. Available: http://www.momentix.com/downloads/references/manual/5491/Aterrell%20fcc.pdf [accessed December 31, 2001].

Smithson R. No date. Stories: Men and the health care delivery system. The fathers network. [Online]. Available: http://www.fathersnetwork.org/554.html.

Smits H, Furletti M and Vladeck B. 2002 (February). Palliative Care: An Opportunity for Medicare. New York City: Institute for Medicare Practice, Mount Sinai School of Medicine. [Online]. Available: http://www.mssm.edu/instituteformedicare/pdfs/palliative_care_0202.pdf [accessed June 14, 2002].

Soderstrom L, Martinson I. 1987. Patients' spiritual coping strategies: A study of nurse and patient perspectives. *Oncology Nursing Forum* 14(2):41.

Solomon MZ. 1993. How physicians talk about futility: Making words mean too many things. *Journal of Law, Medicine, and Ethics* 21(2):231–237.

Solomon MZ. 2001. Institutional accountability in end-of-life care. In: Solomon MZ, Heller KS, Romer AL, eds. *Innovations in End-of-Life Care: Practical Strategies and International Perspectives*, vol. 2. Larchmont, NY: Mary Ann Liebert, Inc. Pp. 137–142.

Solomon, MZ. In press. Research to improve end-of-life care in the United States: Toward a more behavioral and ecological paradigm. In: Portenoy R, Bruera E, eds. *Issues in Palliative Care Research*. New York: Oxford University Press.

Solomon MZ, Guilfoy V, O'Donnell L, Jackson R, Jennings B, Wolf S, Nolan K, Donnelley S, Koch-Weser D. 1997. *Faculty Guide: Decisions Near the End of Life*. Revised by Solomon MZ, Fins JJ, Crigger B, Heller KS. Newton, MA: Education Development Center, Inc. [Online]. Available: http://www.edc.org/CAE [accessed July 9, 2002].

Solomon, MZ, Romer AL, Heller KS. 2000b. *Innovations in End-of-Life Care: Practical Strategies and International Perspectives*, vol. 1. Larchmont, NY: Mary Ann Liebert, Inc.

Solomon MZ, Sellers DE, Heller KS, Dokken D, Levetown M, Rushton C, Truog R, Fleischman A. 2000c (October). New research in pediatric end-of-life care. Presented at The American Society of Bioethics and Humanities Annual Meeting, Salt Lake City.

Solomon MZ, Dokken D, Fleischman A, Heller KS, Levetown M, Rushton CH; Sellers D, Truog, R [for the Initiative for Pediatric Palliative Care (IPPC)]. 2001a. *Enhancing Family-Centered Care for Children With Life-Threatening Conditions: Background and Goals*. Newton, MA: Education Development Center. [Online]. Available: http:// www. pediatricpalliativecare.org [accessed March 31, 2002].

Solomon MZ, Romer AL, Heller KS, Weissman DE. 2001b. *Innovations in End-of-Life Care: Practical Strategies and International Perspectives Volume 2*. Larchmont, NY: Mary Ann Liebert, Inc.

Solomon MZ, Dokken DL, Fleischman AR, Heller K, Levetown M, Rushton CH, Sellers DE, Truog RD [for the IPPC]. 2002. The initiative for pediatric palliative care (IPPC): Background and goals. Newton, MA: Education Development Center, Inc. [Online]. Available: www.ippcweb.org [accessed June 20, 2002].

Sommer D. 2001 (September 8). Statement presented on behalf of the Pediatric Chaplains Network to the IOM committee on Care of Children Who Die and Their Families, Open Meeting. Washington, DC.

Sourkes, B. 1980. Siblings of the Pediatric Cancer Patient. In: Kellerman J. ed. *Psychological Aspects of Childhood Cancer*. Springfield, IL: Charles C. Thomas. Pp. 47–69.

Sourkes B. 1982. *The Deepening Shade: Psychological Aspects of Life-Threatening Illness*. Pittsburgh: University of Pittsburgh Press.

Sourkes B. 1995a. *Armfuls of Time: The Psychological Experience of the Child with a Life-Threatening Illness*. Pittsburgh: University of Pittsburgh Press.

Sourkes, B. 1995b. A Life of My Own: The Adolescent's Psychological Experience of Life-threatening Illness. Fifth annual Ruth A. Succop Lecture, Children's Hospital of Pittsburgh and University of Pittsburgh.

Sowards KA. 1999. What is the leading cause of infant mortality? A note on the interpretation of official statistics. *American Journal of Public Health* 89(11):1752–1754.

Speck PW. 1998. Spiritual issues in palliative care. In: Doyle D, Hanks GWC, MacDonald N, eds. *Oxford Textbook of Palliative Medicine*. Oxford: Oxford University Press. Pp. 515–525.

Spiro H. 1992. What is empathy and can it be taught? *Annals of Internal Medicine* 116:843–846.

Spragens LH, Wenneker M. 2001 (July). Creating a Compelling Business Case for Palliative Care. Presentation at Center to Advance Palliative Care Seminar, Oakland, CA. The Bard Group, LLC. [Online]. Available: http://www.capcmssm.org/content/42/index.html? topic=3 [accessed July 20, 2001].

Stahlman MT. 1990. Ethical issues in the nursery: Priorities versus limits. *Journal of Pediatrics* 116:167–170.

Stanfield J. 2000. Faith, healing and religious treatment exemptions to child-endangerment laws: Should parents be allowed to refuse necessary medical treatment for their children based on their religious beliefs? *Hamline Journal of Public Law & Policy* 22:45.

Stanford Faculty Development Center. 2002. The End of Life Care Program. [Online]. Available: http://www.stanford.edu/group/SFDP/progeol.html [accessed March 15, 2002].

Stanley BH, Sieber JE eds. 1992. *Social Research on Children and Adolescents: Ethical Issues.* Sage Focus Editions. Newbury Park, CA: Sage Publications.

Starren J, Hripcsak G, Sengupta S, Abbruscato CR, Knudson PE, Weinstock RS, Shea S. 2002. Columbia University's informatics for diabetes education and telemedicine (IDEATel) Project. *Journal of the American Medical Information Association.* 9:25–36.

State MW, King BH, Dykens E. 1997. Mental retardation: A review of the past 10 years. Part II. *Journal of the American Academy of Child & Adolescent Psychiatry.* 36(12):1664–1671.

Stedman's Medical Dictionary, 26th edition. 1995. Baltimore: William and Wilkins.

Steinberg A. 1998. Decision-making and the role of surrogacy in withdrawal or withholding of therapy in neonates. *Clinical Perinatology* 25(3):779–790.

Stepanek MTJ. 2001. *Heartsongs.* Alexandria, VA: VSP and Hyperion Books.

Stepp LS. 2002, January 2. Adolescence: Not just for kids. By some definitions, it ends at 34. Aren't we stretching it just a bit? *Washington Post,* p. C01

Stevens B, Yamada J, Ohlsson A. 2001. Sucrose for Analgesia in Newborn Infants Undergoing Painful Procedures. [Online]. Available: http://www.nichd.nih.gov/cochrane/Stevens/ Stevens.HTM [accessed March 10, 2002].

Stevens MM. 1998. Psychological adaptation of the dying child. In: Doyle D, Hanks GWC, MacDonald N, eds. *Oxford Textbook of Palliative Medicine,* 2nd ed. Oxford: Oxford University Press. Pp. 1045–1055.

Stevens MM, Jones P, O'Riordan E. 1996. Family responses when a child with cancer is in palliative care. *Journal of Palliative Care* 12(3):51–55.

Stiller CA. 1988. Centralisation of treatment and survival rates for cancer. *Archives of Disease in Childhood* 63(1):23–30.

Stoll BJ, Kliegman RM. 2000a. Overview of morbidity and mortality. In: Behrman RE, Kliegman RM, Jenson HB, eds. *Nelson Textbook of Pediatrics,* 16th ed. Philadelphia: WB Saunders. Pp. 451–454.

Stoll BJ, Kliegman RM. 2000b. The high-risk infant. In: Behrman RE, Kliegman RM, Jenson HB, eds. *Nelson Textbook of Pediatrics,* 16th ed. Philadelphia: WB Saunders. Pp. 474–486.

Stone P, Phillips C, Spruyt O, Waight C. 1997. A comparison of the use of sedatives in a hospital support team and in a hospice. *Palliative Medicine* 11:140–144.

Strauss D, Eyman RK, Grossman HJ. 1996. Predictors of mortality in children with severe mental retardation: The effect of placement. *American Journal of Public Health* 86(10): 1422–1429.

Strauss D, Kastner TA. 1996. Comparative mortality of people with mental retardation in institutions and the community. *American Journal of Mental Retardation* 101(1):26–40.

Strauss D, Kastner T, Ashwal S, White J. 1997. Tubefeeding and mortality in children with severe disabilities and mental retardation. *Pediatrics* 99(3):358–362.

Stroebe MS, Stroebe W, Hansson R, eds. 1993. *Handbook of Bereavement: Theory, Research, and Intervention.* New York: Cambridge University Press.

Stroebe MS, Hansoon RO, Stroebe W, Schut H, eds. 2001a. *Handbook of Bereavement Research: Consequences, Coping, and Care.* Washington, DC: American Psychological Association.

Stroebe MS, Hansson RO, Stroebe W, Schut H. 2001b. Future directions for bereavement research. In: Stroebe MS, Hansoon RO, Stroebe W, Schut H, eds. *Handbook of Bereavement Research: Consequences, Coping, and Care.* Washington, DC: American Psychological Association. Pp. 741–766.

Stroebe MS, Schut H. 2001c. Models of coping with bereavement: A review. In: Stroebe MS, Hansoon RO, Stroebe W, Schut H, eds. *Handbook of Bereavement Research: Consequences, Coping, and Care.* Washington, DC: American Psychological Association. Pp. 375–403.

Stroul BA, Pires SA, Armstrong MI, Meyers JC. 1998. The impact of managed care on mental health services for children and their families. *Future Child* 8(2):119–133.

Strunk BC, Cunningham PJ. 2002 (March). *Treading Water: Americans' Access to Needed Medical Care, 1997–2001.* Tracking Report No. 1. Washington, DC: Center for Studying Health System Change.

Stuber M. 1992. Psychotherapy issues in pediatric HIV and AIDS. In: Stuber M, ed. *Children and AIDS.* Washington, DC: American Psychiatric Press.

Sullivan MC. 2001. Lost in translation: How Latinos view end-of-life care. *Last Acts Electronic Newsletter.* [Online]. Available: http://www.lastacts.org [accessed February 22, 2001].

Sulmasy DP. 1992. Physicians, cost control, and ethics. *Annals of Internal Medicine* 116(11): 920–926.

Sulmasy DP. 1995. Managed care and managed death. *Archives of Internal Medicine* 155: 133–136.

Sulmasy DP. 2000. Commentary: Double effect—intention is the solution, not the problem. *Journal of Law, Medicine, and Ethics* 28(1):26–29.

Sulmasy DP, Dwyer M, Marx E. 1995. Knowledge, confidence, and attitudes regarding medical ethics: How do faculty and housestaff compare. *Academic Medicine* 70(11):1038–1040.

Sulmasy DP, Geller G, Levine DM, Faden R. 1993. A randomized trial of ethics education for medical house officers. *Journal of Medical Ethics* 19(3):157–163.

Sumner L. 2001. Pediatric care: The hospice perspective. In: Ferrell BR, Coyle N, eds. *Textbook of Palliative Nursing.* New York: Oxford University Press. Pp. 556–569.

Support Organization for Trisomy 13/18 and Related Disorders. 2001 (September 8). Statement presented by Kenneth McWha to the IOM committee on improving palliative and end-of-life care for children and their families, Open Meeting. Washington, DC.

SUPPORT Principle Investigators. 1995. The study to understand prognoses and preferences for outcomes and risks of treatment. *Journal of the American Medical Association* 274(20):1591–1598.

Swarm RA, Cousins MJ. 1998. Anaesthetic techniques for pain control. In: Doyle D, Hanks GWC, MacDonald N, eds. *Oxford Textbook of Pallative Medicine,* 2nd ed. Oxford: Oxford University Press. Pp. 390–413.

Taddio A, Ohlson A. 1997. *Lidocaine–Prilocaine Cream (EMLA) to Reduce Pain in Male Neonates Undergoing Circumcision.* [Online]. Available: http://www.nichd.nih.gov/cochrane/Taddio/Taddio1.htm [accessed March 10, 2002].

Tang S, Yudkowsky BK, Siston AM. 2000. *Children's Health Insurance Status and Public Program Participation: State Reports, 1999 and 2001 Estimates.* Elk Grove Village, IL: Division of Health Policy Research, AAP.

Teddell JS, Litwin SB, Berger S. 1996. Twenty-year experience with repair of complete atrio-
    ventricular septal defects. *Annals of Thoracic Surgery* 62:419–424.
Teno JM, Neylan Okun S, Casey V, Welch LC. 2001. Toolkit of Instruments to Measure End
    of Life Care (TIME)—Resource Guide: Achieving Quality of Care at Life's End. [Online].
    Available: http://www.chcr.brown.edu/pcoc/resource guide/resourceguide.pdf [accessed
    March 31, 2002].
Thayer P. 2001. Spiritual care of children and parents. In: Armstrong-Daley A, Zarbock S,
    eds. *Hospice Care for Children*, 2nd ed. Oxford: Oxford University Press. Pp. 172–189.
Thibault GE. 1994. The use of clinical models for end of life decision making in critically ill
    ICU patients. In: Field MJ, ed. *Summary of Committee Views and Workshop Examining
    the Feasibility of an Institute of Medicine Study of Dying, Decisionmaking, and Appro-
    priate Care*. IOM Committee for a Feasibility Study on Care at the End of Life. Wash-
    ington, DC: Institute of Medicine.
Thibault GE. 1997. Prognosis and clinical predictive models for critically ill patients. In: Field
    MJ, Cassel CK, eds. *Approaching Death: Improving Care at the End of Life*. Washing-
    ton, DC: National Academy Press. Pp. 358–362.
Thornes, R. (on behalf of the Joint Working Party on Palliative Care for Adolescents and
    Young Adults). 2001. *Palliative care for young people aged 13–24*. [Online]. Available:
    http://www.act.org.uk/pages/viewpointasp?Active=F3.
Thorns A, Sykes N. 2000. Opioid use in last week of life and implications for end-of-life
    decision-making. *Lancet* 356(9227):398–399.
Tilly J, Wiener JM. 2001. State pharmaceutical programs for older and disabled Americans.
    Health Affairs 20(5):223–232.
Timmermans S. 1997. High touch in high tech: The presence of relatives and friends during
    resuscitative efforts. *Scholarly Inquiry for Nursing Practice* 11(2):153–168; discussion
    169–173.
Tobin DR, Lindsey K. 1998. *Peaceful Dying: The Step-by-Step Guide to Preserving Your
    Dignity, Your Choice, and Your Inner Peace at the End of Life*. Reading, MA: Perseus
    Books.
Tolle SW, Tilden VP. 2002. Changing end-of-life planning: The Oregon experience. *Journal
    of Palliative Medicine* 5(2):311–317.
Tolle SW, Tilden VP, Nelson CA, Dunn PM. 1998. A prospective study of the efficacy of the
    physician order form for life-sustaining treatment. *Journal of the American Geriatrics
    Society* 46:1–6.
Tommiska V, Heinonen K, Ikonen S, Keroll P, Pokela M, Renlund M, Virtanen M, Fellman
    V. 2001. A national short-term follow-up of extremely low birth weight infants born in
    Finland in 1996–1997. *Pediatrics* 107(1):e2. [Online]. Available: http://www.mindfully.
    org/Health/Low-Birth-Weight.htm [accessed September 27, 2001].
Trafford A. 2001 (June 20). Children of denial: Recent advances in end-of-life care haven't
    reached the youngest patients. *Washington Post*, p. A01.
Traugott I, Alpers A. 1997. In their own hands: Adolescents' refusal of medical treatment.
    Archive of Pediatrics & Adolescent Medicine 151:922–927.
Truog RD. 2000. Addressing ethical conflicts in the ICU. *Forum*, August 2000. [Online].
    Available: http://www.rmf.harvard.edu/publications/forum/v20n4/fv20n4-a3/index.html
    [accessed October 22, 2001].
Truog RD, Brett AS, Frader J. 1992. The problem with futility. *New England Journal of
    Medicine* 326:1560–1564.
Truog RD, Burns JP, Mitchell C, Johnson J, Robinson W. 2000. Pharmacologic paralysis and
    withdrawal of mechanical ventilation at the end of life. *New England Journal of Medi-
    cine* 342:508–511.

Truog RD, Cist AF, Brackett SE, Burns JP, Curley MA, Danis M, DeVita MA, Rosenbaum SH, Rothenberg DM, Sprung CL, Webb SA, Wlody GS, Hurford WE. 2001. Recommendations for end-of-life care in the intensive care unit: The Ethics Committee of the Society of Critical Care Medicine. *Critical Care Medicine* 29(12):2332–2348.

Tsai E. 2002. Should family members be present during cardiopulmonary resuscitation? *New England Journal of Medicine* 346(13):1019–1021.

Tucson (Arizona) Unified School District. 1996. Emergency Life-Sustaining Care for Students: Board Policy 5527. Governing Board Policies Series 5000. Adopted September 3, 1996. [Online]. Available: http://www.tusd.k12.az.us/contents/govboard/gbpol5000/pol5527.html [accessed April 16, 2002].

Tulsky JA, Chesney MA, Lo B. 1996. See one, do one, teach one? House staff experience discussing do-not-resuscitate orders. *Archives of Internal Medicine* 156(12):1285–1289.

Twycross R, Lichter I. 1998. The terminal phase. In: Doyle D, Hanks GWC, MacDonald N, eds. *Oxford Textbook of Palliative Medicine*, 2nd ed. Oxford: Oxford University Press. Pp. 977–994.

Ubel P, Goold S. 1997. Recognizing bedside rationing: Clear cases and tough calls. *Annals of Internal Medicine* 126:74–80.

U.S. Census Bureau. 2001. Resident population estimates by age and sex, April 1, 1990, to July 1, 1999. [Online]. Available: http://eire.census.gov/popest/archives/national/nation2/intfile2-1.txt [accessed March 31, 2002].

USDHEW (U.S. Department of Health and Human Services). 1977. *Research Involving Children: Report and Recommendations*. Washington, DC: The National Commission for the Protection of Human Subjects of Biomedical and Behavioral Research.

USDHHS (U.S. Department of Health and Human Services). 1993. *Institutional Review Board Guidebook*, Chapter 6, Special Classes of Subjects, Section C, Children. Washington, DC: Office of Human Research Protections. [Online]. Available: http://ohrp.osophs.dhhs.gov/irb/irb_chapter6.htm#g4 [accessed December 17, 2001].

USGAO (U.S. General Accounting Office). 2001a (September). *Medicaid and SCHIP: States' Enrollment and Payment Policies Can Affect Children's Access to Care*. GAO-01-883. Washington, DC: USGAO.

USGAO. 2001b. Testimony Before the Committee on Health, Education, Labor and Pensions, U.S. Senate: Pediatric Drug Research: Substantial Increase in Studies of Drugs for Children, but Some Challenges Remain. Statement of Janet Heinrich, Director, Health Care–Public Health Issues, May 8, 2001. GAO-01-705T.

Vachon, M. 1976. Stress reactions to bereavement. *Essence* 1:23.

Vaidya VU, Greenberg LW, Patel KM, Strauss LH, Pollack MM. 1999. Teaching physicians how to break bad news: A 1-day workshop using standardized parents. *Archive of Pediatric Adolescent Medicine* 153(4): 419–422.

Van Eys J, E. Mohnke, eds. 1985. *Life, faith, hope and magic: The chaplaincy in pediatric cancer care*. Houston, TX: University of Houston.

Vazirani RM, Slavin SJ, Feldman JD. 2000. Longitudinal study of pediatric house officers' attitudes toward death and dying. *Critical Care Medicine* 28(11):3740–3745.

Vernon DD, Dean JM, Timmons OD, Banner W Jr, Allen-Webb EM. 1993. Modes of death in the pediatric intensive care unit: Withdrawal and limitation of supportive care. *Critical Care Medicine* 21(11):1798–1802.

Vertrees JC, Pollatsek JS. 1993. Paying for pediatric inpatient care. Final report of the Universal Access for Children Reimbursement Study Project, conducted for NACHRI. Alexandria, VA: Solon Consulting Group Ltd.

Vetto JT, Elder NC, Toffler WL, Fields SA. 1999. Teaching medical students to give bad news: Does formal instruction help? *Journal of Cancer Education* 14(1):13–17.

Vintzileos AM. Egan JF. 1995. Adjusting the risk for trisomy 21 on the basis of second-trimester ultrasonography. *American Journal of Obstetrics & Gynecology* 172(3):837–844.

Vizza CD, Yusen RD, Lynch JP, Fedele F, Patterson GA, Trulock EP. 2000. Outcome of patients with cystic fibrosis awaiting lung transplantation. *American Journal of Respiratory Critical Care Medicine* 162(3 Pt 1):819–825.

von Gunten CF. 2000. Palliative care and home hospice program, Northwestern Memorial Hospital. In *Programs in Palliative Care: Nine Case Studies*. New York: Milbank Memorial Fund and Robert Wood Johnson Foundation. Pp. 161–182 [Online]. Available: http://www.milbank.org/pppc/0011pppc.html [accessed March 31, 2002].

von Gunten CF. 2001. Discussing do-not-resuscitate status. *Journal of Clinical Oncology* 19(5):1576–1581.

Wagner HP, Dingeldein-Bettler I, Berchthold W, Luthy AR, Hirt A, Pluss HJ, Beck D, Wyss M, Signer E, Imbach P. 1995. Childhood NHL in Switzerland: Incidence and survival of 120 study and 42 non-study patients. *Medical and Pediatric Oncology* 24(5):281–286.

Waisel DB, Truog RD. 1995. The cardiopulmonary resuscitation-not-indicated order: Futility revisited. *Annals of Internal Medicine* 122(4):304–308

Walco GA, Cassidy RC, Schechter NL.1994. Pain, hurt, and harm—the ethics of pain control in infants and children. *New England Journal of Medicine* 331(8):541–544.

Walco GA, Sterling CM, Conte PM, Engel RG. 1999. Empirically supported treatments in pediatric psychology: Disease-related pain. *Journal of Pediatric Psychology* 24(2):155–167.

Wall SN, Partridge JC. 1997. Death in the intensive care nursery: Physician practice of withdrawing and withholding life support. *Pediatrics* 99(1):64–70.

Wallston KA, Burger C, Smith RA, Baugher RJ. 1988. Comparing the quality of death for hospice and non-hospice cancer patients. *Medical Care* 26(2):177–182.

Walsh, RA, Girgis A, Sanson-Fisher RW. 1998. Breaking bad news 2: What evidence is available to guide clinicians? *Behavioral Medicine* 24(2):61–72.

Warady BA, Carr B, Hellerstein S, Alon U. 1992. Residential summer camp for children with end-stage renal disease. *Child Nephrology & Urology* 12(4):212–215.

Washburne, CK. 2000. Zink the Zebra: Teaching the Acceptance of Our Differences. [Online]. Available: http://www.zinkthezebra.org/ [accessed March 31, 2002].

Wass H. 1984. Concepts of death: A developmental perspective. In: Wass H, Corr CA, eds. *Childhood and Death*. Washington, DC: Hemisphere Publishing.

Wear D. 2002. Face-to-face with it: Medical students' narratives about their end-of-life education. *Academic Medicine* 77:271–277.

Webb M. 1997. *The Good Death: The New American Search to Reshape the End of Life*. New York: Bantam Books.

Weeks JC, Cook EF, O'Day SJ, Peterson LM, Wenger N, Reding D, Harrell FE, Kussin P, Dawson NV, Connors AF Jr, Lynn J, Phillips RS. 1998. Relationship between cancer patients' predictions of prognosis and their treatment preferences. *Journal of the American Medical Association* 279(21):1709–1714.

Weil K. 1996. *Zink the Zebra*. Milwaukee: Gareth Stevens Publishing.

Weil L. 2001 (September 9). Statement and discussion with the IOM committee on improving palliative and end-of-life care for children and their families, Open Meeting. Washington, DC.

Weir RF. 1983. The government and selective nontreatment of handicapped infants. *New England Journal of Medicine* 309:661–663.

Weir RF. 1992. *Selective Nontreatment of Handicapped Newborns: Moral Dilemmas in Neonatal Medicine*. New York: Oxford University Press.

Weisman SJ, Bernstein B, Schechter NL. 1998. Consequences of inadequate analgesia during painful procedures in children. *Archives of Pediatric Adolescent Medicine* 152(2):147–149.

Weissman DE, Block SD. 2002. ACGME requirements for end-of-life training in selected residency and fellowship programs: A status report. *Academic Medicine* 77:299–304.

Weissman DE, Block SD, Blank L, Cain J, Cassem N, Danoff D, Foley K, Meier D, Schyve P, Theige D, Wheeler HB. 1999. Recommendations for incorporating palliative care education into the acute care hospital setting. *Academic Medicine* 74(8):871–877.

Weissman DE, Griffie J, Gordon D, Dahl JL. 1997. A role model program to promote institutional changes for management of acute and cancer pain. *Journal of Pain Symptom Management* 4(5):274–279.

Weithorn LA, Campbell SB. 1982. The competency of children and adolescents to make informed treatment decisions. *Child Development* 53:1589–1598.

Wenger NS, Kanouse DE, Collins RL, Liu H, Schuster MA, Gifford AL, Bozzette SA, Shapiro M. 2001. End-of-life discussions and preferences among persons with HIV. *Journal of the American Medical Association* 285(22):2880–2887.

Whitfield JM, Siegel RE, Glicken AD, Harmon RJ, Powers LK, Goldson EJ. 1982. The application of hospice concepts to neonatal care. *American Journal of Disabled Children* 136(5):421–424.

Whitten P, Doolittle G, Hellmich S. 2001. Telehospice: Using telecommunication technology for terminally ill patients. *Journal of Clinical Monitoring and Computing* 6(4). [Online]. Available: http://www.ascusc.org/jcmc/vol6/issue4/whitten2.html [accessed April 16, 2002].

WHO (World Health Organization). 1990. *Cancer Pain Relief and Palliative Care*. WHO Technical Report Series 804. Geneva: WHO.

WHO. 1998. *Cancer Pain Relief and Palliative Care in Children*. Geneva: WHO.

Wijdicks EF. 2001. The diagnosis of brain death. *New England Journal of Medicine* 344(16):1215–1221.

Williams DL, Gelijns AC, Moskowitz AJ, Weinberg AD, Ng JH, Crawford E, Hayes CJ, Quaegebeur JM. 2000. Hypoplastic left heart syndrome: Valuing the survival. *Journal of Thoracic and Cardiovascular Surgery* 119(4 Pt 1):720–731.

Williams DG, Hatch DJ, Howard RF. 2001a. Codeine phosphate in paediatric medicine. *British Journal of Anaesthesia* 86:413–421.

Williams MA, Lipsett PA, Shatzer JH, Rushton CH, Berkowitz ID, Mann SL, Lane K, Knapp JC, Humphreys SL, Zaeske R, Haywood C. 2001b. Experiential, interdisciplinary training in end-of-life care and organ donation. *Critical Care Medicine* 28 (Suppl):A204.

Williams MA, Rushton CH, Grochowski E, Shatzer JH, Berkowitz ID, Mann SL, Lane K, Zaeske R, Haywood C, Lipsett PA. 2002 (January). Family attitudes about organ donation. *Critical Care Medicine* 29:A82. Presented at the 31st Conference of Society for Critical Care Medicine.

Williamson-Noble E. No date. Alexander: A Windflower's Story. [Online]. Available: http://www.wish.org/home/frame_aboutus.htm [accessed March 31, 2002].

Willinger M, Hoffman HJ, Wu KT, Hou JR, Kessler RC, Ward SL, Keens TG, Corwin MJ. 1998. Factors associated with the transition to non-prone sleep positions of infants in the United States: The National Infant Sleep Position Study. *Journal of the American Medical Association* 280:329–339.

Wing B. 1997 (April 15). Presentation to the National Committee of Vital and Health Statistics Subcommittee on Health Data Needs, Standards, and Security. [Online]. Available: http://ncvhs.hhs.gov/97041516.htm [accessed March 20, 2002].

Wisconsin's BadgerCare program. [Online]. Available: http://www.dhfs.state.wi.us/badgercare/ [accessed March 31, 2002].

WMA (World Medical Association). 1964. *Declaration of Helsinki: Ethical Principles for Medical Research Involving Human Subjects.* Adopted June 1964, Helsinki, Finland, and most recently amended October 2000. [Online]. Available: http://www.wma.net/e/policy/17-c_e.html [accessed December 17, 2001].

Wolfe J, Grier HE, Klar N, Levin SB, Ellenbogen JM, Salem-Schatz S, Emanuel EJ, Weeks JC. 2000a. Symptoms and suffering at the end of life in children with cancer. *New England Journal of Medicine* 342:326–333.

Wolfe J, Klar N, Grier HE, Duncan J, Salem-Schatz S, Emanuel EJ, Weeks JC. 2000b. Understanding of prognosis among parents of children who died of cancer: Impact on treatment goals and integration of palliative care. *Journal of the American Medical Association* 284(19):2469–2475.

Wolfe J. 2001 (June 11). Statement and discussion with the IOM committee on improving palliative and end-of-life care for children and their families, Open Meeting. Washington, DC.

Wood AJ. 2001. Racial differences in the response to drugs—pointers to genetic differences. *New England Journal of Medicine* 344(18):1393–1396.

Woolf SH, Grol R, Hutchinson A, Eccles M, Grimshaw J. 1999. Potential benefits, limitations, and harms of clinical guidelines. *British Medical Journal* 318:527–530.

Wooten B. 2001. Written, unpublished responses to survey of bereaved parents developed and distributed by J. Hilden and H. Janes-Hodder for Children's Oncology Group Parent Advocates Group. Used with permission.

Worden JW, Monahan JR. 2001. Caring for Bereaved Parents. In: Armstrong-Daley A, Zarbock S, eds. *Hospice Care for Children,* 2nd ed. New York: Oxford University Press. Pp. 137–156.

Wordsworth, W. 1798. We Are Seven. *The Complete Poetical Works.* London: Macmillan and Co., 1888. [Online]. Available: www.bartleby.com/145 [accessed July 20, 2001].

Wright JL, Klein BL. 2001. Regionalized pediatric trauma systems. *Clinical Pediatric Emergency Medicine* 2:3–12.

Wyeth-Ayerst Laboratories. 1999. *Prescription Drug Benefit Cost and Plan Design Survey Report.* Albuquerque, NM: Wellman Publishing, Inc.

Yaster M, Krane E, Kaplan R, Cote C, Lappe D. 1997. *Pediatric Pain Management and Sedation Handbook.* St. Louis: Mosby.

Young KD, Seidel JS. 1999. Pediatric cardiopulmonary resuscitation: A collective review. *Annals of Emergency Medicine* 33:195–205.

Yudowsky BK, Tang SS, Siston AM. 2000 (October). Pediatrician Participation in Medicaid: Survey of Fellows of the American Academy of Pediatrics. [Online]. Available: http://www.aap.org/statelegislation/med-schip/Wholedpc.pdf [accessed July 12, 2001].

Zacharias M. 1998. Pain relief in children: Doing the simple things better. *British Medical Journal* 316:1552–1560.

Zeltzer L. 1980. The adolescent with cancer. In: Kellerman J, ed. *Psychological Aspects of Childhood Cancer.* Springfield, IL: Charles C. Thomas.

Zucker MB, Zucker HD, eds. 1997. *Medical Futility and the Evaluation of Life-Sustaining Interventions.* Oxford: Cambridge University Press.

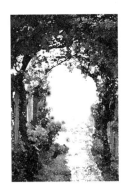

STUDY ORIGINS AND ACTIVITIES

In Summer 1999, the Institute of Medicine's Board on Health Sciences Policy recommended that IOM undertake a study to investigate care for children who die and their families. With funding from a mix of public and private agencies, the IOM began the study in Fall, 2000. The broad objectives were to 1) develop recommendations to strengthen the knowledge base for compassionate and effective care for dying children and their families; 2) inform health care providers, researchers, medical and nursing educators, state and federal policy makers, insurers, and others about these recommendations; and 3) encourage thoughtful discussion of what constitutes good end-of-life care for children and their families.

The IOM appointed a committee of 14 experts to oversee the study. That committee met 5 times between April 2001 and February 2002. Its task was to develop a report that

- described the major causes and settings of death for children;
- reviewed what is known about 1) the medical and other services provided to dying children and their families and 2) the education of physicians and other professionals who care for gravely ill children;
- assessed the state of knowledge about clinical, behavioral, cultural, organizational, legal, and other important aspects of palliative and end-of-life care for children and their families;
- examined methods for communicating information, determining family and child/patient preferences, resolving conflicts, and evaluating the quality of palliative and end-of-life care as experienced by children and their families; and
- proposed a research and action agenda to strengthen the scope and application of the knowledge base for providing effective and compassionate care for children who die and their families.

The committee arranged for seven background papers, which are readable online (www.nap.edu) as Appendixes B through H. It also conducted a one-day meeting to hear views from family support and advocacy organizations and health care groups, and it invited written statements from additional organizations. In addition, the committee met for a half-day with parents whose children had died from or were living with life-threatening medical problems. Both meetings were open to the public. The agendas and participants are listed below as are additional groups that submitted written statements to the committee.

Public Meeting
Lecture Room, National Academy of Sciences
2101 Constitution Avenue NW, Washington, DC.
Saturday, September 8, 2001
AGENDA

8:30 a.m.   Welcome and Introductions
                       Richard Behrman, M.D., Chair

8:40-9:20 a.m   Panel 1

The Compassionate Friends, Inc.
Patricia A. Loder

Candlelighters: Childhood Cancer Foundation
Ruth Hoffman

National Organization of Parents of Murdered Children
Jean Lewis

9:20-10:00 a.m.   Panel 2

SIDS Alliance
Deborah Boyd

MISS - Mothers in Sympathy and Support
Richard K. Olsen

Hygeia
Michael R. Berman, M.D.

10:20-11:00 a.m.   Panel 3

National Tay-Sachs & Allied Diseases Association
Carol and Eric Zimmerman

Support Organization for Trisomy 13/18 and Related Disorders
Kenneth McWha, M.D.

National Organization for Rare Disorders
Diane Dorman

11:00-11:30 a.m.   Panel 4

Make-a-Wish Foundation
Michele R. Atkins

1:15-2:00 p.m.   Panel 5

American Academy of Pediatrics (AAP)
G. Kevin Donovan, M.D., M.L.A.

Critical Care Section, AAP
M. Michele Moss, M.D.

2:00-2:40 p.m.   Panel 6

American Psychological Association/Society of Pediatric Psychology
Daniel Armstrong, Ph.D.

American Board of Pediatrics
Ernest F. Krug III, M.D.

3:10-3:50 p.m.   Panel 7

National Association of Children's Hospitals and Related Institutions
Susan Dull, R.N., M.S.N., M.B.A.

National Hospice and Palliative Care Organization
Stephen R. Connor, Ph.D.

National Association of Pediatric Home and Community Care
Dorothy Page, F.N.P., M.S.N.

3:50-4:30 p.m.   Panel 8

Pediatric Chaplains Network
The Reverend Dane R. Sommer

Child Life Council
Christina Brown

National Association of Social Workers
Mirean Coleman, M.S.W.

4:30 p.m.   Adjourn

Additional groups submitting written statements
American Academy of Hospice and Palliative Medicine
American Association of Colleges of Nursing
American Association of Critical Care Nurses
American Board of Pediatrics Program Directors Committee
American College of Emergency Physicians
American Society of Pediatric Hematology/Oncology
Children's Oncology Group End-of-Life Subcommittee
Hospice and Palliative Nurses Association
National Association of State Emergency Medical Services Directors
Organization of Neonatal-Perinatal Training Program Directors

Public Meeting
Room 150, National Academy of Sciences
2101 Constitution Avenue NW, Washington, DC.
Sunday, September 9, 2001

PARTICIPANTS

Winona Kittiko   Tina Heyl-Marinueau
Atlanta, Georgia   Weymouth, Massachusetts

Rose and Gary Conlon   Deborah Dokken
Fremont, California   Chevy Chase, Maryland

Les Weil   Rosario and Salvador Avila
Milwaukee, Wisconsin   Palo Alto, California

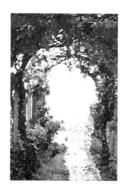

Appendices B through H
(pages 449 through 664)
are available online
http://www.nap.edu/catalog/10390.html

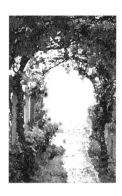

COMMITTEE
BIOGRAPHICAL STATEMENTS

Chair
Richard E. Behrman, M.D., J.D., is Executive Chair, Federation of Pediatric Organizations, Education Steering Committee. He serves as Consultant to the Lucile Packard Foundation for Children's Health and Sr. Advisor for Health Affairs at the David and Lucile Packard Foundation. He is also Clinical Professor of Pediatrics at Stanford University and the University of California, San Francisco. He previously held positions as Chairman of the Boards of Lucile Packard Foundation for Children's Health and the Lucile Packard Children's Hospital and Director of the Center for the Future of Children. Prior to holding these positions, he served as Vice President of Medical Affairs and Dean of the School of Medicine at Case Western Reserve University. Dr. Behrman also served as Professor and Chairman of the Departments of Pediatrics at Case Western Reserve University and at Columbia University. His areas of special interest include perinatal medicine, intensive and emergency care of children, the provision and organization of children's health and social services, and related issues of public policy and ethics. Dr. Behrman has published extensively in critically reviewed scientific journals and is Editor-in-Chief of *Nelson Textbook of Pediatrics* and the journal, *The Future of Children*. He is a member of the Institute of Medicine (IOM) and has served as chairman of two IOM committees concerned with child welfare.

Grace H. Christ, D.S.W., is an Associate Professor at Columbia University School of Social Work and has clinical and research interests in the fields of psychosocial oncology, end-of-life care, social work education and research, and childhood bereavement. Among other publications, she is the founder of the *Journal of Psychosocial Oncology* and author of *Healing Children's Grief*, published in 2000 by Oxford University Press. She is currently a

Senior Faculty Scholar with the Project on Death in America and is a recipient of the National American Cancer Society's Distinguished Service Award. She was formerly Director of Social Work at Memorial Sloan Kettering Cancer Center.

Francis Sessions Cole, M.D., is Director of Newborn Medicine, Vice Chair of the Department of Pediatrics, Park J. White M.D. Professor of Pediatrics, and Professor of Cell Biology and Physiology at Washington University School of Medicine, St. Louis, Missouri. His research interests focus on the molecular basis of the susceptibility of the newborn infant to infection and, more recently, on the contribution of genetic variation in the surfactant protein B gene to risk of respiratory distress syndrome in newborn infants. He has produced more than 70 publications on these topics. Dr. Cole is also committed to excellence in education and has received numerous teaching awards including Clinical Teacher of the Year Award and Washington University's Distinguished Faculty Award. He has facilitated the formation of community outreach programs for medical students including the Perinatal Project and Students Teaching AIDS to Students (STATS). He is a member of the Society of Pediatric Research, the American Society for Clinical Investigation, and the American Pediatric Society.

Harvey R. Colten, M.D., is VP and Senior Associate Dean for Translational Research at Columbia University Health Sciences, and previously served as Chief Medical Officer at iMetrikus, Inc., a health services company that provides Internet-based, interactive health management solutions for patients with chronic illness. In the past, he has served as Professor of Pediatrics at Harvard Medical School and Chief of the Division of Cell Biology, Pulmonary Medicine, and Director of the Cystic Fibrosis Program at Children's Hospital Medical Center, Boston; Chair of the Department of Pediatrics and Professor of Molecular Microbiology at Washington University School of Medicine, St. Louis, Mo.; and Dean of the Medical School and Vice President for Medical Affairs at Northwestern University. He is also a Fellow of the American Association for the Advancement of Science, the American Academy of Allergy and Immunology, and the American Academy of Pediatrics. He is a member of the Institute of Medicine and is a past Vice-Chair of its Council.

Joanne Hilden, M.D., is currently Chair, Department of Pediatric Hematology/Oncology at The Children's Hospital at The Cleveland Clinic. Dr. Hilden was formerly the Director of Oncology Research and Children's Oncology Group (COG) Responsible Investigator at Children's Hospitals and Clinics, St. Paul. She founded and co-chairs the COG Task Force on

End-of-Life Care. She is involved in clinical care and teaching medical trainees about end-of-life care and the delivery of bad news. Dr. Hilden is a member of the American Society of Clinical Oncology (ASCO), and served on the ASCO Subcommittee on Cancer Care at the End of Life which produced the group's position statement on care of the dying and carried out a survey of the country's oncologists regarding end of life care. She is a Faculty Scholar of the Project on Death in America. Dr. Hilden is also a member of the Minnesota Commission to Improve End-of-Life Care and she is a certified trainer for the American Medical Association's EPEC project to educate physicians about end-of-life care. She is a Fellow in the American Academy of Pediatrics and a member of the American Society of Pediatric Hematology/Oncology. She led the preparation of a paper on end-of-life issues in pediatric oncology that was included in the 2001 IOM report *Improving Palliative Care for Cancer*.

Pamela Hinds, B.S.N., Ph.D., is the Director of Nursing Research at St. Jude Children's Research Hospital in Memphis, Tennessee. She has expertise in the care of children with cancer and in developing effective team care to meet immediate and long-term needs of children and their families. Her research focuses on decision-making in pediatric oncology, coping and adolescents, and the experience of pediatric oncology nurses, among other topics. Among other publications, she authored the chapter on "End-of-life decision-making by pediatric oncology patients, their parents, and their health care professionals" in the *Oxford Textbook of Palliative Nursing Care* (Ferrell and Coyle, editors). She is co-chair of the Nursing Research Committee for the Children's Oncology Group and is co-chair of the Palliative Care Initiative at St. Jude Children's Research Hospital. She also serves on the Institutional Review Board and the Pain and Symptom Management Committee at St. Jude and is member of the Oncology Nursing Society.

Angela R. Holder, LL.M., is currently Professor of the Practice of Medical Ethics at Duke University Medical Center. Ms. Holder was formerly Clinical Professor of Pediatrics (Law) at Yale University School of Medicine, where she taught a required first-year medical school course on law, medicine, and ethics entitled, "Professional Responsibility." Her primary research interests involve legal and ethical issues of children and adolescents in the health care system, but she has also studied issues of human subjects research, malpractice, confidentiality, and legal and ethical issues in human reproduction. She served on the IOM Committee on the Effects of Medical Liability on the Delivery of Maternal and Child Health Care which produced the report *Medical Professional Liability and the Delivery of Obstetrical Care* (1989).

Haiden A. Huskamp, Ph.D., is an Assistant Professor of Health Economics in the Department of Health Care Policy at Harvard Medical School. Her primary areas of research are: 1) the economics of mental health and substance abuse (MHSA) treatment; 2) the economics of the pharmaceutical industry; and 3) the financing of end-of-life care services. Dr. Huskamp recently served as principal investigator for a study funded by the Robert Wood Johnson Foundation to study the impact of Medicare financing methods on the provision of services to patients at the end of life. Her teaching areas include health care policy and health economics. She received her Ph.D. from Harvard University.

Robert Kliegman, M.D., is Chairman of Pediatrics at the Medical College of Wisconsin and has interests in general and community pediatrics, pediatrics education, neonatology, and public health. He completed residency training in general pediatrics at Babies' Hospital in New York, New York; and he completed neonatology and metabolism fellowships at Case Western Reserve University in Rainbow Babies and Children's Hospital. He is the co-editor of *Controversies in Perinatology* and *Nelson Essentials of Pediatrics*. Dr. Kliegman has been a child advocate working with the American Academy of Pediatrics, municipal, state, and federal governments, and the George Washington University Health Policy Institute-Packard Foundation Roundtable for Children. He served on the IOM committee that produced the report *Approaching Death: Improving Care at the End of Life* in 1997.

Marcia Levetown, M.D., works as a Pain and Palliative Care Education Consultant in Galveston, TX. She also serves as a Clinical Associate Professor of Pediatrics and Internal Medicine at the University of Texas Medical Branch at Galveston. She received her medical degree at the Medical College of Virginia, completed a pediatric residency at Baylor College of Medicine in Houston, and a fellowship in Pediatric Critical Care at Children's National Medical Center in Washington, D.C. Her experience in the PICU led her to establish the award-winning Butterfly Program, a program designed to meet the needs of children living with life-threatening conditions and their families. She is a Project on Death in America Faculty Scholar and Chair of the Children's International Project on Palliative and Hospice Services. She is the Principal Editor of the *Compendium of Pediatric Palliative Care* and author of numerous articles, chapters and curricula on pediatric palliative care issues. Dr. Levetown is a member of the ethics committees of the American Academy of Pediatrics, the National Hospice and Palliative Care Organization and the American Academy of Hospice and Palliative Medicine. She is also a founding board member of the Texas Partnership for End-of-Life Care.

Neil L. Schechter, M.D., is Director of the Pain Relief Program at the Connecticut Children's Medical Center, and Professor of Pediatrics and Head of the Division of Behavioral and Developmental Pediatrics at the University of Connecticut School of Medicine and St. Francis Hospital. His clinical and research experience covers the entire range of pain experience and treatment in children including pain during routine pediatric care and pain of children with advanced illnesses. He was one of the pediatric representatives on the AHCPR Clinical Guideline Panel on Acute Pain Management and was a member of the WHO Expert Committee that developed guidelines on cancer pain and palliative care for children. He is the senior editor of the major textbook on pain management in children. He is the chair of the Special Interest Group on Pain in Children of the Ambulatory Pediatric Association and has been a member of numerous committees at the local, state, and national levels which advocate for pain control and behavioral medicine research including the Supportive Care Committee of the Children's Cancer Study Group, the Executive Council of the Society for Developmental and Behavioral Pediatrics, and the Task Force on Pain in Children of the American Pain Society, among others. In 1998, he received the Jeffrey Lawson Award for Advocacy in Children's Pain Relief of the American Pain Society.

Barbara Sourkes, Ph.D., is the first Kriewall-Haehl Director of Pediatric Palliative Care at the Lucile Packard Children's Hospital and Associate Professor of Pediatrics and Psychiatry, Stanford University School of Medicine. Dr. Sourkes was previously at the Montreal Children's Hospital and McGill University, and at the Boston Children's Hospital and Dana-Farber Cancer Institute of Harvard Medical School. She has published three books: *The Deepening Shade: Psychological Aspects of Life-Threatening Illness* and *Armfuls of Time: The Psychological Experience of the Child with a Life-Threatening Illness* (1982, 1995, University of Pittsburgh Press); and *Les enfants en deuil (Bereaved Children)* with Michel Hanus, M.D. (Frison-Roche, Paris, 1997). She was the recipient of the Charles A. Corr Award for Literature from Children's Hospice International in 1999. Dr. Sourkes, a child psychologist, has consulted nationally and internationally on the psychological aspects of pediatric life-limiting illness, palliative care and bereavement. In addition to her clinical activities, research, publications, committee and board memberships, Dr. Sourkes is on the editorial boards of the *Journal of Clinical Psychology in Medical Settings* and *The American Journal of Hospice & Palliative Care* and has served as consultant for films on children with life-threatening illnesses.

Lizabeth H. Sumner, R.N., B.S.N., has been involved in hospice care for over 22 years and is currently the Children's Program Director of San Diego

Hospice. She created the regional Children's Program for terminally ill children in 1987 in partnership with San Diego Children's Hospital / Health Center. The program includes several components such as an "Early Intervention Program" Perinatal Hospice, an innovative program that supports parents through pregnancy and birth of babies diagnosed with life-threatening conditions. The Children's Program also provides services such as counseling and play therapy to support healthy children grieving the loss of a parent, sibling, or classmate. Ms. Sumner has consulted statewide and nationally with other hospices developing programs for dying and bereaved children. She has spoken at numerous local, national and international meetings on the topic of end-of-life care for children. Ms. Sumner has published both academic and popular articles and book reviews in nursing journals, textbooks, and newspapers, as well contributing as an expert resource for various publications. Most recently, she authored the chapter "Pediatric Care: The Hospice Perspective" in the *Textbook of Palliative Nursing* (Ferrell and Coyle, editors), and has a chapter in *Hospice Care for Children* (Armstrong-Dailey and Zarbock, editors). She is a member of the ChIPPS (Children's International Project on Palliative and Hospice Services) workgroup, serves on the Ethics Committee of the San Diego Children's Hospital, and participates in other collaborative initiatives.

Joseph Wright, M.D., M.P.H., is Medical Director for Advocacy and Community Affairs at Children's National Medical Center (CNMC) in Washington DC. He is also an Associate Professor of Pediatrics, Emergency Medicine, and Prevention and Community Health at the George Washington University Schools of Medicine and Public Health and practices pediatric emergency medicine in the Emergency Medicine and Trauma Center at Children's. Administratively, Dr. Wright is founding Director of the Center for Prehospital Pediatrics in the Division of Emergency Medicine at CNMC, and also serves as the State Medical Director for Pediatrics within the Maryland Institute for Emergency Medical Services Systems. His major areas of academic interest include injury prevention and health services research, and he is currently developing a comprehensive program of pediatric prehospital research in the District of Columbia. He has received recognition for his advocacy work throughout his career including the Shining Star award from the Los Angeles-based Starlight Foundation acknowledging his outstanding contributions to under-served communities, and induction into Delta Omega, the national public health honor society. He has authored and co-authored many publications, serves on several national advisory boards, including the American Academy of Pediatrics Committee on Injury, Violence and Poison Prevention, and lectures widely to professional and lay audiences.

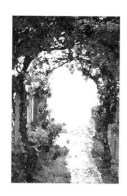

INDEX*

---

*Index does not include Appendices.